Dr. V. S. Palekar's CLINICAL DIAGNOSIS FOR MEDICAL UNDERGRADUATES

Dr. V. S. Palekar's

CLINICAL DIAGNOSIS FOR MEDICAL UNDERGRADUATES

DR. (MRS.) SHAILA PALEKAR
M.D. (Paediatrics), M.D. (General Medecine)

MUMBAI
POPULAR PRAKASHAN

POPULAR PRAKASHAN PRIVATE LIMITED
301, Mahalaxmi Chambers
22, Bhulabhai Desai Road
Mumbai - 400026
Website: www.popularprakashan.com

First Published 1992
Revised Second Edition, 1998
Reprinted, 1999
Reprinted, 2001
Reprinted, 2002
Reprinted, 2004
Reprinted, 2006
Reprinted, 2008
Reprinted, 2009
Reprinted July 2011
Reprinted April 2013

(3561)

ISBN 978-81-7154-799-9

PRINTED IN INDIA

By Rama Printer, 4743/23, Ansari Road, Darya Ganj, New Delhi - 110002
and Published by Harsha Bhatkal for Popular Prakashan Pvt. Ltd.
301, Mahalaxmi Chambers, 22, Bhulabhai Desai Road
Mumbai - 400026

Foreword

Clinical Diagnosis for Medical Undergraduates fills a long felt need of the students in Indian Universities. While there is a plethora of textbooks on the subject, it has not been dealt with from the point of view of a clinician who would actually handle the cases. The methodological approach starting with history taking and leading upto diagnosis is the main characteristic of this book.

As far as the C.N.S. is concerned, the presentation of the symptomatology and the signs has been different from the books usually used by the students. It is clinically oriented and more in tune with the bed-side clinic which is the common mode of teaching in most medical schools even today. Treatment is included under certain disease ailments.

The book was originally conceived and designed by Dr. V. S. Palekar and the first draft prepared when he suddenly expired. This unfinished task has been completed by Dr. (Mrs.) Shaila Palekar, M.D. (Paediatrics), who followed up her years of practice as a paediatrician by obtaining a second M.D. in General Medecine.

While the book does not aim at being a complete textbook, it covers most cases which an undergraduate student would be expected to handle with sufficient discussion and use of diagrams and photographs.

N.H.Wadia
M.D., F.R.C.P. (London)
F.A.M.S., F.A.Sc., F.N.A.

Preface

Perhaps no practising consultant would think of sitting down and writing a textbook for the undergraduate students. He will have least inclination and little time to do this. But realising that the immense knowledge and experience gained in the course of practice would be of great help to the students, late Dr. V. S. Palekar, thought of jotting down the findings of the clinical examination done on a large number of patients. This book has emerged out of these notes and jottings. It was his ambition to extend this knowledge to innumerable students who studied under him both at the Seth G.S. Medical College and Grant Medical College in Bombay from 1963 to 1983. Unfortunately he did not live long enough to complete the work and after 1983 it was left to me to complete what he intended to do.

In my opinion, the interface that exists between purely clinical practice and academic pursuits ultimately provides nourishment to the intellect and widens the knowledge of the medical students and practitioners. I have therefore tried to strike a delicate balance between the two approaches in this book. I feel confident that the students will be benefited by this endeavour.

Our emphasis has, of course, been to understand the clinical implications of symptoms and signs of each disease and to appreciate its patho-physiology and thus to make the otherwise humdrum task more meaningful and an interesting pursuit.

We have also tried to explain the system with appropriate illustrations which are specially drawn by Mr. Sawant, the medical artist. I am thankful to him. Dr. (Mrs.) Meena Behrani and Dr. (Mrs.) Laxmi Nadkarni have been of great assistance to me in going through the manuscript minutely and critically. I cannot express adequate thanks to them. I am grateful to Dr. K. Ramamoorthy and Dr. N.H. Wadia who spared valuable time from their busy schedule to go through the manuscript and gave me valuable suggestions. I feel honoured by the Foreword given by Dr. N.H. Wadia and the Introduction given by Dr. K. Ramamoorthy to this book.

I sincerely thank members of my family, innumerable friends, and Mr. Ramdas Bhatkal of Popular Prakashan who encouraged me to complete the task.

Bombay
June 1991

Shaila Palekar

Preface to Revised Second Edition

The response received by the first edition of *Clinical Diagnosis* was beyond my expectations. Hence the revised second edition. Certain points have been elaborated now and the fresh photographs have been added.

I must express my gratitude to Dr. Sunil G. Dalvi for his constant encouragement and Dr. Mrs. Suruchi Dalvi for helping me for the fresh photographs and correction of proofs. I sincerely thank members of my family, innumerable friends, and Mr. Ramdas Bhatkal of Popular Prakashan who encouraged me to complete the task.

Mumbai
April 1998

Shaila Palekar

Introduction

This book has been written by the two authors from the point of view of the undergraduate medical student in particular. The book offers a very practical approach in clinical diagnosis which is the baseline for further patient management.

The book has been written by Dr. V. S. Palekar, an astute physician, who made a mark as a good clinician in Bombay. Due to his untimely death, the burden of revising and completing the book fell on his wife Dr. (Mrs.) S.V. Palekar who is a practicing paediatrician herself. She has also successfully passed the second M.D. in General Medicine after years of practice as a paediatrician and she has done an excellent job.

The use of diagrams, photographs, charts and tables has made the book more presentable.

I would unequivocally and strongly recommend this book to all medical undergraduates.

K.Ramamoorthy, M.D.

Contents

Section I : History Taking and Physical Examination

1. Introduction

The main aim of every physician is to cure his patient or at least to relieve the patient's suffering to the best of his ability. For this he has to institute either curative or palliative treatment which will be guided by his diagnosis.

To arrive at a correct diagnosis, a physician has to follow a set routine path. This will consist of the interview or history taking, physical examination and the necessary investigations depending upon the findings during the examination.

The aim of this book is to discuss the basic art of history taking and physical examination. The student should always strive to take a good history as this will very often point to the system involved (i.e., C.N.S., R.S., C.V.S., etc.). Not only that, with experience one can have a precise idea of the nature of the lesion and its anatomical site in the affected system, by proper evaluation and interpretation of the patient's complaints.

Eliciting a good history is an art. Some have a natural flair for it, while others have not. This interview between the patient and the examiner not only paves the way towards the diagnosis, but also marks the beginning of the patient-doctor relationship which is an extremely important factor in the treatment of the patient. Hence all of us must strive to obtain as precise a history as possible while gaining the confidence of the patient at the same time.

Certain points must be remembered while eliciting the history. The patient should be encouraged to narrate his symptoms in his own way and in his own native tongue as far as possible. Very few patients are good narrators. Either they go on rambling about irrelevant matters or they are too worried or shy to describe their complaints properly. Though leading or direct questions should be avoided, a gentle prodding is very often required to elicit the proper symptomatology. So also quite a few patients tend to give a history in quasimedical terms like "I had flu" or "heartburn" or "liver swelling", without understanding anything about the disease or anatomical organs involved. A careful questioning to elicit the description of these symptoms is always necessary.

For eliciting the history, the points to be asked in special interrogation, should include past history, personal history and family history. Direct questioning is usually necessary. For this the knowledge of the examiner regarding the disease comes into the picture. It is not expected of the patient to volunteer precise and relevant information without direct questioning for instance the examiner will have to ask about past history of fever and joint pains in childhood to a patient who has come at the age of forty for congestive cardiac failure due to rheumatic valvular disease.

In short, how to question a patient and how to elicit proper history is a matter of judgement which can be acquired after prolonged practice. How much importance to give to a particular symptom and which one to ignore will be understood only after gaining the necessary experience.

HISTORY TAKING

The history of the patient should be taken in the following manner :

1. Preliminary data : Name, age, sex, address, occupation;
2. Chief complaints;
3. Onset, duration, progress;
4. Special inquiry;
5. Past history;
6. Personal history;
7. Family history.

1. Preliminary Data

Name : One usually starts the interview by asking the name of the patient. This is usually the opening question in any interview. Obviously one should know his patient's name, but the judicious use of either the first name or the surname while conducting the interview puts the patient in a more responsive frame of mind.

Age and Sex : The importance of knowing the age is that certain disease processes are common at certain age groups. In general degenerative and atherosclerotic disorders occur at a later age, while congenital diseases are common at a younger age. However, a congenital abnormality can manifest rarely at a later age—for example syringomyelia.

Certain diseases are more common in a particular sex. Haemophilia clinically manifests only in males, so also myocardial infarction is more frequent in them. On the other hand rheumatic mitral stenosis for no apparent reason is more common in females; thyrotoxicosis also is more common in females.

Address : Not only the residence but also the area from which the patient hails and the duration of his stay there should be recorded. For instance — lathyrism is common in persons who have been staying in North India for a long time. People staying in urban areas develop allergic lung diseases more commonly due to the polluted atmosphere, while goitre is common in the foothills of Himalayas because of the low iodine content of the water in that area. Diseases like tuberculosis, gastrointestinal infections are common among people staying in the slums and overcrowded areas.

Occupation : Occupation of a patient can in some cases straightaway point towards the etiological factors in diagnosis. Some of the obvious examples are pneumoconiosis in coal workers and silicosis in persons engaged in mining, sand blasting or in quarries. Byssinosis is common in textile workers while asthma is common in people working in bakeries or printing industry, due to exposure to allergens like flour or gum acacia. Lead poisoning, causing either abdominal or neurological complaints is seen in plumbers. People working in chemical factories can get cirrhosis due to chemical necrosis of liver. Policemen get varicose veins as they have to stand for a long time.

2. Chief Complaints

Under this heading the main complaint or complaints of the patient should be inquired. A patient should be asked as to what his complaint is and how long he has been suffering from it. If there are more than one complaints then they should be recorded in chronological sequence.

Complaints should be recorded as far as possible in non-medical terms or in the patient's own words. For instance, if a patient complains of a shooting type of pain in the trigeminal nerve area, it should be recorded as the pain in that particular area of the face (mandibular, maxillary, etc) and the term trigeminal neuralgia should be avoided.

So also description of the complaints should be avoided at this stage. It is necessary only to enumerate complaints under this heading. For example, if a patient has more than one complaint then recording should be as follows :

1. Breathlessness on exertion — 1 month
2. Cough with expectoration — 2 weeks
3. Hemoptysis — 1 day

3. Onset Duration Progress

After recording chief complaints a detailed inquiry about various symptoms recorded should be carried out. This is necessary as the same symptoms, for instance, breathlessness may be due to diseases of either cardiac or respiratory system. However, when a patient is made to give a detailed description, the examiner would know that, when the breathlessness is exertional it is more likely to be cardiac in origin. Dyspnea which is paroxysmal and associated with wheezing and which is brought upon by allergic irritation associated with cough is more likely to be due to respiratory system involvement.

Though direct questioning has always been frowned upon, quite often it is needed to elaborate the symptomatology. However, questions should be framed in such a manner that a patient gives descriptive answers rather than yes or no.

Progress of a disease should be studied carefully. A disease process may start and remain stable or be slowly or rapidly progressive. Inquiry about improvement of a disease process either spontaneously or due to treatment is quite often omitted due to oversight of an examiner.

Classically, inquiry under this heading includes only a description of the onset, duration and progress of the chief complaints. However, it is seldom enough to come to a definite diagnosis. A patient needs to be asked about various other symptoms which are related to a main complaint or the examiner's knowledge of a disease process will prompt him to ask a patient seemingly unrelated questions.

For instance, if a patient complains of cough with expectoration, it is obvious that the history will never be complete without asking him about fever and its description. But when a patient complains of weakness in the legs, the history is not complete without asking him about lifting of heavy weights. This obviously entails a knowledge of etiological process causing paraplegia.

4. Special Inquiry

After elaborate inquiry of onset, duration and progress of the chief complaints special inquiry should always be conducted in a systematic manner.

A detailed description of points to be inquired into under this heading is given in chapters dealing with various systems.

Psychological make up of the patient should be assessed from his mode of giving history; his insight, concern,overconcern, or approach toward his illness have important bearing in management.

5. Past History

This should include an enumeration of all illnesses since childhood and those disease processes which have a bearing on the present complaint should be elaborated in detail. This will entail a knowledge of various etiological factors. It is impossible to enumerate all the relevant point here as in certain diseases a very obscure point for a beginner will clinch the diagnosis (for example injections of sera in acute demyelinating process affecting the C.N.S.).

At the end of this chapter a comprehensive list has been given of those points which should be inquired into when a particular system is affected. Though by no means complete, it will be a useful guideline for a student. (Table-1).

Not only the disease processes but also a history of injuries or previous operations should be inquired into. For example, a minor head injury a few months ago may be the cause of a subdural hematoma causing pressure symptoms in the brain, while a surgical operation a few years ago may bring a patient with intestinal obstruction at present.

6. Personal History

Socio-Economic Status : It is important to assess the social and economic background of patient. The stress and strain of life may produce certain symptoms which may not have a physical background. Certain diseases like gout and diabetes are common in the well-to-do, while diseases like pulmonary tuberculosis and intestinal infections are common among people living in overcrowded dwellings and insanitary conditions.

Diet, frequency of micturition, bowel habits should be recorded.

Type of Work : Sedentary habits, work causing mental anxiety or heavy physical activity predispose to certain ailments and inquiry into these matters should be conducted.

Drugs and Addictions : Use of self medications or abuse of drugs can lead to various ailments. Aspirin can cause hematemesis as a sensitivity reaction or it can lead to toxic poisoning in children. Excessive use of purgatives may be the cause of various gastrointestinal problems.

Alcohol and consumption of tobacco in any form (smoking, chewing tobacco, snuff or its use as tooth powder or paan masala) are the most common addictions which can cause various ailments. Details of these habits should be gone into. Not only the quantity of alcohol but its quality should be noted, as the cheaper variety contains methyl alcohol causing additional toxic effects. The amount of tobacco or alcohol is as important as the number of years of consumption.

Diet : Details about a patient's diet should be inquired into. Excessively spicy food may cause gastritis or can be one of the etiological factors in peptic ulcer. Excessive caloric intake causing obesity may predispose a patient to maturity onset diabetes or atherosclerotic vascular diseases. Low caloric intake leads to malnutrition and can be an etiological factor in cirrhosis of liver. Diet which has very poor content of proteins can lead to hypoproteinemia.

7. Family History

The health of close family members should be inquired into. In certain diseases like haemophilia one may have to check the history of male members of two or three generations.

History of marriage amongst blood relations (i.e., consanguinity) is important in cases of heredofamilial diseases like cerebellar ataxia, mental retardation, epilepsy, etc.

It is always wise to start this inquiry by asking whether any other member of the family has a similar complaint. This automatically paves the way for further questioning regarding the health of the family members. The ages of the living members, their state of health or if deceased, the cause of death and age at death should be inquired into and recorded. H/o hypertension, ischemic heart disease and diabetes mellitus in parents and sibs leading to death at younger age is important.

Again as mentioned before a knowledge of the various disease processes is essential to elicit a good family history. Certain diseases are inherited and have a very strong heredofamilial transmission like Huntington's chorea or muscular dystrophies or phenyl ketonuria. While some others like coronary artery disease, retinitis pigmentosa have only some degree of genetic influence. Diabetes, hypertension in other members of the family and parents is also important.

Infections and/or drug ingestions by the mother especially in the first fourteen weeks of pregnancy should be inquired as they can cause anomalies of heart, mental retardation or congenital anomalies of limbs of the foetus.

METHOD OF PHYSICAL EXAMINATION

History taking is followed by physical examinaiton of a patient.

Complaints narrated by the patient may point towards an affection of a particular system or systems or they may not give any clue as to which system is affected, for example fatigue or loss of weight. In either case, a set method of examination must be followed as described below:

I. General Examination:

This should precede the systemic examination. It has been described in detail in the next chapter.

General examination can lead to what is described as 'spot diagnosis'. The exophthalamic stare of a patient suffering from thyrotoxicosis or the shuffling gait of parkinsonism are two classic examples. However, a stepwise general examination should never be omitted so as not to miss any associated complications or any other associated or unrelated pathology.

II. Systemic Examination :

The system which is apparently affected should be examined first.

All the major systems, i.e., Cardiovascular, Respiratory, Alimentary and Central nervous system should be examined one after the other. Detailed description of these systemic examinations is given in later chapters.

Table I

	Past history	Personal history	Family history
Cardiovascular system	• Cyanosis since birth • Fainting spells • Squatting especially after exertion • Rheumatic fever • Syphilis • Hypertension • Diabetes • Thyroid disorders • Tuberculosis (may cause pericardial effusions)	Addiction to tobacco in any form —Alcoholism —Socio-economic state —Nocturnal frequency of micturition. Polyuria — polydypsia	• H/o. coronary artery disease • H/o. diabetes in family members • H/o. cerebrovascular accidents • H/o. consanguinity, mother having German measles in the first trimester of pregnancy • H/o. hypertension in sibs & parents.
Respiratory system	• Whooping cough • Influenza • Bronchopneumonia following measles • Allergic manifestations like hay fever • Recurrent upper respiratory tract infections • Operations on the upper respiratory tract • Chronic ear infections • Tuberculosis	• Smoking • Occupation — which can cause pneumoconiosis • Socio-economic factors causing overcrowding and undernutrition	• Pulmonary tuberculosis • Family H/o. allergy asthma
Alimentary system	• Chronic diarrhoea in childhood (can give rise to malabsorption syndromes) • Dysentry • Jaundice • Hematemesis or melena • Malaria • Kala azar • Worm infestations • Tuberculosis	• Alcohol • Dietary habits (like type of food), hurried meals irregular food habits • Stress and strain due to socio-economic or other factors • Ingestion of tobacco or smoking • Occupation — whether working in chemical factory • Ingestion of drugs	• Jaundice in siblings • Pulmonary tuberculosis • Familial polyposis of colon • Sanitary conditions at home • H/o. Ca colon in other members
C.N.S.	Trauma • Could be mild or indirect • Birth injuries • Kernicterus • Febrile convulsions in childhood • H/o. infections like encephalitis or meningitis in childhood • Hypertension • Diabetes • Syphilis • Inj. of vaccines and sera • Rheumatic fever • H/o conjunctivitis	• Smoking or addiction to tobacco & alcohol • Exposure to heavy metals like lead due to occupation • Ingestion of kesari dal • Bladder control • Change of behaviour as noticed by relations • Right-handed or left-handed	• Mental retardation • Epilepsy • Cerebellar diseases • Myopathies • Migraine • Consanguinity
Urinary system	• Hematuria in childhood Suggestive of acute nephropathy in childhood • Repeated upper respiratory tract infections	• Socio-economic factors causing overcrowding leading to UTI • H/o. drug ingestions • Exposure to toxic materials due to occupation	• Polycystic kidneys

2. General Examination

General Examination : This is conducted at the start of the examination of a patient and should always precede the systemic examination.

Various points to be noted are as described below. However with practice and experience, quite a few of them become apparent when the examiner is eliciting the history. However,a step by step examination should always be conducted so as not to be misled by initial impressions.

The following method should be adopted when a complete general examination has to be done.

(1) Posture of the patient;
(2) Build of the patient;
(3) State of nutrition;
(4) Facies;
(5) Head and neck;
(6) Examination of mouth and oral cavity;
(7) Skin and hair;
(8) Extremities;
(9) Joints;
(10) Genitalia;
(11) Hernial sites;
(12) Temperature.

1. POSTURE : Posture or the attitude of a patient should be observed when he is lying down (decubitus) and also when he is standing up whenever possible.

The attitude of a patient in these two positions can provide a clue as to the system involved and sometimes the nature of the disease process.

The following description has classified various postures observed in various systemic disorders. Though most important in the diagnosis of central nervous disorders, certain postures point towards affection of other systemic involvement.

(a) Posture due to CNS involvement: (i) Photophobic attitude : In this condition, the patient is seen lying curled up, i.e., legs are flexed over the trunk, the spine is bent with concavity anteriorly and the patient turns away from any source of light or disturbance. He resents any attempt to be straightened for examination.

This posture is assumed by patients who are suffering from inflammation or irritation of meninges.

Sometimes instead of curling in the midline as described above, a patient may show a lateral curling of the body — pleurosthotonus.

(ii) Opisthotonus : A patient in bed is seen to have a characteristic arching of the back due to extreme spasm of back muscles. The back is arched in such a way that in extreme cases the weight of the body is supported by the head and feet.(Plate 2.1).

This is classically seen when the patient is suffering from either tetanus or strychnine poisoning; or whenever there is spasm of back muscles as in meningitis or pre-paralytic poliomyelitis.

(iii) Hemiplegic attitude : This depends upon the stage of the disease in which the patient is observed. In acute stage, the patient is seen lying down flat in bed with eyes, head and neck turned towards one side. The damage to the brain or the lesion in the brain is on the side towards which the eyes and the head are pointing. On the opposite side, the cheek is flapping in and out with respiration and the nasolabial furrow is obliterated. The extremities on paralysed side are flaccid and without any movement and the leg is externally rotated with a foot drop. (Plate 2.2)

It is not possible to examine such a patient in standing position at this stage.

In the established stage of hemiplegia, rotation of the eyes, head and neck disappear. The face is asymmetrical and nasolabial furrow on the affected side is absent or poorly marked. The upper extremity is flexed at the elbow and slightly pronated. The fingers are flexed at the metacarpophalangeal joints and extended at the interphalangeal joints. The shoulder is adducted and internally rotated. The lower extremity is extended at the hip and knee joints and there is a plantar flexion of the foot.

All these abnormalities are better observed when the patient is made to stand. In addition to this, the trunk is found to be bent on the side of paralysis.

(iv) Due to brain stem lesions: Head is turned one side and there is flexion of limbs on the same side.

(b) Postures due to cardiovascular and respiratory involvement: These will be discussed together as most of the abnormal postures adopted by the patient are due to dyspnea in most cases.

(i) Orthopneic posture: This attitude is assumed by the patient when there is a marked dyspnea.

The patient is either propped up on two or three pillows or he is made to sit upright. He is unable to lie down and will immediately become uncomfortable and sit up if asked to do so.

The posture is adopted to relieve respiratory distress. In this position the diaphragm is at the lower level than when lying down so that the vital capacity is relatively increased. Also the accessory muscles of respiration, both intercostal as well as back muscles can act much better in this position.

Cardiac causes: Left ventricular failure; Pericardial effusion; Corpulmonale.

Respiratory causes: Emphysema; Bronchial asthma; Massive pleural effusion; Pneumothorax.

(ii) Forward kneeling posture: In extreme conditions of dyspnea, the patient bends forward and usually prefers to sit up in bed with a support on his lap on which he kneels. The hands usually hold the sides of the support so as to render further assistance to the respiratory muscles by providing a fixed point at their point of insertion.

This position is also known as Mohammed in prayer position and is seen usually in patient suffering from massive pericardial effusion, severe congestive cardiac failure or aortic aneurysm.

(Rarely the same position is assumed by patients suffering from pancreatic carcinomas and abdominal aortic aneurysms so as to relieve pain caused by pressure on the spine.)

2. BUILD OF THE PATIENT : Build of the patient should be examined for:

(a) type of constitution;

(b) height and span.

(a) **Constitution:** Also known as diathesis, constitution is important, as certain diseases are common in certain types of constitutions.

The three main types of individual variations are:

(i) Normosthenic: An individual with a normal body build.

(ii) Asthenic: These individuals are slender, their body appearing thin and long, with an elongated neck and a flat chest. The extremities appear longer due to their thinness and the fingers are usually slender.

(It was presumed in the past that these individuals are more prone to pulmonary tuberculosis).

(iii) Sthenic : These are short individuals with a rounded thick muscular chest, short neck and stumpy stocky extremities. The fingers are also fairly thick.

In between these three main types, there are many variations in which there is an exaggeration of the main features. Various types of constitutions are described according to these variations. However, it can be said that no definite correlation between any constitution and certain diseases exists, except probably in disorder which is described as Marfan's syndrome.

Marfan's syndrome: This is a hereditary disorder of the connective tissues. It is associated with abnormalities of the eye (dislocation of lens) and the cardiovascular system; so the diagnosis is important. (Plate 2.3)

The stature is abnormally long and the span is greater than the height. The distance between the symphysis pubis and the heels is greater than the body above. Ratio of upper segment to lower segment is less than one. The fingers are long, thin and slender and the palate is high arched. There is deformity of the chest either the pigeon breast (outward displacement) or the pectus excavatum (inward displacement) variety.

(b) **Height and span:** Normal individuals vary greatly in their height and unless there is a gross abnormality, an individual should not be classified either as a giant or dwarf.

Height depends on various factors, most important of which are hereditary and constitutional factors. Racial influence on height is present and so also males on an average are taller than females.

Normally the height (that is from the top of the head to the soles) is equal to the span, i.e., the distance between the tips of the fingers when the hands are stretched perpendicular to the body. Similarly, the distance between the top of the head and symphysis pubis is roughly the same as the distance between the symphysis pubis and the soles of the feet(Upper segment/lower segment ratio is 1:1).

Gigantism or excessive height may rarely be without any apparent cause but usually the reason is some endocrine disorder. Hyperpituitarism (over activity of pituitary gland either due to a tumour or hypersecretion) before puberty when the epiphyses of the bones are not united is the most common cause, while sometimes hypogonadism also results in the same abnormality.

Dwarfism is a term applied to the condition where individuals are excessively short. Infantilism is a term applied to these individuals who in addition to lack of height, have genital hypoplasia.

A rough classification of various causes of dwarfism can be made as follows:

(I) Racial: Certain races like pygmies of Africa have a very short height though otherwise they are quite normal in all other respects.

(II) Congenital: (i) Certain metabolic defects like glycogen storage disorders result in retarded growth. (Plate 2.4).

(ii) Achondroplasia: This is usually heredofamilial and the affected persons have short and bowed legs and arms. The hands are small and thick and the face has a peculiar appearance which is easily recognised due to its flat nose. The sexual development is normal. Ratio of upper segment to lower segment is infantile, i.e., more than 1. (Plate 2.5)

(iii) Bone diseases like Osteogenesis imperfecta: These individuals have excessive fragile bones which are liable to multiple fractures. Their sclera is usually blue which provides easy diagnostic clue. (Plate 2.6)

(iv) Chondrodystrophies: Diseases caused by abnormalities in the skeletal growth.

(III) Endocrine: Pituitary hypothalamic axis defects (Frohlich's syndrome), pituitary defects (pituitary dwarfs), thyroid hypofunction since birth (cretinism) and gonadal abnormalities all can give rise to dwarfism which have their own typical appearances. (Plate 2.7)

(IV) Childhood diseases: (i) Severe malnutrition with or without any chronic disease like tuberculosis may result in stunted growth.

(ii) Cardiac diseases, either congenital or rheumatic affection can result in dwarfism.

(iii) Conditions like renal rickets, coeliac disease and juvenile diabetes also result in this condition.

3. STATE OF NUTRITION : There is a rough correlation between height and weight. Many charts of average weight in correlation to height and age are available. However, these charts should be interpreted in proper perspective.

The state of nutrition is judged mainly by deposition of fat all over the body. However, when examining a patient clinically, the condition of the skin, the muscle mass and the distribution and the amount of subcutaneous fat should be taken into consideration. A patient with oedema and ascites may look obese, but if attention is paid to his upper extremities and cheeks this mistake can easily be avoided.

Excessive deposition of fat results in obesity while a lack of it is known as either emaciation or in its extreme state of cachexia. Obesity is most commonly the result of over-eating though it may also be a familial characteristic. Patients who are overweight are more prone to cardiovascular diseases, osteoarthritis and diabetes. Other causes of obesity are various endocrine disorders like Frohlich's syndrome, Cushing's syndrome, myxodema and hypogonadism.

An under-weight patient will show a lack of subcutaneous fat. This may be due to leanness which is normal for that particular person. However, emaciation of recent onset can be judged by laxity of the skin along with usually a shallow appearance.

Cachexia is a term applied to severe loss of weight. Here the patient is seen to have an appearance of severe wasting along with anaemia. It is usually a result of a severe infection or a malignant process in the body. Severe uncontrolled diabetes also may result in such an appearance. (Plate 2.8)

4. FACIES : Appearance of the patient's face can suggest an underlying disease immediately leading to a quick or "spot" diagnosis or it may suggest a disease process which can be confirmed by further examination.

Examination of the face includes :

(a) General appearance;
(b) Eyes;
(c) Nose;
(d) Ears;
(e) Lips (and perioral area);
(f) Skin over the face;
(g) Salivary glands.

(a) **General appearance:** General appearance of the face is altered characteristically in many disorders.

The accompanying table enumerates these disorders.

(I) Endocrine disorders: (i) Cretinism, (ii) Myxodema, (iii) Thyrotoxicosis, (iv) Acromegaly, (v)Cushing's syndrome.

(II) Congenital disorders: (i) Mongolism, (ii) Hypertelorism, (iii) Congenital hemolytic anaemia e.g., thalassemia.

(III) Renal diseases: (i) Nephrotic syndrome, (ii) Acute nephritis.

(IV) Infective diseases: (i) Measles, smallpox, (ii) Congenital syphilis, (iii) Leprosy, (iv) Tetanus, (v) Hippocratic facies.

(V) Central nervous system disorders:

(i) Parkinsonism, (ii) Facial Palsy, (iii) Myasthenia gravis, (iv) Myopathies, (v) Tabes dorsalis.

(VI) Cardiovascular diseases: (i) Mitral stenosis, (ii) Congenital cardiac lesions.

(VII) Respiratory diseases: Chronic obstructive lung disease.

(VIII) Miscellaneous : e.g., Hemangiona (Plate 2.24).

(I) Endocrine disorders:

(i) Cretinism: The facial features are coarse and the skin is dry and pale. The nose is broad and flat, the lips are thick, the eyes widely set and the tongue is thick and protruding out of the mouth. The expression is devoid of intelligence or may have a somnolent appearance. (Other associated features are a short stature, hoarse cry and protruberent abdomen with umbilical hernia. The child has delayed milestones and subnormal intelligence.)

(ii) Myxodema: In this condition, the face is dull and expressionless with periorbital puffiness. The skin is dry and pale and on palpation may feel cool and is always rough and doughy. The eyebrow hair become sparse, the loss being more pronounced in the outer one-third area. The hair over the head also becomes dry and sparse. The tongue is large in some patients and a malar flush is seen in a few patients. (Plate 2.9)

(iii) Thyrotoxicosis: The most characteristic features of thyrotoxic face are large protrudent eyes (exophthalmos) which give a peculiar staring look. (Plate 2.10)

Eyes have a staring look due to wide palpebral fissures associated with infrequent blinking. Lid lag is present and in more advanced cases the retraction of the upper eyelids makes the white sclera visible over the upper border of the cornea. There is a failure of convergence and the brow cannot be wrinkled on upwards gaze. Emotional play of the facial muscles is excessive and the skin is moist and warm with excessive sweating.

The hair is silky and thin and sometimes there is a loss of hair from both the temporal areas of the scalp.

(The eye signs described above, that is, staring look, lid lag and lid retraction are due to sympathetic over-stimulation and these diminish after correction of thyrotoxicosis.)

Malignant exophthalmos is sometimes seen in these patients where there is marked proptosis and congestive changes leading to chemosis, conjunctivitis, periorbital swelling which results in corneal ulceration, optic neuritis or optic atrophy.

(Exophthalmic ophthalmoplegia is a term applied to the weakness of ocular muscles which accompanies thyrotoxicosis.)

(iv) Acromegaly: The most prominent feature of this condition is prognathism or prominent lower jaw. This along with the coarse features characterised by large and prominent forehead and cheek bones, large and flat nose, lips and ears gives a typical simian or apelike appearance to the face. The teeth are separated from each other due to over growth of lower jaw and sometimes this prognathism is so marked that it interferes with mastication. Hands are broad and spade like. (Plate 2.11a & 2.11b)

(v) Cushing's syndrome: The classical abnormality of the face in this condition is described as "moon face". The face appears rounded due to deposition of fat in its upper part. The face also appears flushed or plethoric and sometimes has the presence of excessive hair and acne. (Plate 2.12).

(II) Congenital disorders:

(i) Mongolism: The shape of the head of the "Mongol" (Down's syndrome) is oval and the size is small with a sloping forehead. Ears are oval and low set and the lobules are small in size. The eyes are slanting upwards and outwards due to the presence of a medial epicanthic fold which is the most characteristic diagnostic feature. (Plate 2.13)

The bridge of the nose is depressed and a coarse, fissured heavy enlarged tongue is seen lolling out of the partly opened mouth. The iris shows grey white specks of depigmentation. The expression of the face is that of a mentally retarded child.

(The other associated features of a mongol are broad and simian hands with a single transverse crease. The fingers are short and curved inwards due to the middle phalanx being hypoplastic. The stature is usually short and other congenital abnormalities specially in the cardiovascular system are often present.) (Plate 2.14)

(ii) Hyperteleorism: The face in this condition is characterised by a low forehead with a vertical groove (which is produced by an enlargement of the lesser wing of the sphenoid bone), wide set eyes with a depressed nasal bridge and prominent frontal bossing.

Significance: Usually associated with mongolism, or mongoloid facies.

(iii) Congenital hemolytic anaemia: Face looks mongoloid, eyes are slanting; there is epicanthic fold and malar prominence is present due to high cheek bones. (Plate 2.15).

(III) Renal disease:

(i) Nephrotic syndrome : In this condition, the face is swollen up and the skin is puffy and loose.

The oedema is most marked around the eyes so that they appear narrow like slits. Pallor is a very commonly associated feature. (Ref. Plate 5.1 — Chapter 5).

Hypoprotinaemia due to any other cause may also give rise to a similar facial appearance. The appearance in myxodema and nephrotic syndrome may cause confusion, but the dryness of the skin and other features in myxodema differentiate these two conditions.

Rarely urticaria may simulate these facies but this condition is usually associated with plethora and itching.)

(ii) Acute nephritis: The face in this condition shows pallor and puffiness around the eyes, especially the lower eyelids. However, these changes are present in the early morning and may disappear by evening to a great extent.

(IV) Infective diseases:

(i) Measles: "Measly face" as it is known commonly has very typical appearance. The patient usually a child appears ill, there is conjunctivitis with watering of the eyes. The typical red maculopapular rash appears on the face, first on the forehead and then spread downwards.

(Koplik's spots are small, red irregular lesions with blue white centres appearing on the mucous membranes of the mouth one or two days before the onset of the rash.)

(ii) Congenital syphilis: The typical facial appearance of a patient affected by this disorder includes frontal bossing along with a saddle nose due to the sunken bridge of the nose. The maxillae are poorly developed. The dental abnormalities include Hutchinson's teeth (which is a term applied to widely spaced, centrally notched, peg shaped central incisors) and 'mulberry molars' (which have poorly developed multiple cusps instead of the normal four). Corneal opacities due to interstitial keratitis complete the clinical appearance.

(iii) Leprosy: 'Leonine' facies is a term applied to the classical advanced form of lepromatous leprosy.

Due to the thickening of the skin, the face appears typically swollen and corrugated. The hair of the eyebrows, specially the outer one-third is lost and the eye-lashes are scanty or absent. The nose is depressed due to the destruction of the bridge of the nose.

(iv) Tetanus: Due to the sustained spasm of the facial muscles the face assumes a typical appearance described as 'risus sardonicus'. The angles of the mouth are lifted due to the spasm of facial muscles and the eyes are partially closed with elevation of the eye-brows. The 'lockjaw' or inability to open the mouth is present along with this appearance. (Plate 2.16)

(v) Hippocratic facies: This is a term applied to the facial appearance of a moribund patient. It was first described by Hippocrates and denotes a very grave prognosis. The eye-balls are sunken, skin is dry and parched, nose is pinched and lips are dry and may be cracked. Usually it is associated with muttering delirium.

(V) Central nervous system disorders:

(i) Parkinsonism: 'Mask like face' is the most apt description of a fully developed parkinsonism face. The term is derived from the lack of the normal play of expressions on the patient's face due to rigidity of the small muscles of the face. In addition the palpebral fissures are wider than usual and the eyes have a staring appearance due to infrequent blinking and paucity of the spontaneous ocular movements. (Plate 2.17)

(ii) Facial palsy: In unilateral lower motor neurone type of facial palsy, the face is asymmetrical due to weakness of muscles on one side, (Ref. to Plate 15.3b, Chapter 15).

On the affected side the forehead is smooth and there is an inability to close the eye; any attempt to do so results in the eye-ball rolling upwards, this is called Bell's phenomenon. There is an excessive lacrimation from the affected eye. The nasolabial furrow on the paralysed side is absent or much less prominent than on the normal side and the cheeks flap in and out with respiration. There is drooping of the angle of the mouth with dribbling of saliva.

(iii) Myasthenia gravis: Due to the progressive weakness of the muscles, the features of myasthenia are always more prominent at the end of the day rather than in the morning.

The eyes are partly closed due to the drooping eyelids and the mouth hangs open due to weakness of the jaw muscles. The retractors of the angles of the mouth are affected more than the elevators giving rise to a peculiar sneering smile of myasthenia. (Plates 2.18a, 2.18b).

(iv) Myopathies: Facioscapulohumeral muscular dystrophy affects the facial muscles giving rise to a characteristic pouting appearance of the face with a peculiar transverse smile. The eyelids may show drooping and the facial muscles show a particular atrophy.

(v) Tabes: In advanced cases of tabes, the eyelids are retracted due to excessive action of sympathetic system. The forehead is wrinkled to compensate for this drooping and inequality of the small pupils adds to the peculiar appearance.

(VI) Cardiovascular diseases:

(i) Mitral stenosis: A typical 'malar flush' that is flushing of the cheeks or sometimes a bluish discolouration is seen in patient having a tight mitral stenosis.

(ii) Congenital cardiac lesions: Cyanosis due to congenital defects in the development of the heart manifests as a central cyanosis and hence the face will manifest this cyanosis in the lips, car lobes and tongue. In advanced or severely cyanotic cases the whole face will have a dusky appearance.

(b) **Eyes:** (i) **Eye-brows:** Loss of hair over the outer one-third of the eye-brows is seen in myxodema and neurosyphilis.

In leprosy the hair over the eye-brows may be totally lost. Rarely the loss of hair over the eye-brows may be part of a generalised absence of hair in rare cases of ectodermal dysplasia.

(ii) **Eye-lids:** Retraction of eye-lids is seen in sympathetic over-action as in parkinsonism and in local irritative diseases of the eye like trachoma.

Drooping of eye-lids can be unilateral or bilateral and it may be incomplete or complete.

Mysthenia is the only condition where there is a variable ptosis of the eye-lids, the weakness increases progressively with repeated use and is more towards the evening.

The drooping of eye-lids can be due to paralysis of the third nerve or the ocular sympathetic nerves. The local diseases of muscle like myopathies can be a cause of this condition Unilateral drooping can be of congenital origin.

(iii) **Palpebral fissure:** Oblique or slanting palpebral fissures are seen in mongolian facies.

Palpebral fissures are wider in parkinsonism, hyperthyroidism and rarely in cervical sympathetic stimulation.

They are narrower in Horner's syndrome and in paralysis of the third nerve.

(iv) **Eye-balls:** Appearance : The eye balls may be either protruded or retracted. Exophthalmos is more commonly seen in thyrotoxicosis but may rarely be congenital. Rarely chronic corpulmonale or patients with oxycephalic skulls may show a similar appearance. Local deposits behind the eye balls in diseases like leukemias or tumours locally may give rise to this condition and rarely thrombosis of the superior sagital sinus may give rise to a mild exophthalmos. Unilateral exophthalmos may occur in local tumours or scurvy. (Plate 2.19) Severe dehydration usually causes enophthalmos and this may be seen in any severe state of shock or Hippocratic facies due to any cause. In diabetic acidosis, this may be an important diagnostic sign. Horner's syndrome also produces enophthalmos. (Plate 2.20)

(v) **Sclera:** The normal colour of sclera is clear white. A generalised muddy or yellowish discolouration is observed in normal persons.

Yellowish discolouration or icterus is diagnostic of jaundice. Bluish colour of the sclera is seen in osteogenesis imperfecta.

(vi) **Conjunctiva:** Conjunctiva are normally checked for presence or absence of pallor which is a correct clinical index for judging the haemoglobin percentage of blood. However, rarely subconjunctival hemorrhages are seen after severe bouts of coughing especially in whooping cough and rarely after vomiting. Convulsions or severe hypertension also may give rise to these hemorrhages.

(vii) **Cornea:** Xerosis or xerophthalmia is present in vitamin A deficiency: Corneal opacities are the most common causes of blindness and in developing countries, vitamin A deficiency, trachoma and small pox are common causes of opacities. Arcus senilis is a greyish white crescent in the outer border of cornea.

Kayser Fleischer ring is seen in patients suffering from Wilson's disease. It is a brownish greenish ring. Usually it is seen by a slit lamp examination but is rarely visible to the naked eye.

(viii) **Unilateral or bilateral** cataracts should be looked for. (Plate 2.21 (a) & (b))

(c) **Nose:** Saddle nose is produced by depression of the bridge of the nose and is seen in congenital syphilis and leprosy.

Rhinophyma is a rare condition where there is a bulbous appearance of the nose due to hypertrophy.

A pinched appearance of the nose is present in children suffering from adenoids (adenoid facies) and rarely in spinal muscular atrophy (tapir mouth). (Plate 2.22)

Alae nasi movements are seen in conditions causing respiratory distress.

(d) **Ears:** Ears may be the site of deposition of gouty tophi. Ears are low set in mongols and mentally retarded children. (Plate 2.23)

Abnormally formed ears are usually associated with congenital urinary anomalies in children.

The ear lobes and the skin over the ears may show thickening as one of the earliest signs of leprosy.

(e) **Lips and perioral area:** Colour of the lips may be bluish due to central cyanosis or they may be pale due to anaemia.

Lips may be dry and parched in severe dehydration and the mucous membrane over the lips then appears wrinkled.

Angular cheilitis produces cracks at the angles of the mouth and is usually due to vitamin B6 deficiency. These are usually dry cracks with scaling but occasionally they show local bleeding.

Severe cheilitis even with ulcers is seen in drug reaction (Exfoliative dermatitis, ie., Steven Johnson's syndrome).

Rhagades are ulcerative fissures at the angles of the mouth and they produce white linear radiating scars. They are due to congenital syphilis.

Marked swelling of the lips is seen in angioneurotic oedema or hemangioma or may be sometimes due to local insect bites. (Plate 2.24)

Ulcers over the lips are common and they may be either infective or due to growths which can be benign or malignant. The infective ulcers can be pyogenic, syphilitic or rarely tuberculous.

Herpes simplex produces vesicular eruptions over the lips and perioral area. They are painful and are seen in patients suffering from pneumonia.

(f) **Skin over the face:** Colour of the skin over the face may present a diagnostic clue. Bluish or dusky discolouration is seen in patients with severe cyanotic heart disease. A flush over the malar area is seen in mitral stenosis while a typical 'ruddy' flush is seen in chronic alcoholics. Flushed cheeks are also seen in high septicemic fevers. A brownish discolouration is seen in Addison's disease.

A typical butterfly rash which extends on the cheeks and the bridge of the nose is seen in patients suffering from lupus erythromatosis. Rarely areas overlying small joints of hands undergo a peculiar brownish pigmentation in pernicious anaemia.

Dry skin with thickening of the subcutaneous tissues is a hallmark of myxodema while the face has a typical puffy appearance due to swelling of the subcutaneous tissues and skin be cause of renal oedema.

Dryness or wrinkling of the facial skin may be the result of old age or dehydration due to any cause. Acne, adenosebaceum and rash in some infective disorders like measles appear over the skin of the face.

Yellowish dull 'sallow hue' is seen over skin of the face in severe anaemia of nutritional origin.

Dull white colour of skin is present in aplastic anemia or anemia due to malignancy.

(g) **Salivary glands:** Bilateral parotid swellings which are painful are seen in patients suffering from mumps and this condition may affect the other salivary glands. Whenever parotid gland is swollen the ear lobule is raised. Occasionaly a huge mass in connection with cervical glands in posterior triangle, may raise the ear lobule. (Plate 2.25)

Bilateral parotid swellings are seen in patients with a history of chronic alcoholism and is a common occurrence in cirrhosis of the liver.

Unilateral or bilateral painful swelling of the parotid glands can be produced due to acute septic parotitis especially in patients suffering from prolonged debilitating diseases. Swelling of parotid or other salivary glands which increases after food may be due to salivary calculus. Parotid tumours are slow growing and may produce a very large unilateral swelling.

Enlargment of all the salivary glands is seen in Mikulicz's syndrome and is sometimes associated with a bloodpicture of lymphatic leukemia with hepatosplenomegaly.

(5) **HEAD AND NECK:** Examination of head should include :

(a) Shape and size of the skull;

(b) Sutures and fontanelles;

(c) Examination of hair distribution.

(a) **Shape and size of the skull:** The skull may be enlarged abnormally in size producing macrocephaly and the size of the brain is proportionately larger with the ventricles being normal in size.

Hydrocephalus is globular enlargement of the skull due to increased size and pressure in the ventricles. This is seen in children before the sutures have united giving rise to an unnaturally enlarged head. The eye balls are pushed downwards with the sclera being visible above the cornea. This is called sunset sign. The fontanelles are bulging and the hair growth is poor. (Plate 2.26 a & b)

Paget's disease results in an abnormally large head due to hypertrophy of the bones.

Microcephaly is an abnormally small size of the head and is due to lack of brain growth. (Plate 2.27)

Abnormal shape of the skull is produced usually by early abnormal closure of sutures. The term craniostenosis is applied to this abnormality and the abnormal shape depends on which sutures close early.

Oxycephaly (Turricephaly) is produced by closure of sagittal and coronal sutures. The head is elongated vertically with a pointed vertex.

The forehead is wide and the eyes are bulging due to shallow orbits. Anteroposterior diameter of the skull is reduced markedly with an increase in the vertical diameter. This condition produces an increased intracranial tension and stunted brain growth if not recognised and treated on time.

Dolicocephaly is produced by early closure of sagittal sutures and the head becomes long and narrow with prominent brow and occiput.

Brachycephaly is produced by premature closure of coronal sutures and the head becomes wider. One side of the skull may be flattened on the occipital side with a corresponding flattening of the opposite forehead producing plagiocephaly. It is usually due to disease in infancy which forces the patient to lie down with his head turned to one side for a prolonged period of time.

Platybasia or basilar invagination is an abnormality in which the extended head is lying on a short neck with a low hair line. Usually it is associated with cranio-vertebral anomalies in which the basilar and condylar portions of the occipital bone are displaced upwards with abnormalities of the cervical spine.

The skull in rickets is usually oblong with prominent frontal and parietal eminence. In congenial syphilis a typical 'hot cross bun' skull may be seen due to prominence of the frontal eminences along with a vertical forehead and sunken bridge of the nose.

Craniotabes is a term applied to the softening of bones which can be indented by fingers with an immediate return to normal position when the pressure is released. This is seen in early rickets. The surface of the skull should always be palpated carefully for any depressed fracture when there is a history of trauma.

Irregular nodules may be felt over the skull surface in certain types of metastatic malignancy. In children, percussion of the skull may yield a typical cracked pot sound in hydrocephalus or in separation of sutures due to raised intracranial tension; this sign is elicited after closure of fontanelles.

(b) **Sutures and fontanelles:** Hydrocephalus in infants produces a separation of all the satures and fontanelles are bulging. Frontal bossing is peculiar, in sense, there is overhanging forehead. (Plate 2.26 (b)

In children, tne fontanelles are tense in meningitis. In dehydration they are sunken and are used as a clinical guide for judging the degree of dehydration.

Early closure of sutures results in various types of skull deformities as described above and their delayed closure is seen in rickets, cretinism, malnutrition and congenital syphilis.

(c) **Examination of hair distribution:** Alopecia or baldness is mostly hereditary and is seen after the age of forty. However, it can be seen very early due to pathological reasons. (Plate 2.28)

Premature balding is seen in endocrine defects like hypopituitarism or hypothyroidism. Sometimes during pregnancy or in the post partum period, ladies develop alopecia.

Following severe infections or in leprosy alopecia is observed. Prolonged anticoagulant administration or thellium reactions can induce alopecia. Therapy with cytotoxic agents also causes this condition.

Rarely collagen disorders like lupus, erythematosis or iron deficiency even without anaemia, can cause premature baldness.

Frontal baldness is one of the diagnostic features of myotonic dystrophy.

(Normal hair on the scalp are classified as anagen or tolagen. Anagen are the growing hair and tolagen are the hair in the resting phase. This is determined by the presence of root sheath and presence of melanin around the tips in growing hair.

Normal scalp has roughly 100,000 hair and the growth cycle is about 2 to 6 years. Resting phase is about three months. Normally about 70 hair are lost daily from the scalp.)

(d) **Examination of the neck:** Examination of the neck should include both inspection and palpation.

Inspection of the neck should be carried out to determine any gross shortening or lengthening or any abnormal positions. Any obvious swelling in the neck should be inspected as usual and presence of any engorged veins or abnormal arterial pulsations should be noted. Position of trachea (though better checked by palpation) should be observed and any abnormal swelling of the thyroid gland should be checked.

Palpation of the neck is usually carried out to find palpable lymph glands which are not obvious on inspection. Any swelling or abnoromal swelling of thyroid gland should be palpated systematically.

(e) **Abnormalities of the neck:**

(I) Shape and size: Physiologically very short neck is seen in short thin persons (hypersthenic individuals) or in very obese persons. Pathologically, especially when associated with a low hair line, it is indicative of cranio-vertebral anomalies (Klippel -Feil syndrome).

A thin long neck is physiological in hyposthenic type of people. Any wasting disease can also give a similar appearance to the neck.

(II) Neck muscles and their abnormalities: Sternomastoid muscles can be congenitally absent on one or either side as a developmental anomaly and this is ascertained by asking the patient to rotate the head on either side against resistance or by asking him to lift the head. The absent sternomastoid will be detected by the absence of the normal prominent contraction.

Spasm of the neck muscles is seen in a variety of conditions. Tetanus in its earliest stages causes spasm of sternomastoids (sometimes even before the 'lockjaw'). Meningitis or cerebral haemorrhage gives rise to neck rigidity due to neck muscle spasms. In advanced cases and especially in children, this results in head retraction.

Torticollis can be of a continuous or of spasmodic variety. Acute torticollis causing deviation of the head on one side, associated with pain, is usually due to inflammation of sternomastoids or trapezies. Spasmodic torticollis results in a chronic jerking of the head with rotation. This is also seen in cranio cervical spasms due to extrapyramidal lesions. (Plate 2.29)

Titubation or nodding of the head results from contraction of both the sternomastoids and is seen in elderly people with atherosclerosis and patients suffering from parkinsonism.

Weakness of sternomastoids and other neck muscles in advanced myopathies causes the head to fall backwards and the patient is unable to lift up his head from the bed when he is in a horizontal position.

Tics and chorea can cause jerky irregular movements of the neck. Tics are usually repetitive and cause the same type of bizarre movements every time while choreiform movements are non-repetitive and disappear during sleep.

(III) Examination of arterial and venous pulsations: This is described along with the examination of the cardiovascular system.

(f) **Examination of neck glands:** Lymph glands in the neck can be inspected when they are enlarged. However a routine palpation must be carried out.

Palpation for lymph glands should be carried out in the anatomical areas of the neck as follows: The posterior cervical region, the submental area, the anterior triangles of the neck and the supraclavicular area should be palpated in turn.

If the lymph nodes are found to be enlarged, their size, shape, consistency, matting and adherence to the skin or deeper structures should be noted. If the consistency is very soft, presence or absence of fluctuation should be looked for. (Plate 2.30)

Common causes of lymphadenopathy in the neck are :

(I) Inflammatory: (a) Acute lymphadenitis following infection in the mouth, head, neck or scalp; (b) Chronic lymphadenitis due to syphilis, tuberculosis.

(II) Due to reticulosis and blood dyscrasias: (a) Hodgkin's disease; (b) Lymphatic leukemia.

(III) Due to malignant diseases: (a) Lymphosarcoma; (b) Secondary deposits in the neck glands.

The following is a short description of the clinical signs associated with these various types of lymphadenopathies.

1. Inflammatory:

(i) **Acute lymphadenitis:** The glands affected with acute inflammation are swollen, painful and tender. They are fixed and the skin overlying them is red in colour and warm to the touch.

As acute lymphadenitis is secondary to the septic focus in the mouth, head, neck or scalp the examination of these areas should be carried out to find it out. Common infection in scalp is lice infestation.

(ii) **Chronic lymphadenitis:** Tubercle infection of the lymph glands in the neck is one of the most common conditions in developing countries causing cervical lymphadenopathy in the posterior traingle of the neck. However the infection can affect any group of glands in the neck. In the initial stages, the glands are firm, discrete and non-adherent to the surrounding structures and their clinical differentiation from other chronic inflammatory glands is difficult. However, in advanced condition, the glands are matted together. If they necrose to form a 'cold abscess' fluctuation can be demonstrated. They very often break through the skin forming a chronically discharging sinus with scarring.

Syphilitic involvement of the neck glands is common and the glands are discrete (not matted), firm, 'shotty' and painless. They are not adherent to the adjacent structures and are most commonly found in occipital and posterior auricular areas.

II. Due to reticulosis and blood dyscrasias:

(i) **Hodgkin's disease:** This disease causes a large swelling of the affected lymph glands which have a typical 'rubbery' consistency. The glands are usually movable due to non-adherence to the surrounding structures. Systemic symptoms like fever, wasting, anaemia and generalised lymphadenopathy may be present along with this cervical involvement.

(ii) **Lymphatic leukemia:** Neck glands are enlarged as a part of the generalised lymphadenopathy present in this disease. The glands are enlarged, firm and non-adherent. Any group of cervical lymph glands can be affected.

III. Due to malignant diseases:

(i) **Lymphosar-coma:** Any particular group of lymph glands in the neck can be involved and a massive enlargement of the affected glands is seen. The glands are tender and invade the surrounding structures and they can ulcerate through the skin. Mediastinal lymphadenopathy is usually associated with this cervical enlargement and usually precedes it (In the new terminology, lymphosarcoma comes under the category of Hodgkin's lymphoma).

(ii) **Secondary deposits in the neck glands:** The gland's involved by this disease process are usually very firm or stony hard in consistency. The distribution of these glands in the neck depends upon the site of the primary malignancy. Virchow's glands are glands present in the supraclavicular fossa on the left side due to deposits from a gastric malignancy.

(g) **Examination of the thyroid gland:** Thyroid gland's examination should consist of both inspection and palpation.

Inspection is ideally carried out by asking the patient to extend his neck. Then he is asked to carry out a swallowing movement when the enlarged thyroid gland will be seen to move upwards and then downwards.

Palpation is ideally carried out by the examiner standing behind the patient and the thyroid should be palpated by fingers of both hands. The usual practice of examining any swelling for its size, shape, consistency, surface and presence or absence of tenderness should be followed. However, particular attention should be given for noting the presence or absence of nodules. Also presence of a thrill should be looked for and if necessary auscultation should be carried out to confirm the bruit.

Any enlargement of the thyroid gland is known as 'goitre'. However, technically a goitre means a non-inflammatory and non-malignant enlargement of the thyroid gland. (Plate 2.31)

Goitres are classified as simple or toxic. They can also be classified as smooth or nodular.

Simple goitres can be either smooth or nodular but they are not associated with any symptoms of thyrotoxicosis. Simple, smooth goitres are found in puberty or pregnancy and usually do not require any surgical interference except for cosmetic reasons. Nodular goitres even if non-toxic should always be treated surgically as they may become malignant at a later date. Toxic goitres are either treated surgically or with radioactive isotope therapy after a course of medical treatment.

Malignancy of the thyroid glands always produces a very hard swelling usually of one lobe which is adherent to the surrounding structures. Hashimoto's disease produces a very firm uniform goitre which is also described as 'rubbery thyroid' because of this peculiar consistency.

6. EXAMINATION OF THE MOUTH AND ORAL CAVITY: Examination of this region should be carried out by noting the various structures as follows :

(a) Lips,
(b) Teeth,
(c) Gums,
(d) Buccal mucosa,
(e) Tongue,
(f) Palate,
(g) Tonsils,
(h) Posterior pharyngeal wall,
(i) Breath.

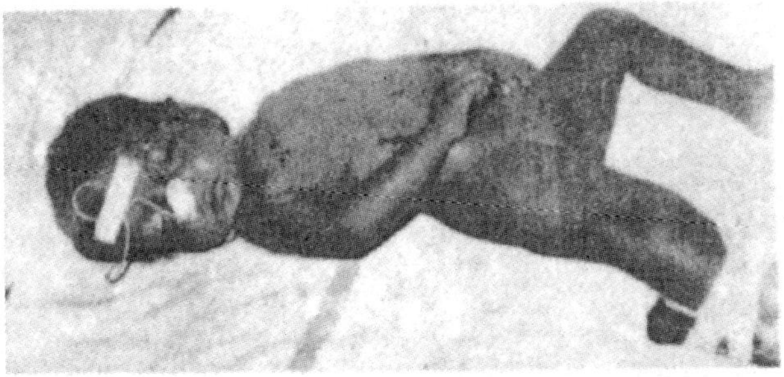

P1.2 1a Opisthotonus
Flexion of head on one side with flexion of contralateral flexion of upper limb.
Also note toxic neck reflex

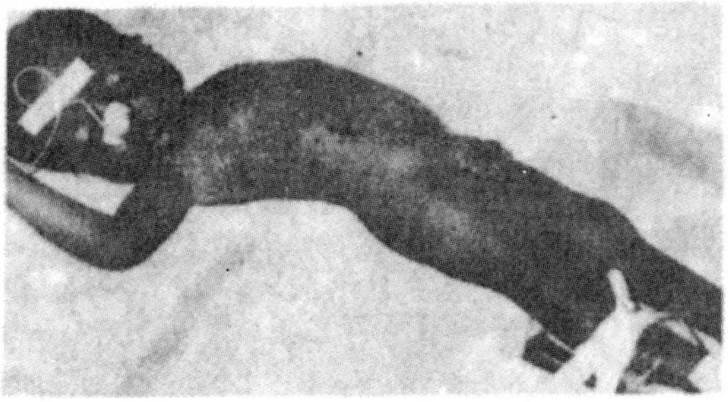

P1. 2.1b Pleurosthotonus
i.e. arching of body on

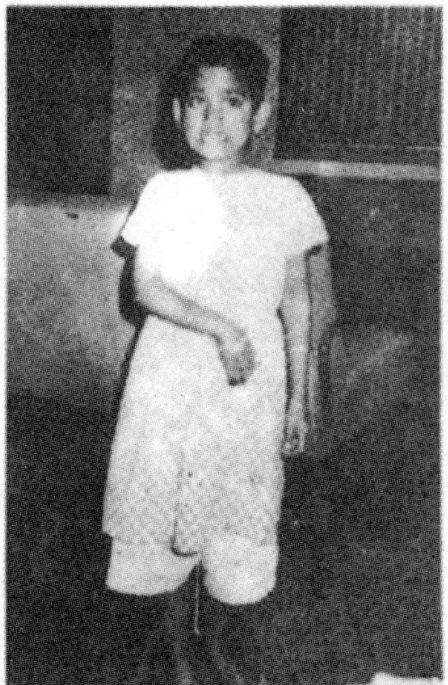

P1.2.2 Hemiplegia
Note the flexed, adducted upper limb

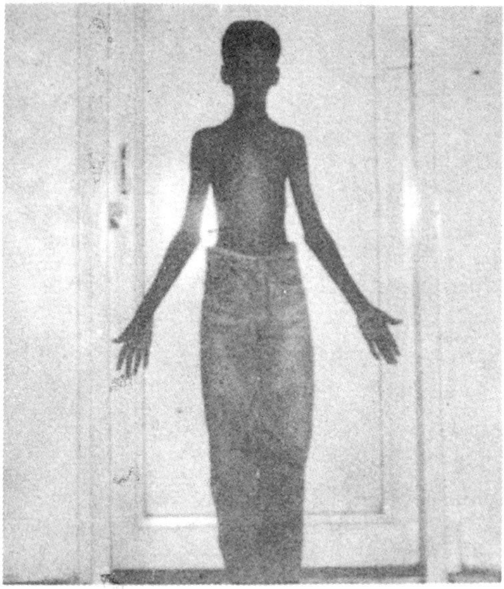

P1.2.3a Seen in a boy aged 11 years.
Note the tall slender build and long fingers

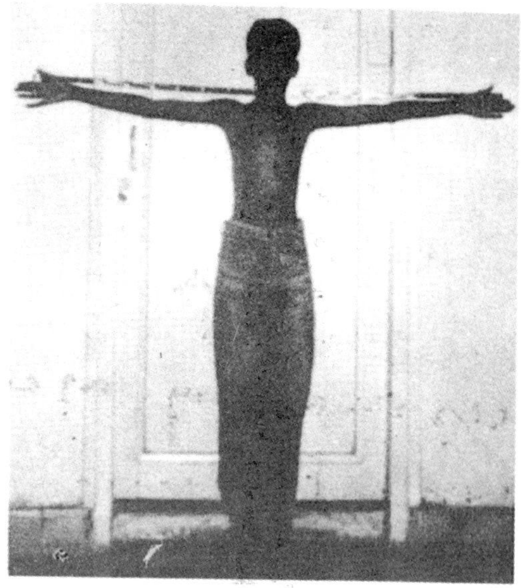

P1.2.3b Note that span is longer than height

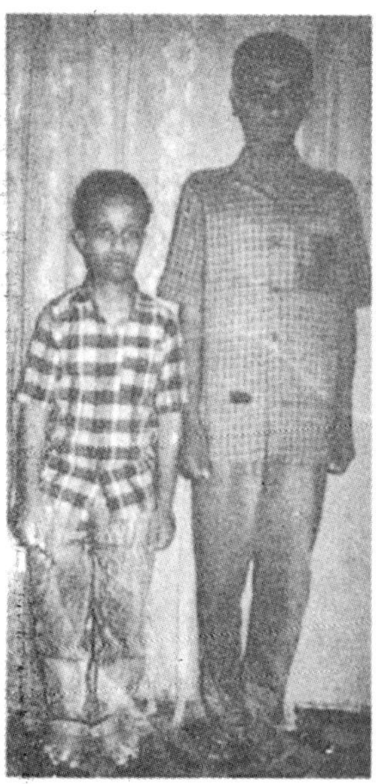

P1.2.4a
Date of Birth
1) Shridhar 31.12.76
20 year - is a primordial dwarf
2) Tushar 21.8.77
19 1/2 years

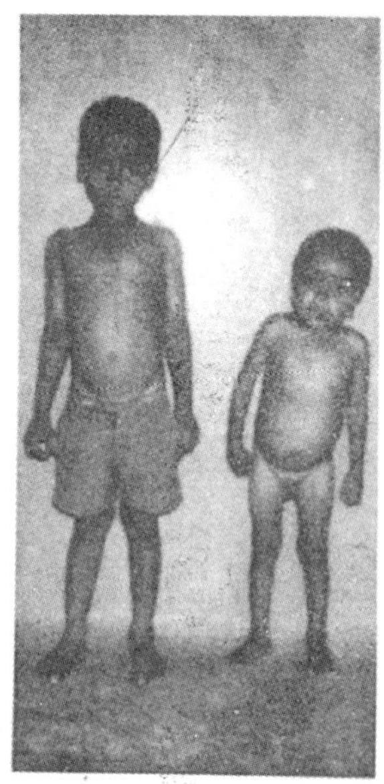

P1.2.4b Both 6 years old

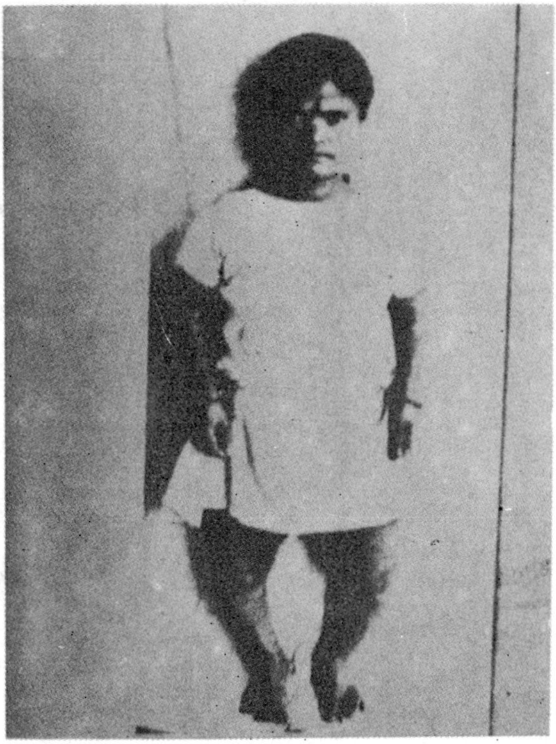

P1. 2.5 Achondroplasia

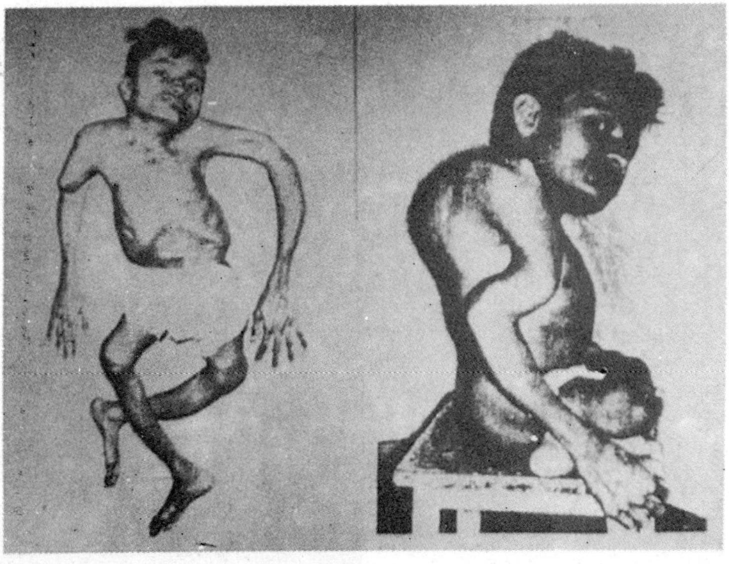

P1. 2.6 Osteogenesis imperfecta

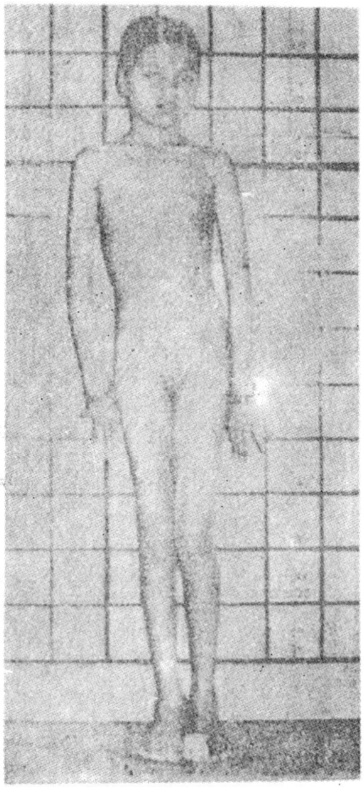

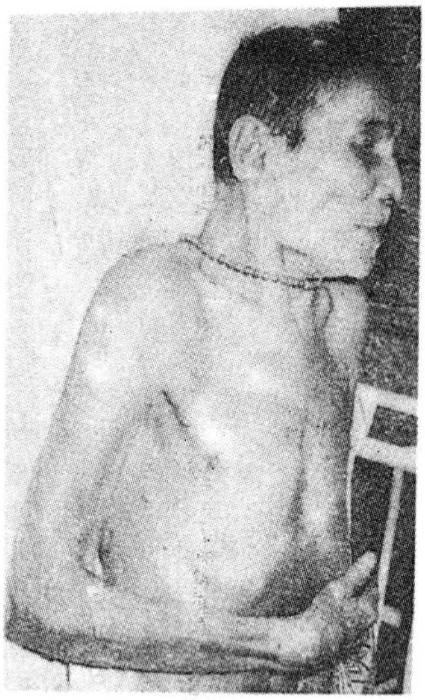

Pl. 2.8 Cachexia

Pl. 2.7 Pituitary dwarf in a girl aged 14 years.
Height is 25 cms. corresponds to that of 8-9 years old child.
Note the absence of secondary sexual characters

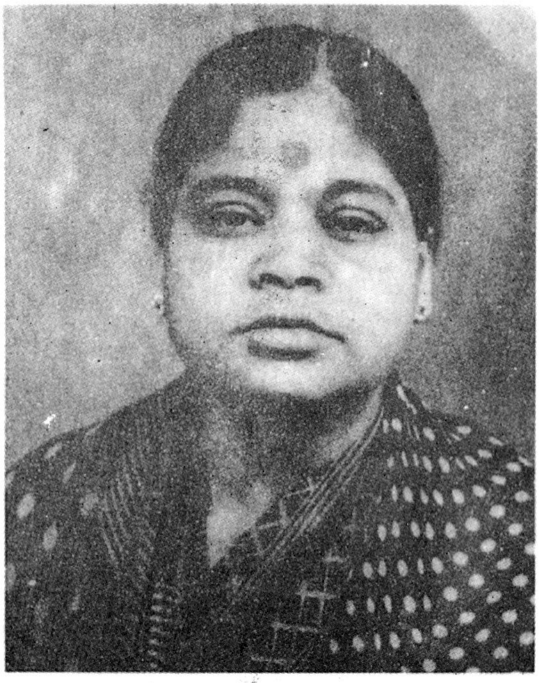

Pl. 2.9 Myxoedema - Note baggy lower eyelids and coarse features

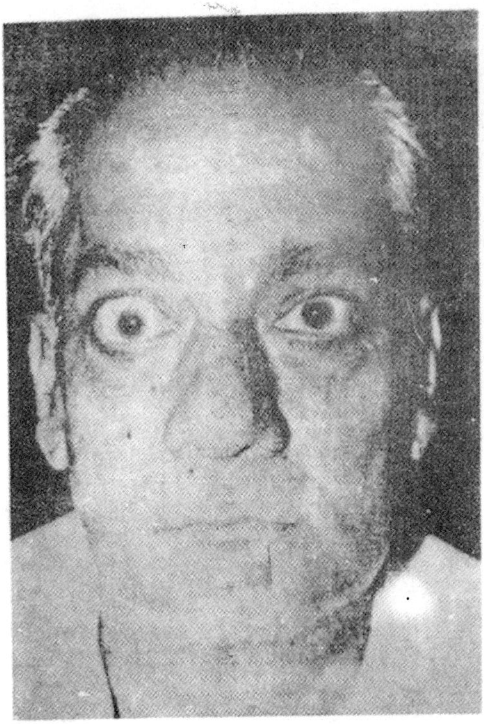

P1. 2.10 Thyrotoxicosis. Note the staring look

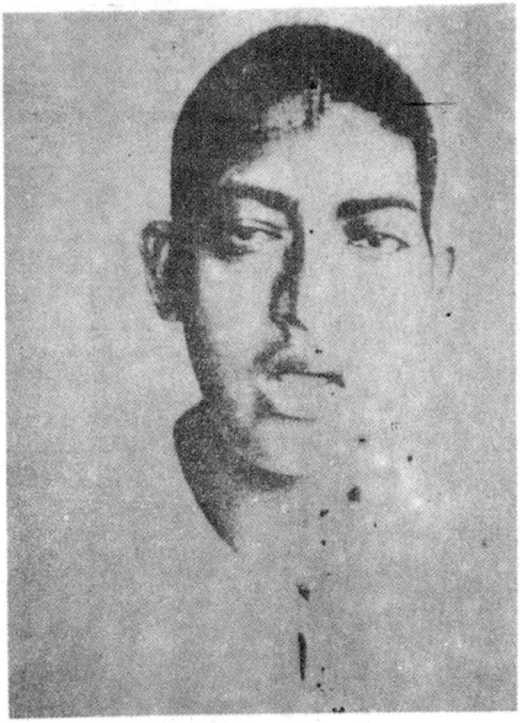

P1.2. 11a Acromegaly. Note coarse broad features prognathism, enlarged nose and orbital plate causing prominent eyebrows

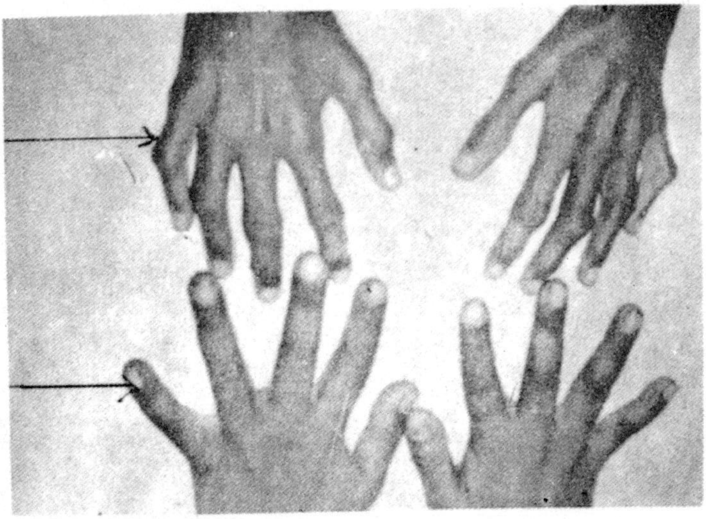

P1. 2. 11b Hands of acromegalic patient as compared with those of normal person

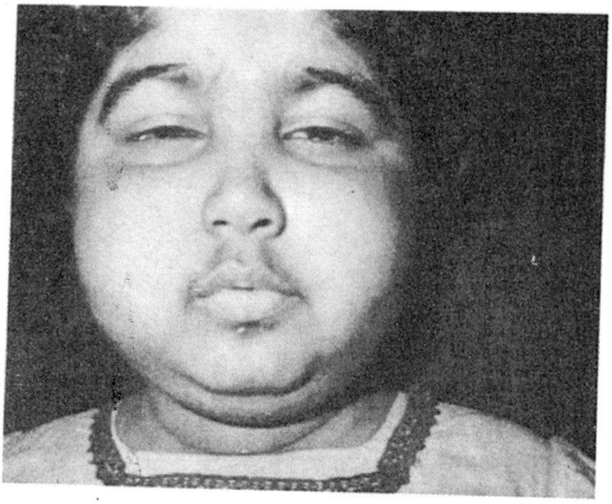

P l. 2.12 Cushing's syndrome

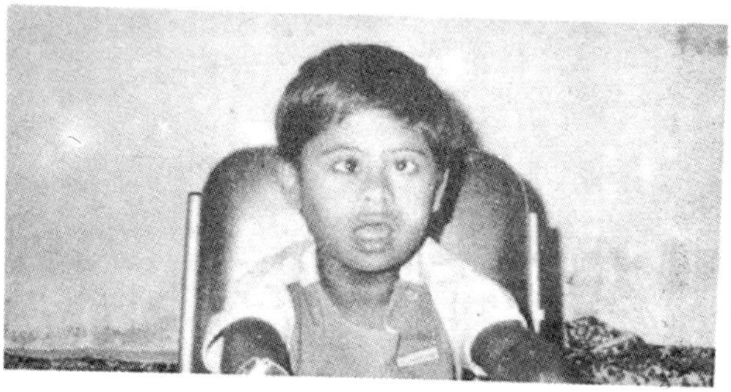

P l. 2.13 Mongolism

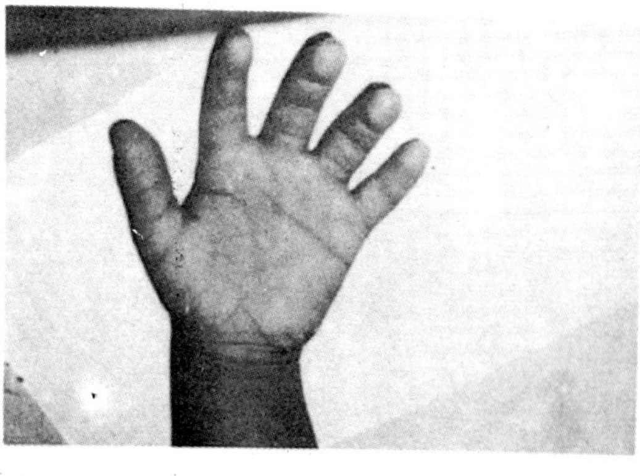

P l. 2.14 Single palmar crease of a mongol child

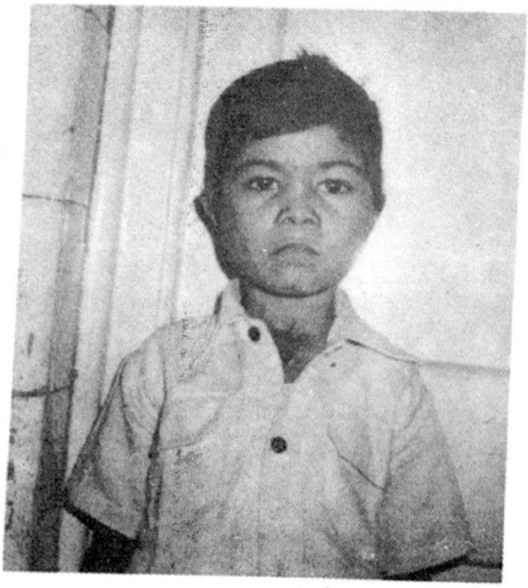

P1. 2.15 Haemolytic face

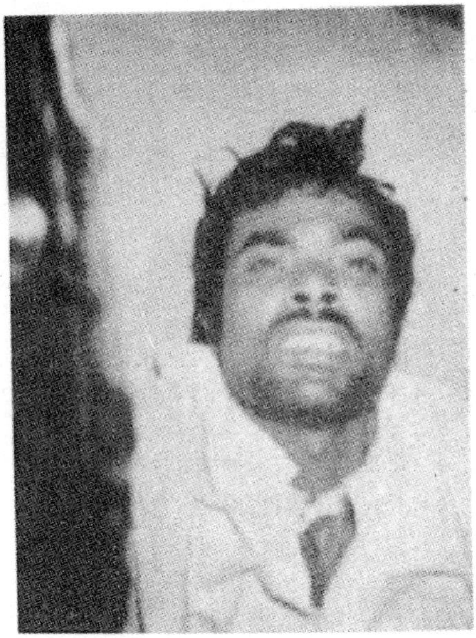

Pl. 2.16 Risus sardonicus

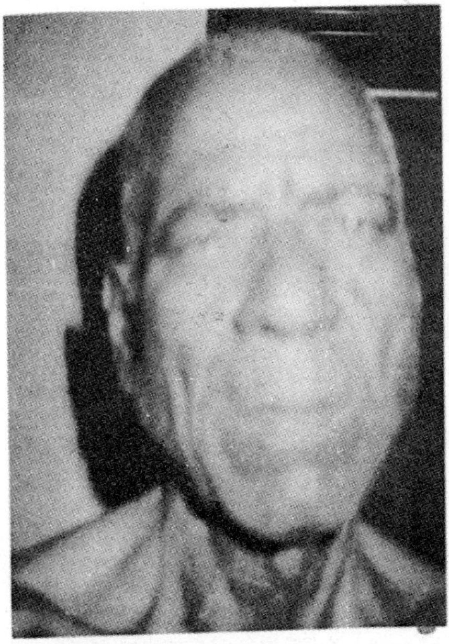

Pl. 2.17a Parkinsonian face

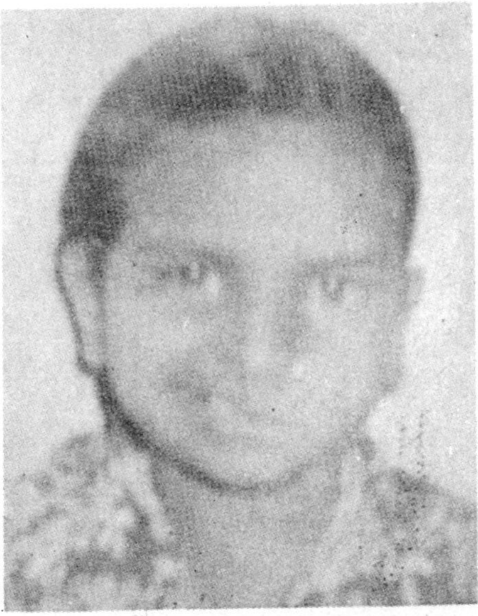

Pl. 2.17b Infranclear facial palsy (L) side
Note absence of naso labial fold

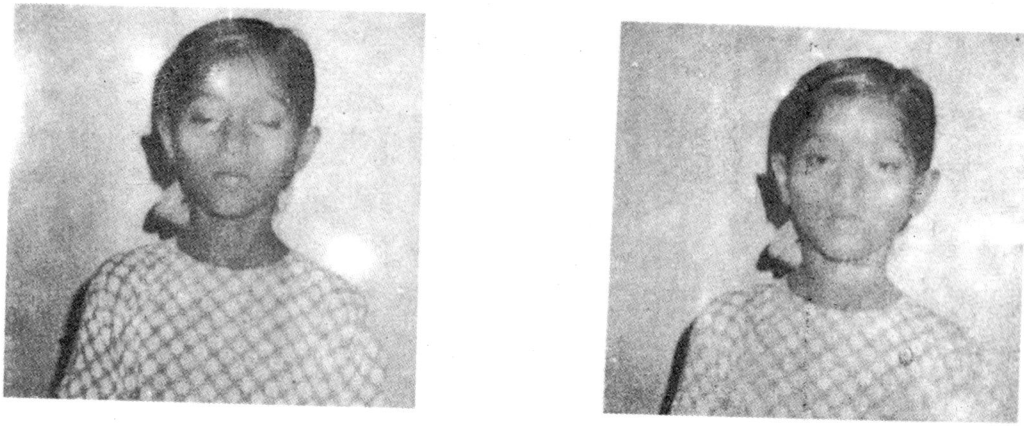

Pl. 2.18(a) Myasthenia gravis (b) after neostigmine test. Note correction of ptosis

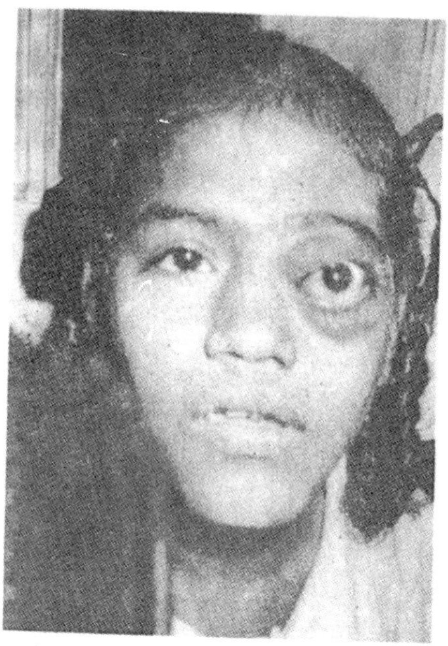

Pl. 2.19 Unilateral exophthalmus

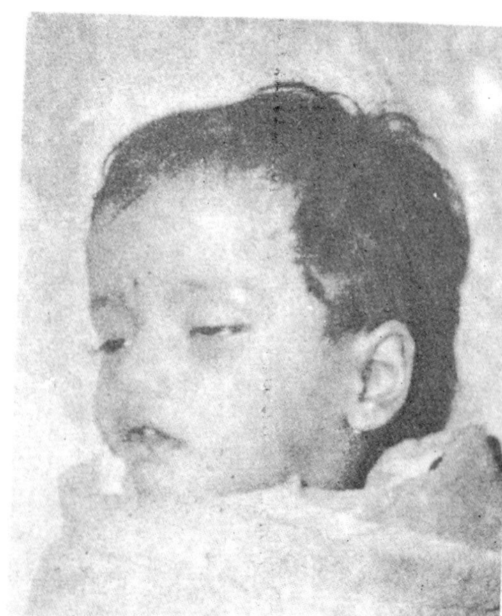

Pl. 2.20 Dehydration - Note sunkem eyeballs

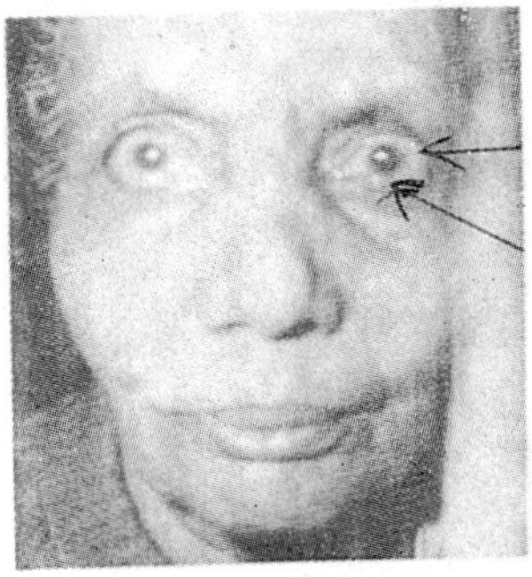
Pl. 2.21(a) Arcus Senilis.

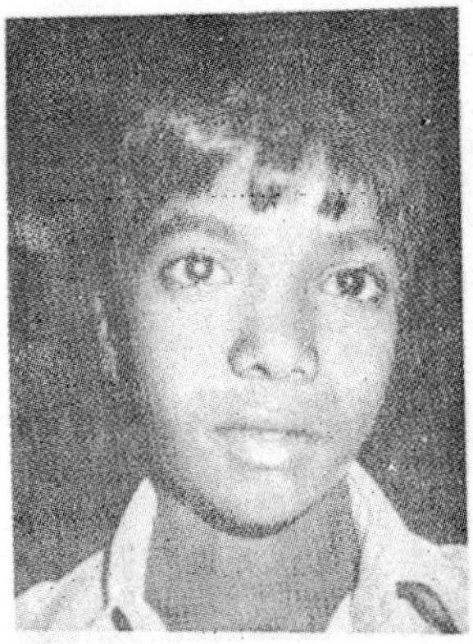
(b) Unilateral cataract

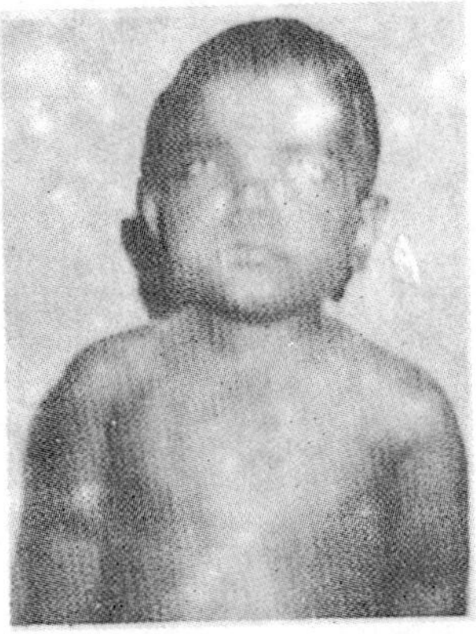
(c) Bilateral cataract

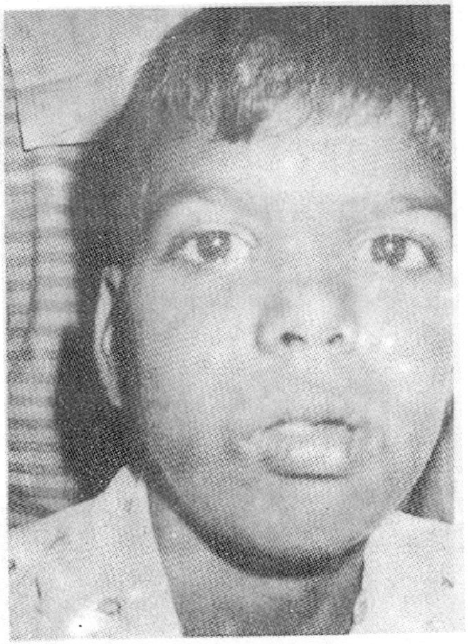
Pl. 2.22 Adenoid facies

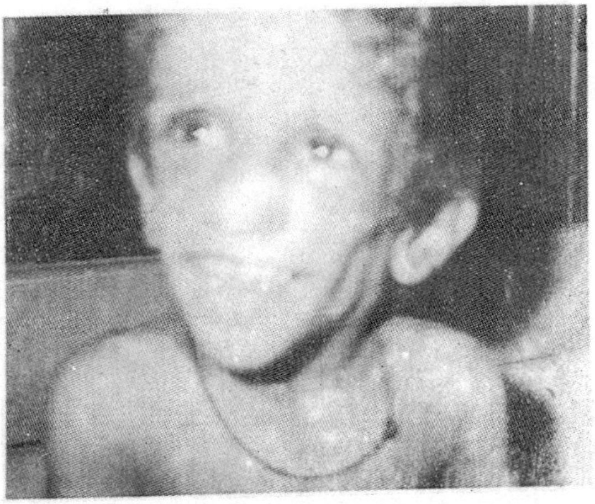
Pl. 2.23 Low set ears suggestive of mental retardation

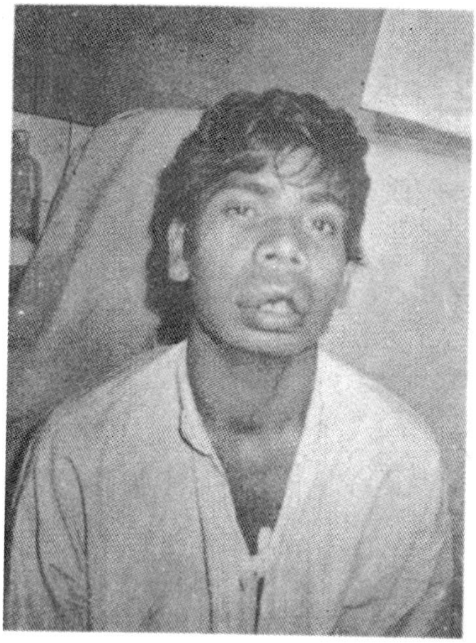

P l. 2.24 Hemangioma upper lip

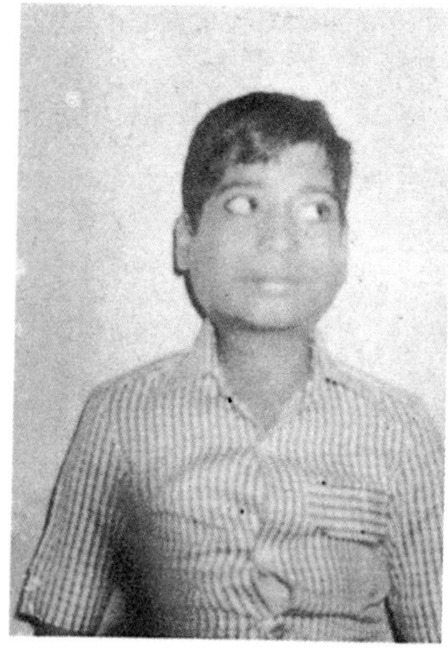

Pl.2.25 Parotid swelling - Note that the ears lobule is lifted by the parotid swelling

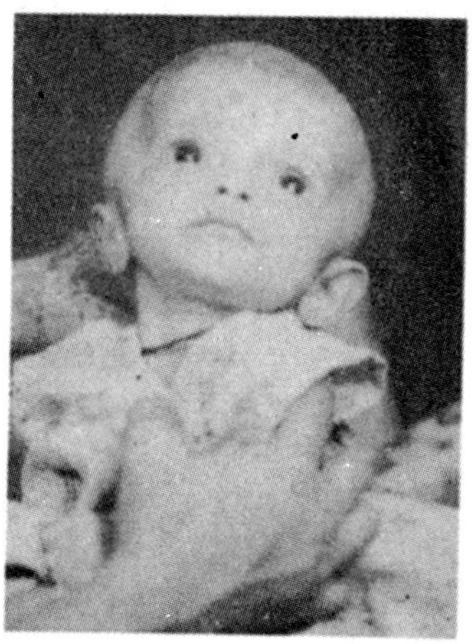

P l. 2.26 (a) Hydrocephalus

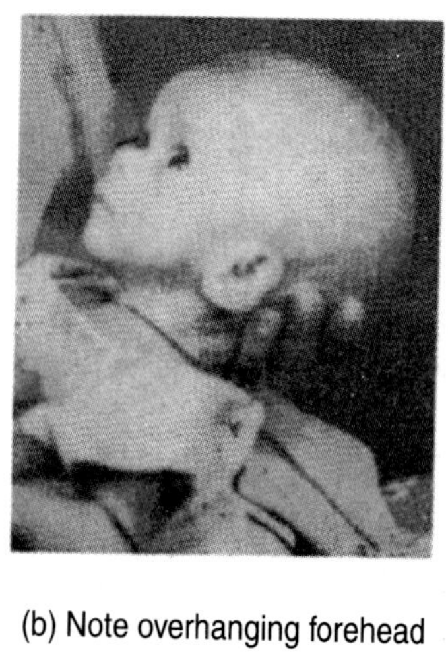

(b) Note overhanging forehead

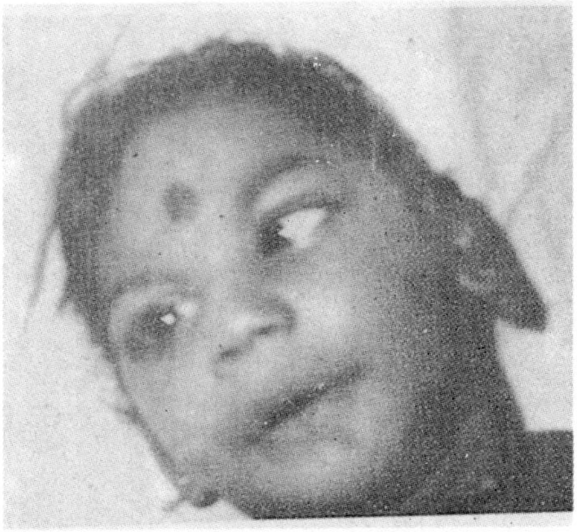

Pl. 2.27 (a) Microcephaly

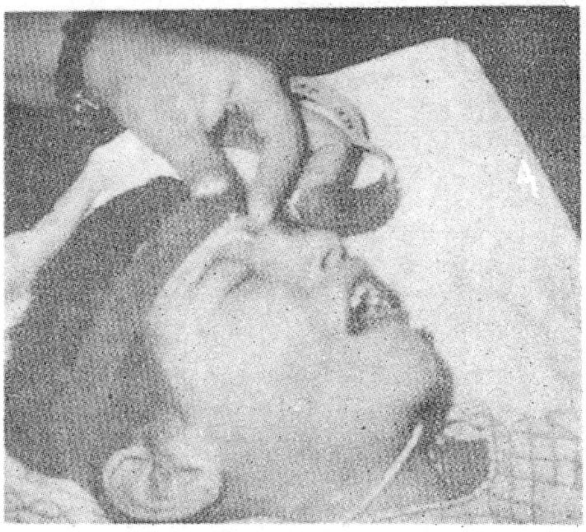

Pl.2.27b Head circumference 16", age 2 years

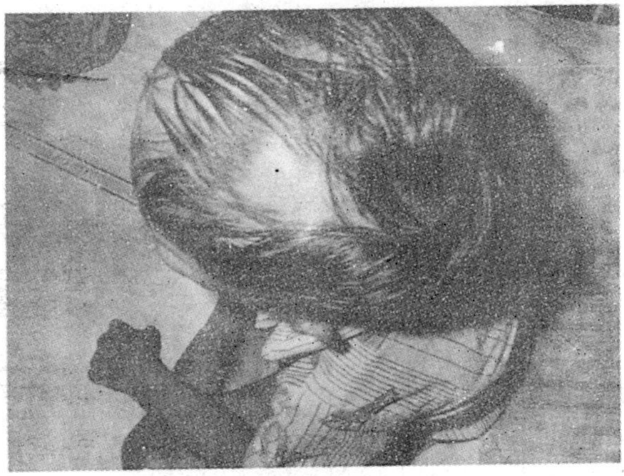

Pl. 2.28 Alopecia

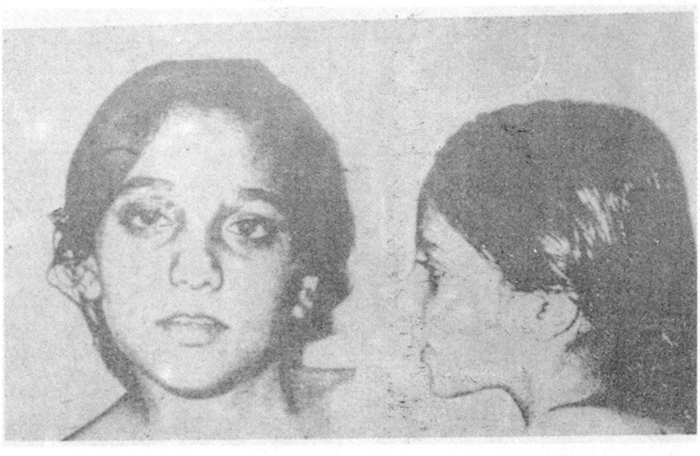

Pl. 2.29 Torticollis

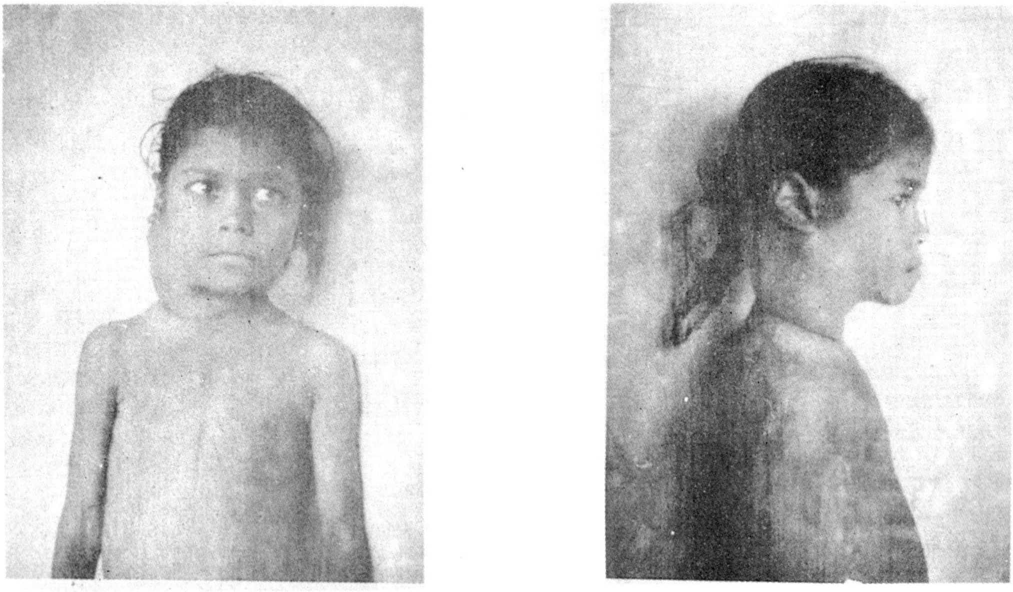

P1. 2.30 Cervical lymphadenitis

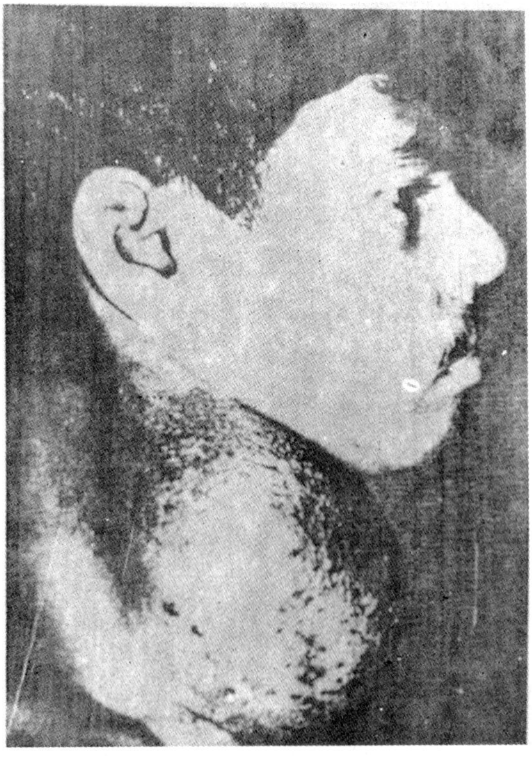

P1. 2.31 Enlarged thyroid

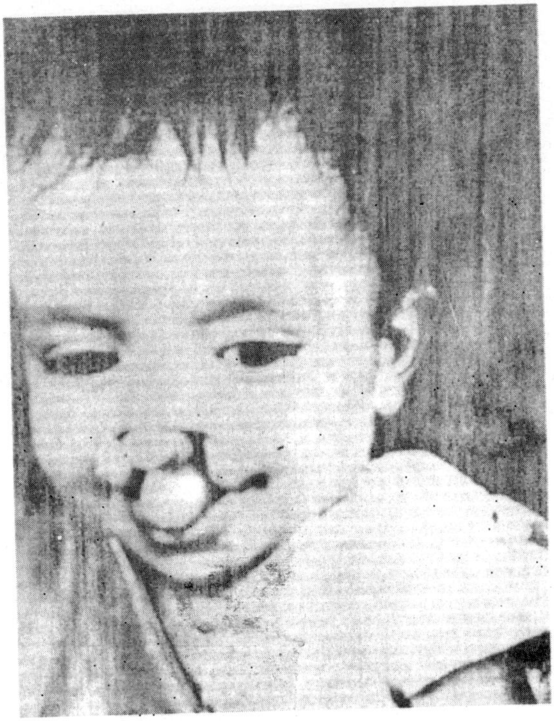

P1. 2.32 Bilateral hare lip and cleft palate

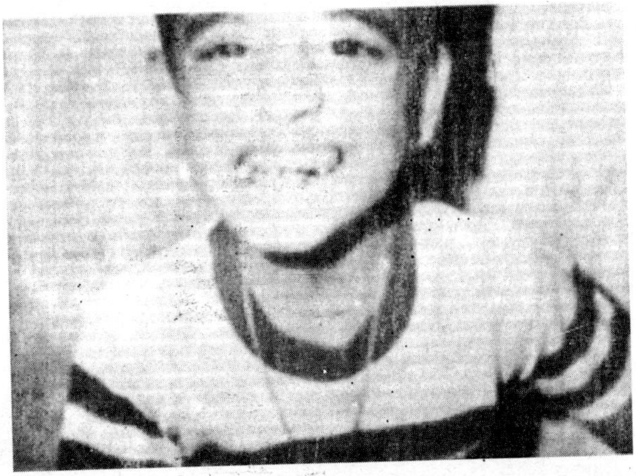

P1. 2.33 Discoloured milk teeth due to administration of antibiotics during infancy

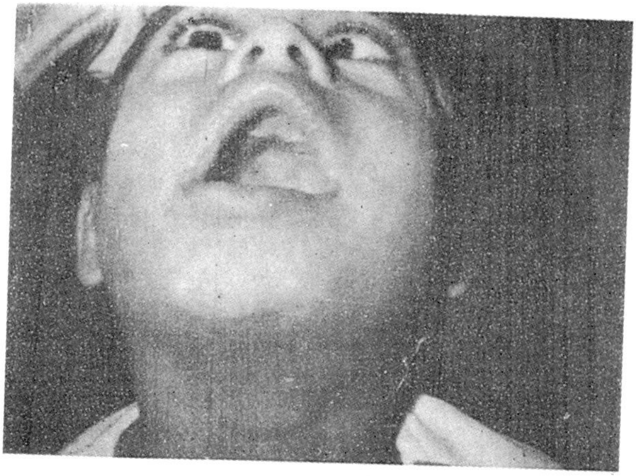

Pl. 2.34 High arched palate

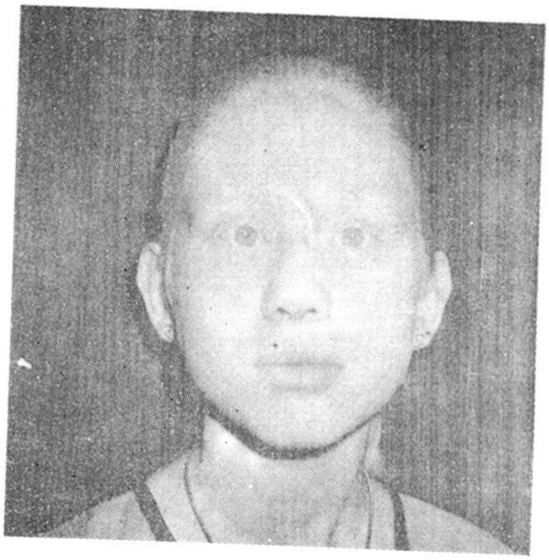

Pl. 2.35 Albinism

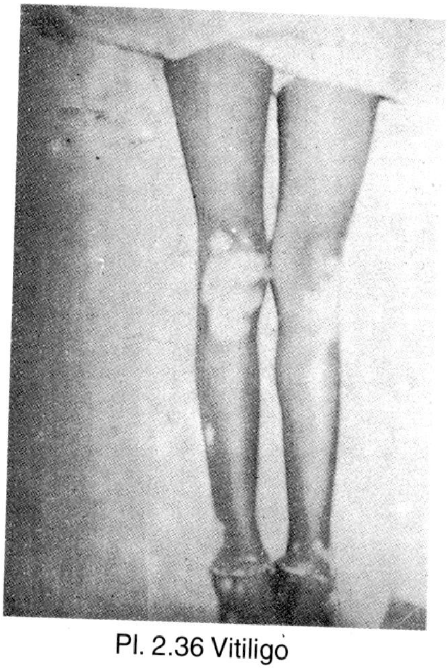

Pl. 2.36 Vitiligo

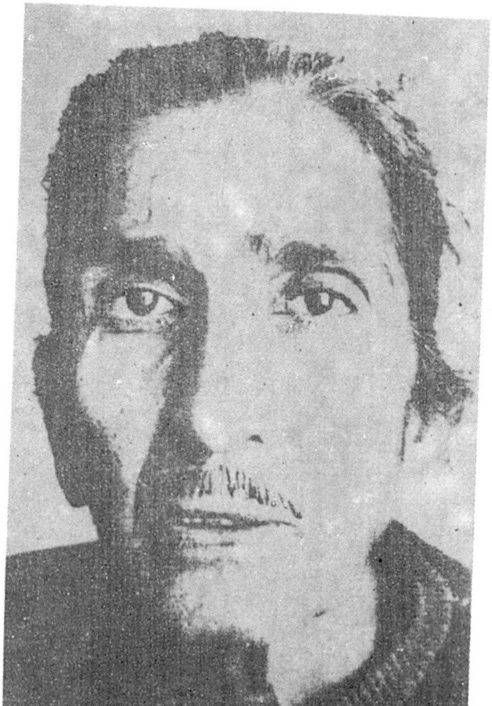

Pl. 2.37 Hirsuitism

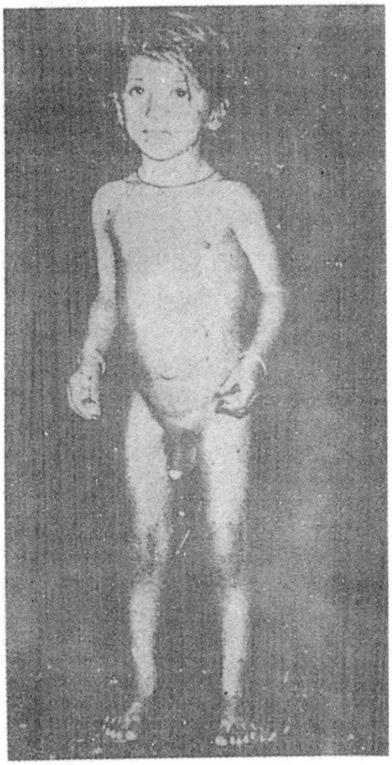

P l. 2.38 Precocious puberty - In a child aged 4 years

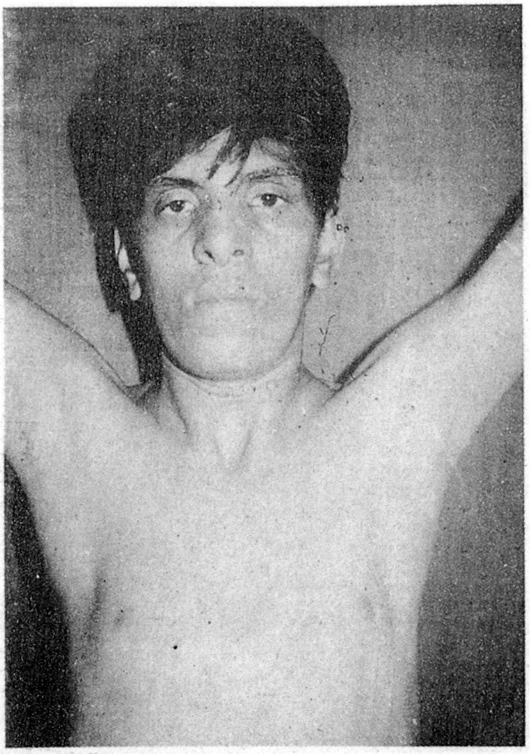

P l. 2.39 Absent sexual hair

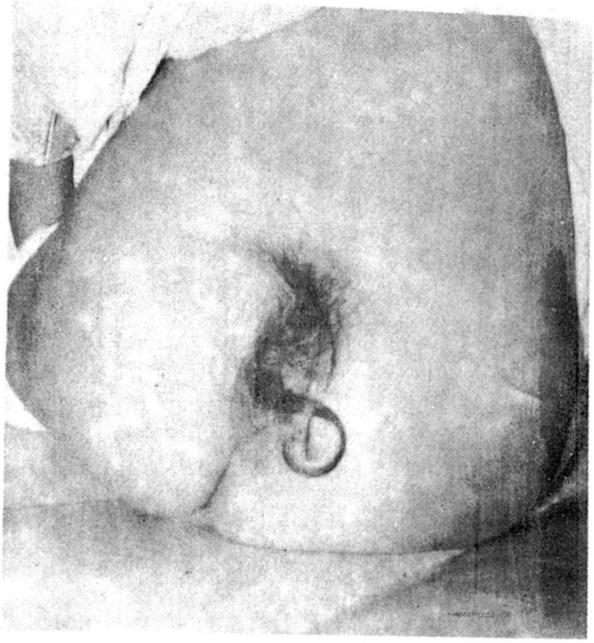

P l. 2.40 Tuft of hair in a case of spina bifida

P l.2.41 Syndyctaly

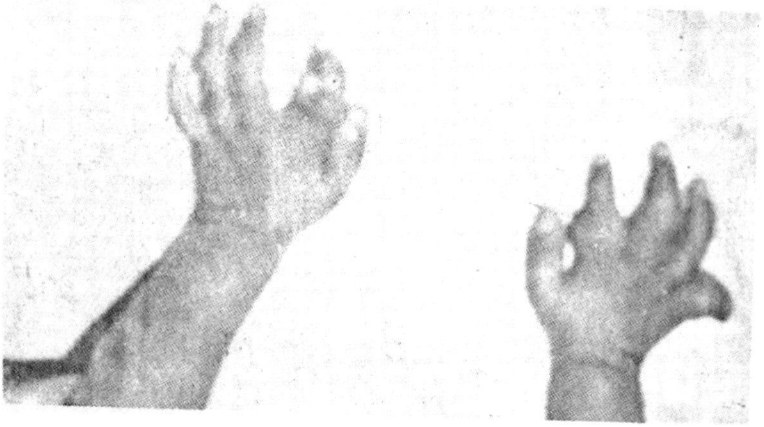

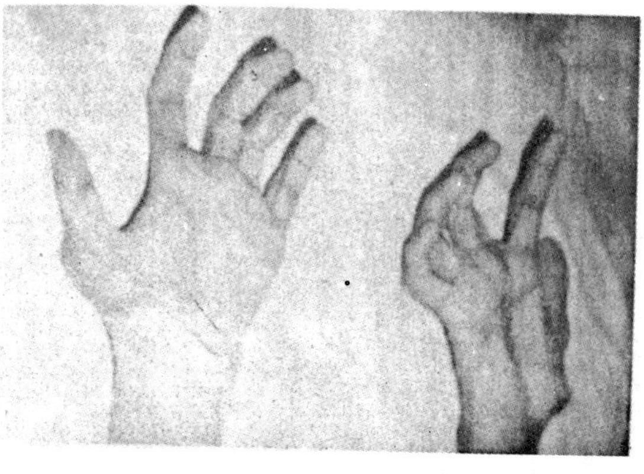

P l. 2.42 Claw hand

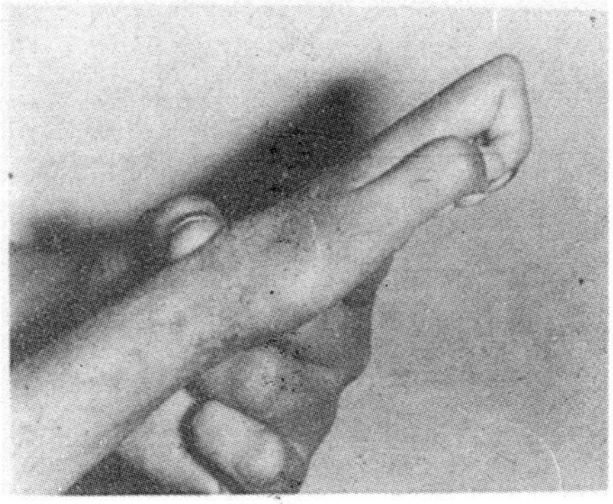

P l. 2.43 Volkman's ischemic contracture

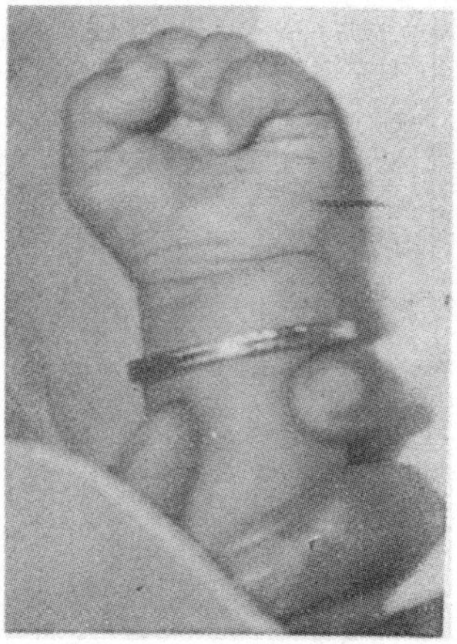

P l. 2.44 Dysplasia of limbs (fingers.

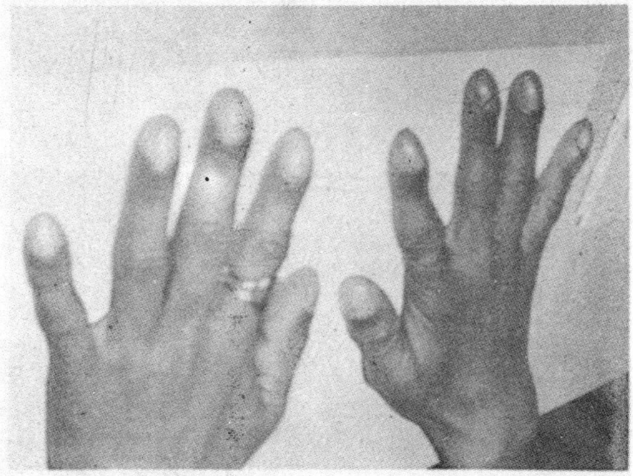

P l. 2.45 Clubbing of fingers

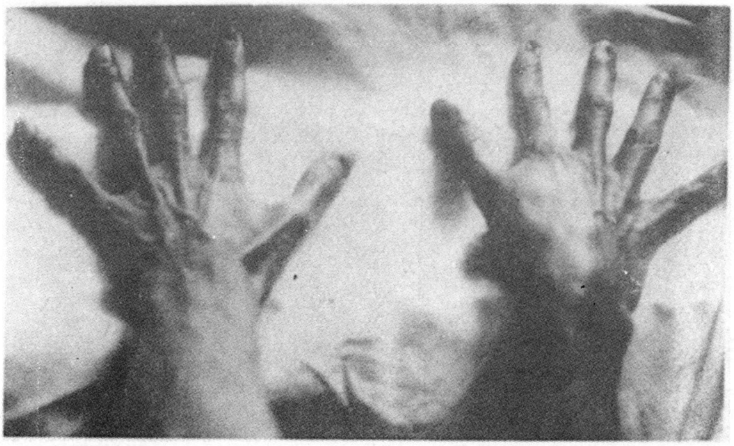

P l. 2.46 Koilonychia

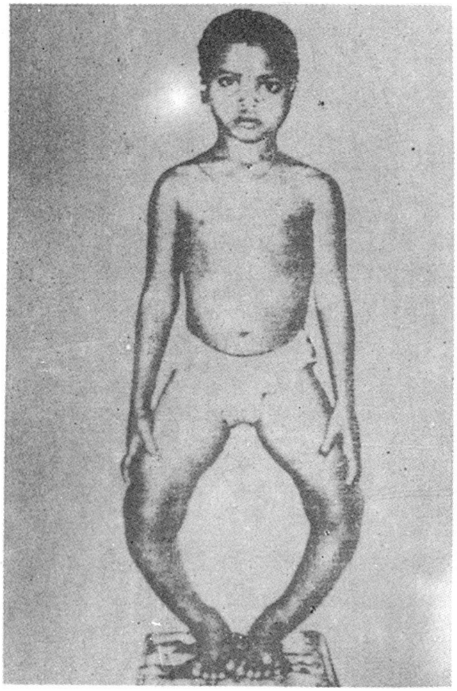

P1. 2. 47 Genu varum

P l. 2.48 Genu valgum

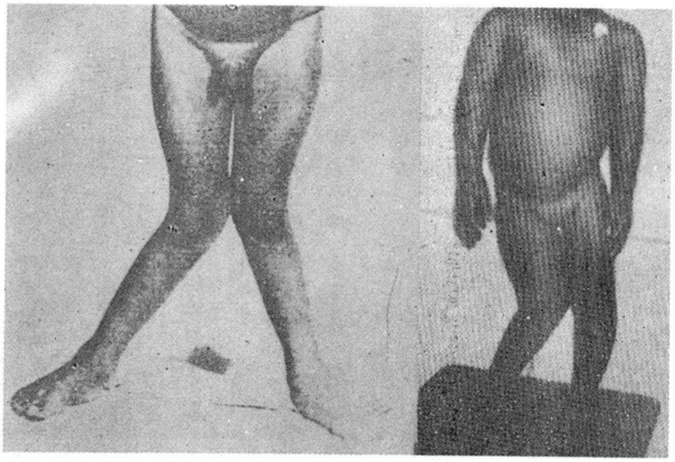

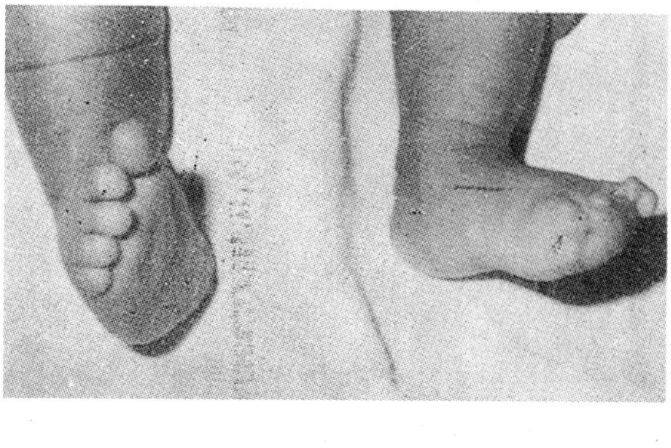

P l. 2.49 Dysplasia of toes

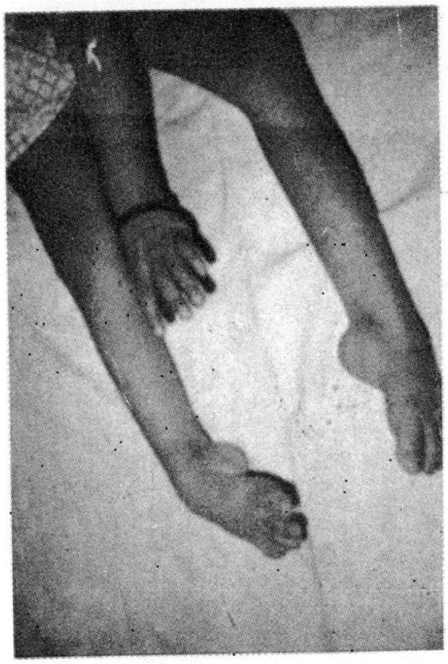

P1. 2.50 Club feet.

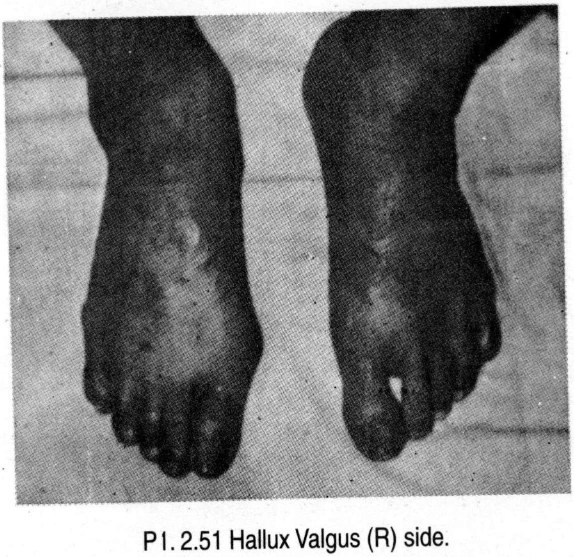

P1. 2.51 Hallux Valgus (R) side.

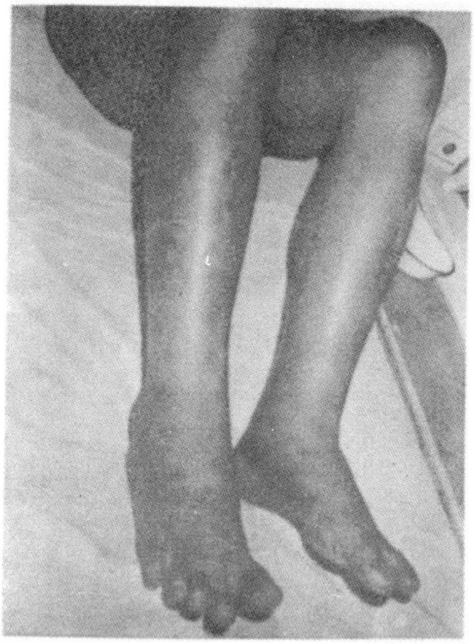

Pl. 2.52 Edema feet

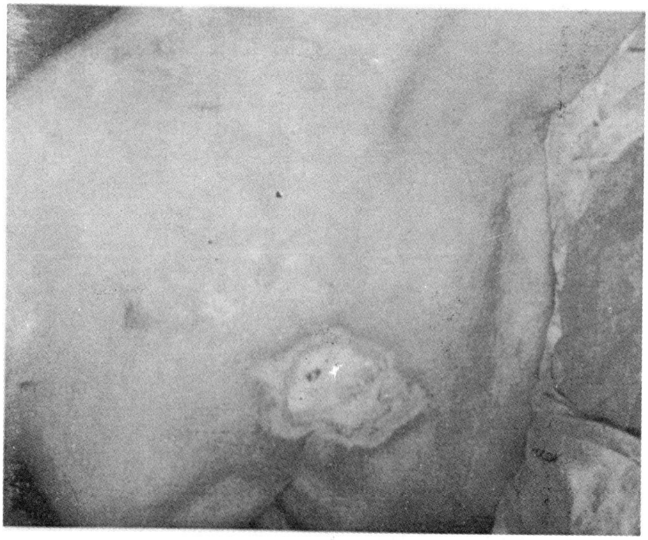

Pl. 2.53 Bed sore

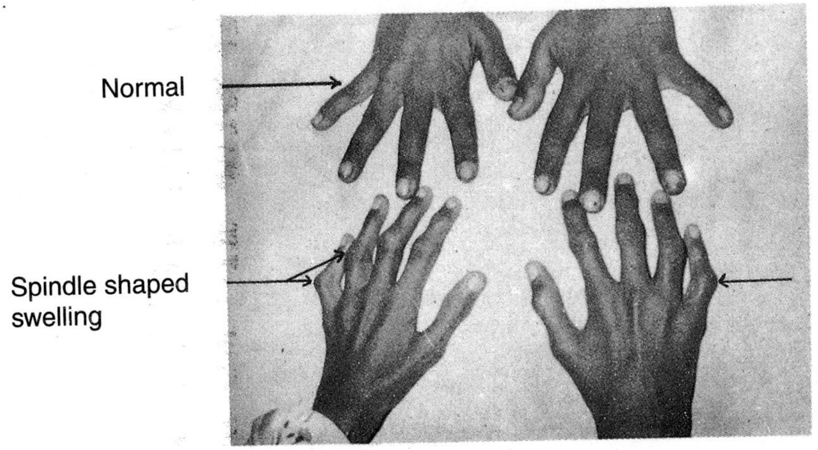

P l. 2.54 Spindle shaped swelling of small joints of hands in acute Rheumatoid arthritis

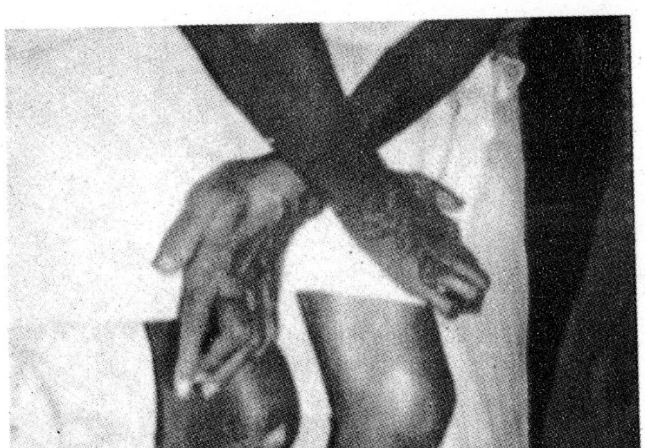

P l. 2.55 Deformities of hands in chronic Rheumatoid arthritis

(a) **Lips:** Lips should be examined to note the presence of any pallor or cyanosis. In anaemic conditions the lips are pale and they appear blue in central cyanosis. They are dry and cracked in dehydration or due to exposure to intense cold or heat. Prolonged fever also results in drying and cracking of the lips. Foam may appear on them in acute pulmonary oedema or in any condition causing convulsions. Inflammation of the lips is known as cheilitis and angular cheilitis is the condition where there are inflammatory cracks at the angles of the mouth. The latter condition though supposed to be due to vitamin B6 deficiency, can occur in anaemia, stomatitis or due to any local inflammation.

Perleche are fissures at the angles of the mouth caused due to severe vitamin deficiency and anaemia. They cause a desquamation which gives a peculiar macerated, wet wrinkled appearance to the anlges of the mouth.

Congenital syphilis produces 'rhagades' which are fissures at the angles of the mouth. They produce radiating white scars after healing.

Lips may be swollen or oedematous following trauma or insect bites or due to angioneurotic oedema.

Ulcers of the lips are seen commonly and they can be infective, syphilitic or malignant. Tumours can also produce local swellings when they affect the lips. Common tumor is hemangioma.

Herpes simplex is known as Herpes labialis when the lesions are found on the lips. They produce vesicular lesions which are extremely tender.

Hare lip is a congenital deformity of the upper lip and is seen as an indentation on the lateral aspect of the midline. It can be unilateral or bilateral and may be associated with a cleft palate. This deformity is obvious but a scar on the upper lip indicating corrective surgery in the past for this condition should be noticed. (Plate 2.32)

(b) **Teeth:** Teeth should be examined for their number, appearance, and any disease process. Caries of the teeth produces a discolouration of the teeth with cavity formation. Irregular and pointed teeth can be the causes of oral ulcerations due to local trauma. Milk teeth may be discoloured and deformed in children when antibiotics have been administered during infancy. (Plate 2.33) Typical deformities of teeth are observed in congenital syphilis.

(c) **Gums:** Pallor of the gums is due to anaemia and excessive redness is due to their inflammation which is known as gingivitis. Cyanosis causes a blue discolouration of the gums which can be easily noticed.

Spongy red hypertrophy of the gums which bleed easily on touch is seen in scurvy while a peculiar hypertrophy of the gums which can cover the lower two-thirds of the teeth can be seen in epileptics on prolonged phenytoin sodium therapy.

Pale bleeding gums without hypertrophy are seen in blood dsycrasias like leukemia,aplastic anaemias and pancytopenia.

Marked ulceration and sloughing of the gums may be present in agranulocytosis. A linear or patchy pigmented line may be seen on the gums in lead or other heavy metal intoxication. Pyorrhoea produces an inflammation of the gums with a foul smelling discharge. Vincent's angina which can affect the whole mouth may cause ulceration and sloughing of the gums.

(d) **Buccal mucous membrane:** This should be examined as a routine if necessary with the help of a spatula.

Stomatitis is inflammation of the buccal mucosa. Deficiencies of vitaminB_6, B_{12} are most common factors leading to stomatitis. It can be caused by trauma due to pointed and irregular teeth, or bad or ill fitting dentures, inflammation, such as thrush, Vincent's angina or aphthous stomatitis. Generalised infections like tuberculosis or syphilis can also cause stomatitis. Due to stomatitis the whole of the buccal cavity is inflamed, tender and firey red. There may be excessive salivation. Mastication and deglutition become painful. Measles like viral infections can also lead to stomatitis. Stomatitis can occur following antibiotic therapy.

Cancrum oris is a severe form of stomatitis and a result of debilitating diseases, especially in children. There is an extensive ulceration of the buccal mucosa with sloughing and eating up of the tissues of the whole cheek from inside.

Pigmentation of the buccal mucosa is common and typical brownish black spots can be observed in patients suffering from Addison's disease. Sometimes similar discoloured spots are seen in patients suffering from pulmonary tuberculosis or chronic debilitating diseases.

Koplik's spots are small bluish white spots with a red base which appear on the buccal mucosa. They are diagnostic of measles and appear a few days before the rash appears.

Leukoplakia affects the buccal mucosa causing white plaques.

Submucous fibrosis in the buccal area produces a difficulty in opening of the mouth due to replacement of the submucous tissue by fibrous tissue. It is seen quite often these days; following frequent use of paan masala. It predisposes to malignancy.

Chronic ulcer in oral cavity is usually pale and should arouse suspecion of malignancy.

(e) **Tongue:** Examination of the tongue has always played a very important part in the clinical examination of any patient.

State of hydration in a patient can be easily judged by examining the tongue. Dehydration immediately results in a dry tongue and in severe dehydration the tongue becomes shrivelled and small.

Furring of the tongue is due to a collection of epithelial cells, micro-organisms and food debris. Though commonly attributed to digestive disturbances it is much more common in persons who breathe through the mouth due to upper respiratory diseases, or are chronic smokers. Severe infection causing fever and dehydration also cause furring and a severe furring known as caking of the tongue is of grave promostic significance.

Morphological changes of the tongue should also be noted.

A large tongue (macroglossia) is seen in patients suffering from acromegaly or cretinism. Mongols have a congenitally large tongue. Primary amyloidosis and local tumours like hemangioma are rare causes of an enlarged tongue.

A fissured (scrotal) tongue has fissures on the dorsal surface and sides. It is a congenital abnormality and the fissures are painless but very commonly food debris collects in them causing local irritation with inflammation.

Median rhomboid glossitis is a congenital abnormality where there is an ovoid area which appears red due to denudation. It is situated in the median posterior portion of the tongue.

Colour changes in the tongue are easily noted. Pallor of the tongue is seen in anaemia and cyanosis also is apparent. A red tongue is seen in vitamin B_6 & B_{12} deficiency. A firey red tongue is seen in scarlet fever due to hypertrophy of the fungiform papillae. A hairy tongue giving rise to a brownish black discolouration is a rare abnormality due to failure of the keratin layer of the papillae to desquamate early.

Geographic tongue is an asymptomatic inflammatory condition of the tongue with rapid growth and loss of the filiform papillae which causes wandering red patches across the surface of the tongue.

The absence of the papillae on the tongue causes what is described as 'bald' tongue. It is usually seen in pernicious anaemia, iron deficiency anaemia, pellagra or syphilis. Rarely congenital hypertrophy of the papillae causes an appearance of swellings at the back of the tongue. This condition is physiological.

Leukoplakia can affect the surface of the tongue causing white translucent patches.

Ulcers of the tongue are common and may be caused by trauma due to sharp teeth or dentures. They may be due to infections like tuberculosis or syphilis. Malignant ulcers of the tongue are usually single and their edges are hard. Multiple small ulcers on the tongue can be produced by dyspepsia and are also a part of the generalised glossitis of vitamin deficiencies.

(f) **Palate:** Cleft palate is a very common deformity where there is a deep rift due to non-fusion of the two sides of the palate.

Palate may be perforated due to syphilitic gummatous involvements. This abnormality is very rarely encountered.

A high arched palate is congenital. It may not have any clinical significance or it may be one of the features of Marfan's syndrome or mongolism. (Plate 2.34)

(g) **Tonsils:** They should be examined for their size and presence of inflammation.

Tonsils are enlarged and fiery red in inflammation. Follicular tonsilitis may cause yellowish spots on the surface of the tonsils. Diphtheritic membranes appear as greyish white patches on the surface and these two conditions sometiems cause confusion in the diagnosis. A peritonsilar abscess (quinsy) causes bulging of the anterior pillar of the fauces and palate on the affected side.

Tonsils may be enlarged rarely in generalised affection of the lymphatic system like lymphoma. Unilateral enlargment of the tonsils may be due to primary malignancy of the tonsils.

(h) **Posterior pharyngeal wall:** The posterior pharyngeal wall appears red in pharyngitis.

There are muliple granular enlargements noted on the posterior pharyngeal wall in a condition called chronic granular pharyngitis which is common in chronic smokers.

Rarely a retropharyngeal abscess will cause a bulge on the surface of the posterior pharyngeal wall.

Multiple ulcers with necrosis may be seen in this area in agranulocytosis.

(i) **Breath:** Described in detail under digestive system.

Alcohol is easily smelt on the breath as it is excreted by the lungs. Paraldehyde can also be smelt on the breath and indicates that the patient had been sedated in the immediate past.

(7) SKIN AND HAIR : Inspection of the skin of the whole body should be carried out routinely.

State of hydration of the skin : A very dry skin is present in dehydration due to any cause. Myxodema causes a peculiar dry and coarse skin which is cold to touch. Vitamin A deficiency also causes a dry skin. The skin in old age is physiologically dry and wrinkled.

Excessive sweating is common during remission in fever, but it is disproportionate in pulmonary tuberculosis and rheumatic fever. Nocturnal sweating is especially common in pulmonary tuberculosis. Hyperthyroidism gives rise to excessive sweating. In anxiety states and in any condition causing severe pain (like myocardial infarct) there is an associated excessive sweating. Shock and hypoglycemia also gives rise to sweating along with a cold clammy pale skin.

Texture of the skin : Normal skin is firm, shiny and elastic. Any alteration from this should be noted.

A very tense and lightly bound skin is seen in scleroderma while the skin is loose and wrinkled in old age and when the person has lost lot of weight over a short period of time.

A thickened skin is seen in acromegaly, thyroid deficiency and vitamin A deficiency. Leprosy also causes a thickening of the skin in its lepromatus veriety. A thick skin is seen over areas of oedema and in malnutrition with hyper-proteinemia. Striae albicantes are produced commonly over the abdominal skin following pregnancy. These are produced due to atrophy of the elastic tissue after stretching. Similar purplish striae over abdomen are seen in Cushing's syndrome.

Pigmentation of the skin : Lack of normal pigment from the skin produces a peculiar whiteness of the affected areas. This will be total in albinism while it is of patchy distribution in vitiligo.

Albinism is congenital in origin and there is a complete lack of pigment from the skin and other epidermal structures like hair. Photophobia and nystagmus are present in this condition because of absence of pigment in the iris. (Plate 2.35)

Leucoderma or vitiligo is an acquired condition where there is a patchy depigmentation producing white patches surrounded by areas of hyperpigmentation, iris is pigmented. (Plate 2.36)

Faint white discoloured patches on the skin are produced by vitamin B complex deficiencies and by fungal infections. Hypopigmented anaesthetic patches are seen in tuberculoid type of leprosy. All these are not well circumscribed and are not surrounded by areas of hyperpigmentation as in vitiligo.

Excessive pigmentation of the skin can be physiological as in Negroes or it may be transitory as after prolonged exposure to sunlight or ultraviolet rays.

Increased pigmentation of exposed parts of the body is a common feature of Addison's disease. Other causes which bring about a similar pigmentation of the skin (but spare the buccal mucosa) are arsenical poisoning, chronic liver disorders, abdominal tuberculosis, malignant disease, causing generalised wasting and vitamin deficiencies like pellagra (pavement or cobble stone pigmentation).

A reddish brown discolouration of the skin is caused by deposition of haemoglobin and its derivatives in hemolytic disorders and kala azar.

'Cafeaulait' spots are brownish black patches which are associated with generalised neurofibromatosis.

Yellowish discolouration of the skin is seen in carotinemia and severe jaundice. Similar yellowish discolouration may also be seen in lipoid storage disorders like Gaucher's disease. The skin in pernicious anaemia also has a peculiar pale lemon yellow appearance.

Heavy metal poisoning can also give rise to characteristic pigmentation. Argyrie (poisoning with silver salts) produce a light gray pigmentation.

Drugs like mepacrine, chloroquine and poisoning by picric acid can produce varying degrees of yellow pigmentation.

Patchy dark pigmentation can be a sequelae of previous allergic rashes or are also seen in 'fixed drug reactions'.

Colour of the skin : Pallor of the skin is present in severe anaemias. Any condition which causes shock or severe peripheral vasoconstriction also give rise to a temporary pallor of the skin.

Excessive redness of the skin is seen in polycythemia vera. Peripheral vasodilation due to any cause like alcohol, hot bath or exposure to heat may give rise to a temporary flushing of the skin.

Cyanosis or bluish discolouration : Cyanosis is a bluish discolouration of the skin as well as mucous membranes. Though patients may complain about this discolouration it is more often a clinical finding.

This discolouration is because of the presence of reduced haemoglobin in the blood. At least 5 gms of reduced (deoxygenated) haemoglobin per 100 ml. of blood has to be present for apparent cyanosis. Hence in severely anaemic patients cyanosis may not be apparent even if a large percentage of the circulating haemoglobin is reduced while it is easily apparent in conditions like congestive cardiac failure and polycythemia vera where the volume of circulating haemoglobin is large.

Cyanosis is of two types : (1) central and (2) peripheral. Central cyanosis is due to the presence of either unsaturated haemoglobin or abnormal haemoglobin in the blood with peripheral areas accompanied by vasoconstriction. Due to combination of these two factors, the haemoglobin is reduced to a greater extent from the normally saturated haemoglobin giving rise to the cyanosis.

Clinically central cyanosis is manifested both in the extremities and lips, conjunctivae and tongue. The conditions are associated with polycythemia and clubbing of fingers. Peripheral cyanosis is seen only in nails and soles of feet. Affected parts are cold to touch.

Causes of cyanosis : I. Central cyanosis :

(a) Mixing of arterial and venous blood due to : (i) congenital heart disease with right to left shunt, Fallot's tetralogy and Eisenmenger's syndrome. (ii) Arteriovenous fistulas in the pulmonary circulation.

(b) Abnormal haemoglobin : (1) Methemoglobinemia, (ii) Sulfhemoglobinemia.

(c) Low oxygen saturation in the atmosphere at high altitudes.

(d) Due to impaired pulmonary function, causing impaired oxygen intake as massive consolidation, fibrosis, atelectasis, emphysema, empyema.

II. Peripheral cyanosis: Clubbing and polycythaemia are not present. (a) exposure to cold leading to sluggish circulation, (b) peripheral circulatory failure, (c) arterial or venous obstruction, (d) severe congestive cardiac failure, (e) differential cyanosis.

Haemorrhagic skin lesions: These are produced due to haemorrhages either in the deep or superficial layers of the skin due to damage to the capillaries.

They are classified as petechiae or purpuric spots when they are small in size (less than 5 mm in diameter) or ecchymoses if larger than 5 mm in size.

These lesions initially are red in colour and gradually change to violet or black then yellow before disappearance.

The common causes of these haemorrhagic lesions are local trauma, infections like meningococcal meningitis, infective endocarditis, haemorrhagic small pox, allergic conditions like Henoch-Schonlein purpura or allergy to drugs, blood dyscrasias like thrombocytopenic purpura, aplastic anaemia or leukemia and haemophilia and vitamin C deficiency.

Common skin lesions: The easiest way of identifying the skin lesions is the **relation of the lesions to the skin surface.**

Table 2.1 gives the classification accordingly and the common skin lesions are described afterwards.

Table 2.1

Flat lesions	Elevated lesions	Depressed lesions
Macule Telangiec- tasis	Papule Vesicle Bulla Pustule Abscess Cyst Plaque Nodule Vegetation Scales Crusts Lichenification	Atrophy Erosion Excoriation Scar Ulcer Sinus

Description of the common skin lesions:
Macule: It is a coloured spot in the skin not raised above the surface of the skin commonly seen in early measles, allergic rashes and in early small pox.

Telangiectasis : It is a small red coloured spot produced due to a capillary hemangioma.

Papule : Papule is a solid lesion usually less than 1 cm in diameter elevated above the skin surface as in measles and allergic rash and early small pox.

Vesicle and Bulla : Vesicle is a circumscribed elevated lesion less than 0.5 mm in size containing clear fluid. The walls may be so thin that the fluid inside can be seen clearly. When the lesion is more than 0.5 cm in size it is known as bulla. Vesicle is seen in eczema, scabies, chicken pox, impetigo, bulla in burns, congenital syphilis, pemphigus, sometimes in insect bites.

Pustule : Pustule is a circumscribed elevated area of the skin which contains pus as in impetigo, chicken pox, small pox and furuncle.

Abscess : It is a large collection of pus which extends to the subcutaneous tissues.

Cyst : Cyst is produced by blocking of the duct of a gland. The gland goes on secreting and the collection of fluid produces a cyst. In a sebaceous cyst a small bluish black punctum can be usually seen in the centre.

Plaque : This is an elevation above the surface occupying a large surface relative to its height above the skin. Very often it is a confluence of papules as in allergic rashes and lichenplanus.

Nodule: Nodule is a palpable, solid, round or oval lesion. It is deeper than a papule and extends in the subcutaneous tissue as in erythema nodosum and rheumatic nodule.

Vegetation: Vegetation is produced by multiple, small, closely packed projected elevations of the papular type.

Scales: Scaling is a visible exfoliation or desquamation of the stratum corneum (the outermost layer of the skin) as in healing impetigo.

Crusts: Crusts are formed when serum, blood or purulent exudates dry on the skin surface. They are yellow when formed from serum, brown or dark red when formed from blood and green when formed from pus.

Lichenification: This is a term applied to describe a thickened skin with prominent surface markings.

Atrophy: In an atrophic skin, the superficial layer remains intact but the inner layers are destroyed and this may result in destruction of hair follicles and sweat glands.

Erosion: The loss of superficial layers of the skin is called erosion.

Excoriation: Excoriation is a term used to describe superficial or deep excavation of the skin usually caused by local trauma like scratching and is also seen around anus in infants with frequent loose motions.

Scar: The replacement of the normal skin by fibrous tissue following an injury or a lesion is known as scarring. There is always a loss of hair follicles and sweat glands in the affected area.

Ulcer: Ulcers are lesions where there is a loss of epidermis and the upper papillary layer of the dermis due to destruction of the layers and not due to trauma.

Sinus: It is a tract in the skin which usually connects an underlying pathological lesion to the surface.

Rashes: Clinical significance of rashes is very great as they are diagnostic of diseases like measles, small pox, etc. They are almost present as a result of haemorrhagic fevers or allergy to drugs.

Whenever a rash is encountered in a patient the type of the skin lesions, whether it is macular, papular or vesicular, etc. should be noted. The progress of the lesion — macular to papular — should be observed and then the patient should be examined to see if various types of rashes are present simultaneously. The areas which are more commonly affected by the rash should be observed and finally the nature of the spread of the rash, whether it is centripetal or centrifugal should also be observed. Associated constitutional symptoms and signs also help in arriving at diagnosis.

Abnormalities of hair distribution: Examination of the hair distribution over the body as a whole should be carried out. Abnormalities of the scalp hair have been already described. The present description will restrict itself to generalised excess or generalised loss of hair.

Excessive hair or hirsutism: Hirsutism without virilism is present in acromegaly and Cushing's syndrome. Rarely hirsutism is seen in porphyris or in patients receiving glucocorticoids, androgens or hydantoin sodium. Presence of excessive hair over the back is one of the constant clinical signs in cretinism. Cretins also have an increased amount of hair on the forearm.

Hirsutism with virilism can occur in testicular ovarian or adrenal tumors. (Plate 2.37) Presence of secondary sexual characters with early growth of hair of adult distribution is found in sexual precocity among children. (Plate 2.38)

Loss of hair : In cirrhosis of liver among males, there is loss of pubic and axillary hair and also hair over the chest. The patient shaves less often due to poor growth of hair over the face. (Plate 2.39)

Hypothyroidism and hypopituitarism can also result in a loss of body hair.

Patch of excessive hair : Tuft of hair over spina bifida occulta is seen often. (Plate 2.40)

8. **EXTREMITIES :** Both upper extremities should be examined for any obvious congenital deformities like polydactaly or congenital absence

of fingers and toes. (Plate 2.41)

A. **Upper extremities:** These should be examined as follows.

Examination of the hand:

(a) **Shape:** Shape of the hand should be noticed first. A rough calloused hand is indicative that the nature of the patient's work is manual. A large broad spade-like hand is suggestive of acromegaly while a broad hand with stubby short fingers is seen in myxodema. A feminine slender hand with very long tapering fingers is seen in Marfan's syndrome and sometimes in patients suffering from hypogonadism.

(b) **Wasting and deformities :** The hand should be examined for any localised muscular wasting or deformities and contractures. Wasting of the small muscles of the hand that is the thenar and hypothenar eminences as well as of palmar and dorsal interossoci should be observed carefully as the patient may not complain about it in the early stages. In advanced wasting of these muscles a typical deformity known as 'claw hand' results where the fingers are extended at the metacarpophalangeal joints and flexed at the inter-phalangeal joints. (Plate 2.42)

The hand may be deformed because of contracture of the palmar fascia and not due to any muscular wasting. This results in a condition known as 'Dupuytren's contracture'.

Volkmann's ischemic contracture is a condition produced by obstruction to the blood supply of the hand due to faulty plastering or bandaging. The wrist is flexed with extension of the metacarpophalangeal joints and flexion of the interphalangeal joints Wrist drop is produced usually by affection of the radial nerve and the hand is then always flexed at the wrist due to paralysis of the extensors of wrist. (Plate 2.43)

Ulnar deviation of the hand is noticed in rheumatoid arthritis.

(c) **Fingers:** Congenital abnormalities like polydactaly and syndactaly and absence of finger or toes should be noted. (Plate 2.44) The fingers should then be examined for presence of clubbing. Clubbing in its earliest stage can be noticed by examining the angle of the base of the nail. (Plate 2.45)

Grades or stages of clubbing: (Fig 2.1) In the 1st stage there is a slight hollowing between the finger pulp and the nail. This angle becomes full in the early stages of clubbing.

In the 2nd stage: There is abnormal mobility of the nails in the nail beds due to spongy thickness of the hypertrophied nail beds.

In the 3rd stage: There is thickening of the nail bed, producing bulbus enlargements of the ends of the fingers.

In the 4th stage: The fingers are markedly enlarged and the nails and bones are also hypertrophied. These changes may be associated with thickening of the ends of the long bones (hypertrophied osteoarthropathy).

Causes of clubbing: Clubbing is due to variety of causes. The main and common causes of clubbing are either congenital or acquired. Congenital clubbing is familial and bears no significance. Acquired clubbing is mainly due to:

(1) Cardiac: (a) Cyanotic heart disease; (b) Infective endocarditis.

(2) Respiratory: (a) Bronchiectasis; (b) Lung abscess; (c) Arteriovenous fistula; (d) Tuberculosis; (e) Bronchogenic carcinoma; (f) Empyema Thoracis.

(3) Hepatic cirrhosis.

(4) Gastrointestinal; (a) Ulcerative colitis; (b) Steatorrhoea.

Cervical rib is a common cause of unilateral clubbing.

Fingers must be examined for presence of localised enlargement of nodes. Heberden's nodes are associated with osteoarthritis and they appear as bony enlargements at the distal interphalangeal joints. Osler's nodes are painful, tender, bluish small sized nodules on the pads of fingers and are a result of embolisation in patients suffering from subacute bacterial endocarditis. Webs of finger should be examined for scabies.

Finally the fingers must be examined for presence of ulcers and colour changes. Trophic ulcers at the tip are very commonly produced by leprosy but syringomyelia or other nervous system

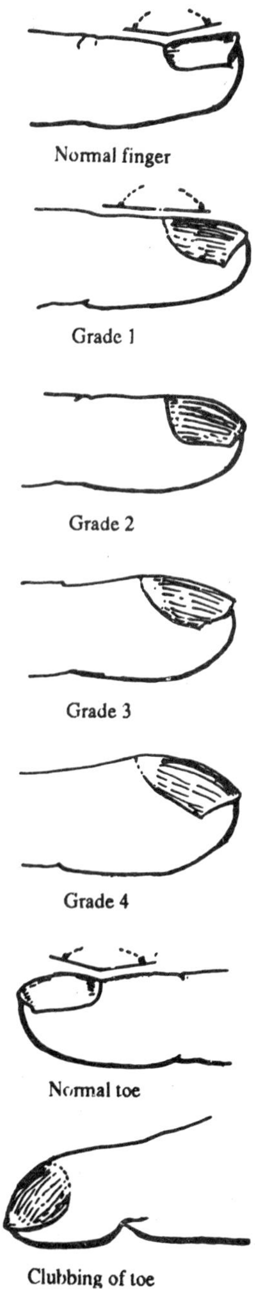

Fig. 2.1
Clubbing of Fingers
To appreciate normal angle between nail bed and nail and to show how the angle changes during various stages of clubbing.

lesions may produce the same. Rarely fingers will be seen to be blanched in the cases of Raynaud's disease when they are exposed to cold. Gangrene of fingers due to obstructive arterial disease (though much more common in toes) produces typical blackening of the skin.

(d) **Colour of the palm:** Palms appear to be very pale in anaemia while in polycythemia they appear to be purple in colour. Cyanosis will impart a blue colour to the palms and jaundice and carotinaemia will make them appear yellow. Liver palms (pink palms) are seen in cirrhotic individuals as well as severe chronic alcoholics. The hypothenar and thenar eminences are bright red with the central area appearing pale in colour.

(e) **Examination of the nails:** Colour of nails is usually the first thing to be noted on examination. Pallor is indicative of anaemia while cyanosis is easily noticed by the blue colour. Rarely silver poisoning or Addison's disease may colour them black. Nails in cirrhosis are opaque and white in colour.

Shape of the nail changes characteristically in many diseases. Koilonychia or spoon shaped deformity of the nails is seen in iron deficiency anaemia while a convexity of the nails is observed in advanced clubbing of the fingers. In acromegaly, the nails are broad while they are long and narrow in hypogonadism and hypopituitarism. (Plate 2.46)

Splinter haemorrhages are seen below the nails in patients suffering from infective endocarditis while capillary pulsations in the nail bed can be demonstrated in persons having aortic incompetence.

Scarring, pitting and brittleness of the nails is seen after any chronic severe illness. They may also be produced by vitamin deficiencies or local infections.

Examinations of the rest of the upper extremities:

Examination of pulse and other arterial pulsations is discussed in the chapter on cardiovascular system.

Abnormal engorgement of veins of extremities should be observed. Similarly, unilateral or bilateral edema of the upper extremities should be noted.

Bones and joints should be checked for any abnormality (see discussion in the section on 'joints'). However, 'frozen shoulder' is a fairly common complaint and any abduction or rotation of the joint is painful. In advanced cases there is wasting of muscles of the shoulder girdle.

Lymphadenopathy should be observed carefully both in axillary and supratrochlear regions.

Presence of rheumatic nodules which appear as painless, discrete, non-tender small nodules should be checked for over the posterior aspect of the elbows and over the tendon sheaths, occiput and spine.

B. Lower extremities: Deformities: Any deformities of legs should be noted. Legs may be either bent outwards (genu varum) due to severe osteoarthritis, osteomalacia. Paget's disease or due to old rickets or they may be bent inwards (genu valgum ie knock knees) as a result of congenital abnormality or rickets. Genu recurvatum is a rare deformity produced by hyperextension of knee joints. (Plate 2.48)

Feet should be examined for absent toes. (Plate 2.49)

Tibiae are bent forwards in rickets or congenital syphilis. The latter condition produces the so-called sabre shaped tibiae due to anteroposterior bowing with thick and round borders.

Deformities of feet are common and may be of clinical significance. Pes cavus or claw foot is seen in conditions like Friedrich's ataxia or peroneal muscular atrophy. In this deformity there is marked upward convexity of the instep of the foot due to exaggeration of the longitudinal arch. The toes are drawn up secondary to the exaggerated curvature. Talipes equinovarus (club foot) is a deformity where there is an adduction of both feet downwards (Plate 2.50) and inwards with a medial concavity. Flat feet are produced by loss of both longitudinal and transverse arches of the feet. Hallux valgus is a deformity of the great toe which is laterally bent. It is seen as a hereditary defect or is sometimes seen in advanced osteoarthritis. (Plate 2.51)

Edema : Edema can be bilateral or rarely unilateral. Mild edema will be evident only by applying pressure by examiner's thumb which produces 'pitting'. The earliest sites where pitting can be demonstrated are the ankle regions over the shins of the legs. (Plate 2.52) Non-pitting edema is present when it is produced by filariasis or rarely due to myxodema.

Causes: 1. Any condition leading to hypoproteinemia, e.g., nephrotic syndrome, malnutrition, cirrhosis of liver. 2. Diminished cardiac output due to congestive cardiac failure or phlebothrombosis or thrombophlebitis — all these lead to diminished circulatory blood volume and oedema as shown in the accompanying chart.

Grades of edema: Gr. 1 Minimum pitting on pressure-edema extending upto ankle. Gr. II Definite pitting on pressure-edema extending to legs. Gr. III Edema all over the body, but no or minimal ascites or scrotal edema. Gr. IV Generalised anasarca with ascites and scrotal edema.

Veins and lymphatics: Posterior aspect of the legs of a patient in standing posture should be examined for varicose veins. Advanced varicosity is associated with chronic ulcers over the medial malleoli. Thrombophlebitis of the superficial veins

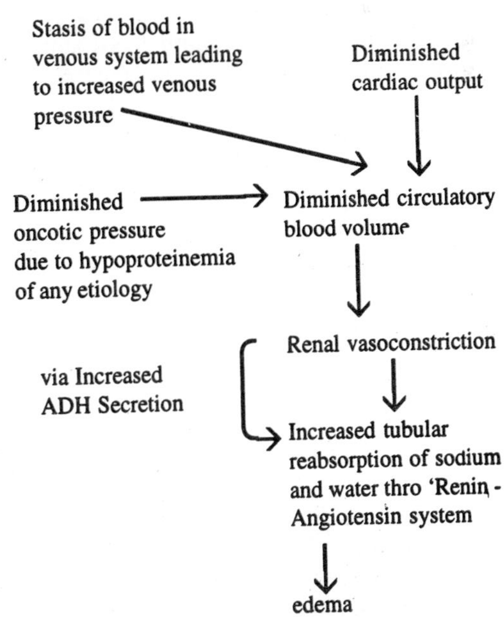

Table 2.2

Differentiation between lymphatic edema and pitting edema:

Edema of lymphatic origion	Edema of any other origin
1. Anywhere depending on obstruction	Dependent parts
2. Usually unilateral	Bilateral or may be unilateral
3. Does not pit on pressure	Pits on pressure
4. Lymph gland palpable	Lymph gland not palpable
5. No response to diuretics	Responds to diuretics

is easy to detect due to the tenderness and redness over the overlying skin. Phlebothrombosis of the deep veins which usually follows prolonged recumbency is more difficult to detect. Homan's sign is usually positive in such cases.

Inflammation of lymphatics is seen as superficial red streaking and is usually due to filarial infection. The pulse in the inferior extremities should be felt successively at all the palpable arteries like dorsalis pedis, posterial tibial, popliteal and femoral pulsations. Diabetic angiopathy, thromboangitis obliterans, atherosclerosis, embolisation from heart all contribute to the cause of absent pulsations in the leg.

Lymphadenopathy and nodules: The inguinal and popliteal lymph gland should be palpated as a routine for any marked enlargements. Erythema nodosum gives rise to painful, oval and rounded tender red swelling on the front of the legs on shins of tibiae.

Ulcers and gangrene: Perforating ulcers of the foot are usually situated on the plantar aspect of the great toe and they are the result of trophic changes in neurological disorders. (Plate 2.53)

Gangrene of the foot is very common in diabetes and the affected part is cold to touch and dark with demarcation.

9. **JOINTS:** Joints are examined when they are affected by a disease process as follows:

They should be checked for their size, shape, movements and inflammatory changes. An inquiry should also be made as to which joints are involved and whether they were involved simultaneously or in any particular serial order.

The common types of arthritis encountered and their brief description is presented here:

(a) **Acute suppurative arthritis:** Usually only a single joint is involved. The affected joint is very markedly swollen, hot, painful, tender and the movements are greatly restricted.

(b) **Rheumatic arthritis:** Arthritis is one of the features of rheumatic fever. Usually the larger joints are involved and the joints affected are very painful, swollen, red and tender. Less frequently the first affection is of the elbows or shoulder joints. Characteristically a fresh joint gets involved when the inflammation of the previously affected joint is subsiding. Hence, the joint pains are also described as 'fleeting' from one to another. The joint inflammation always subsides without any sequelae. There is more periarthritis than arthritis — never suppuration and responds to salicylates.

(c) **Rheumatoid arthritis:** The initial affection is usually of the small joints of the fingers. The proximal interphalangeal joints are involved but the distal interphalangeal joints are spared. Initially there is a soft tissue swelling of the joints which are painful and tender. Early morning stiffness is typical. The accompanying muscular wasting and the swollen joint combine to give the typical 'spindle' shaped deformity of the fingers or the legs when the knee joints are involved. (Plate 2.54) Usually this type of arthritis leads to deformities due to fibrous or bony ankylosis. Ulnar deviation of the hand is another typical feature of this type of arthritis. (Plate 2.55)

(d) **Osteoarthritis:** Knee joints, spine and joints of the fingers are commonly involved in this type of arthritis which usually occurs in elderly individuals. Stiffness of the joints at the beginning of any activity is typical of this type of arthritis. 'Creaking' can usually be demonstrated by movements of the joints, which are usually accompanied by muscular wasting.

(e) **Charcot's joints:** This produces a painless enlargement of the affected joint which can be swollen up to a very great extent. Abnormal movements are possible in the joint without evoking any pain. The ends of the bones forming the joint are destroyed. Usually this disease involves the knee or ankle joints but rarely shoulder joints are affected in a similar fashion in syringomyelia.

(f) **Gout:** The classically involved joint in this is the great toe which becomes very painful and tender with marked erythema and swelling. Initially there are complete remissions from these acute attacks but in later stages the joint remains in a state of chronic inflammation with secondary changes due to gouty deposits.

10. **GENITALIA AND SECONDARY SEXUAL CHARACTERS :** Local examination of the genitalia should be carried out as a part of the general examination.

Infantile or poor development of the male genitalia is present in many endocrine disorders like hypopituitarism, enuchoidism or hypogonadism. Secondary sexual characters like the adult type of male voice, growth of pubic and axillary hair and beard growth are poor or absent in these persons. In females the development of breasts is poor and there is scanty pubic hair along with poor menstruation.

Sexual precocity (sexual development before the age of 8 years) results in early development and growth of secondary sexual characters and genitals. In females hirsutism with precocity is seen in the adrenogenital syndrome.

Local ulcerations due to venereal diseases or scars over the penis due to old ulcerations should be observed. Similarly presence of warts or condylomata should be noted.

Scrotum may be enlarged unilaterally or bilaterally due to presence of hydrocele. Testes should always be palpated to note their size and to examine the presence of normal tenderness. Epididymis should be palpated for presence of thickening which is commonly due to tuberculous or filarial involvement.

Examination of the vulva should be carried out too, for atrophy, edema or presence of venereal ulcers, leukoplakia or condylomata.

11. **EXAMINATION OF HERNIAL SITES:** Routine examination of inguinal, femoral, umbilical region should be carried out for herniae.

12. **TEMPERATURE:** In the normal persons body temperature is always maintained within a very small range.

It is usually measured in centigrade and the instrument used is the clinical thermometer graduated in 0.1 degrees from 35^0 to 42^0 C.

Ideally the oral temperature should be recorded and the thermometer should be inserted in the oral cavity below the tongue and the person should close the mouth and avoid biting the thermometer with his teeth. This reading should not be taken immediately after a hot or cold drink.

The thermometer should be shaken firmly before recording the temperature and the reading should be checked initially. It should be kept in position for at least two minutes so that the recording is accurate.

The temperature can also be recorded per rectum by a rectal thermometer.

The normal body temperature shows a diurnal variation. It is on an average about 36.1^0 C oral in the morning. It rises throughout the day and the peak is reached in the evening between 6 to 10 p.m. The reading can be as high as 37.2^0 C oral in the evening. Then it starts falling until it reaches the lowest reading at about 3 to 4 a.m. This variation is supposed to be the result of physical activity in the day. However, this variation exists in the same manner in people who work at night and sleep in the day time.

Fever: Any rise in temperature above the normal is known as fever of pyrexia. Hyperpyrexia denotes very high temperatures (above 41^0 C).

This procedure of taking oral temperature may not be possible in patients of pediatric age group and in those who have painful oral ulcers or in unconscious or irritable uncooperative patients. Hence either a rectal temperature or a skin temperature can be recorded. Rectal recording is more ideal as the skin may be cold and clammy when the patient with even very high temperature is in shock or is suffering from septic fever. However a rectal temperature recording may be inconvenient.

Rectal temperature is recorded by a special rectal thermometer and reading is usually 0.5^0 to 1^0 C higher than the oral temperature.

Before recording the skin temperature care, should be taken to see that the area is wiped dry. It can be taken either in the axilla or the groin. The arm or the thigh should be firmly apposed over the instruments. The temperature recorded in the axilla or the groin is lower than the oral temperature by about 0.5^0 C.

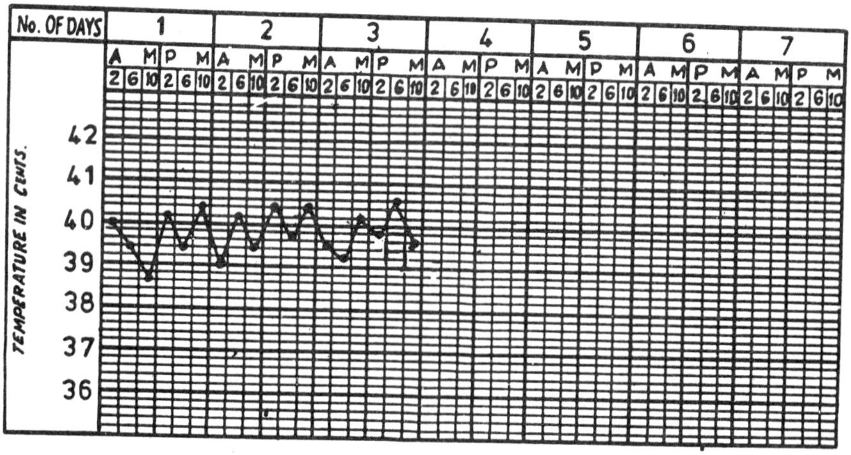

Fig. 2.2 a
Continuous fever

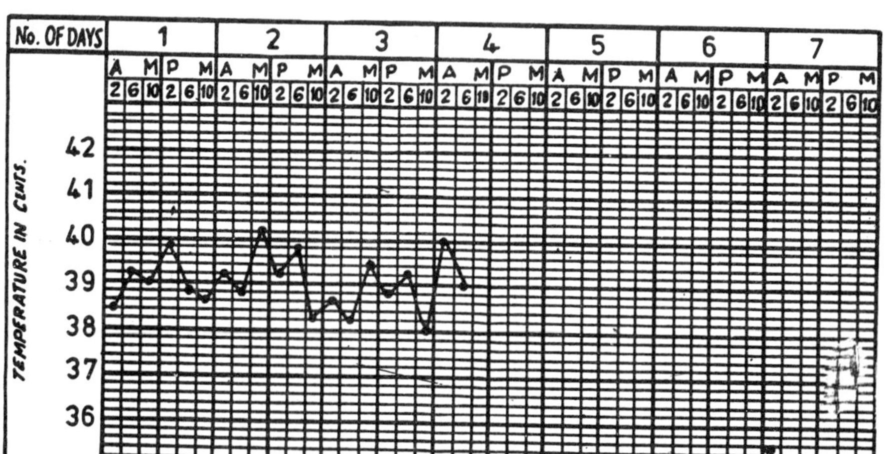

Fig. 2.2 b
Remittent fever

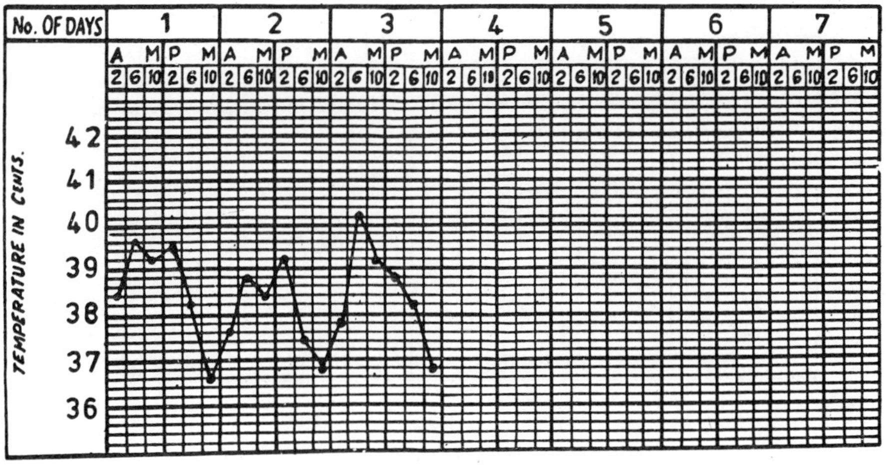

Fig. 2.2 c
Intermittent fever

Types of fever: The rise in temperature occurs in various patterns and depending upon the rise and fall, the fever is classified as follows:

(a) **Continuous fever:** When the temperature is continuously above normal and the fluctuation in the temperature is minimal, it is known as continuous fever (fluctuation less than 0.75^0 C). This variety is seen commonly in typhoid or typhus fever; pleurisy with effusion. (Fig. 2.2a)

(b) **Remittent fever:** The temperature in this variety is always above normal but the fluctuation is fairly significant. (Fluctuation more than 0.75^0 C and does not touch normal). It is known as remittent fever and this does not signify any particular type of infection (Fig. 2.2b)

(c) **Intermittent fever:** When the fever comes down and the temperature is normal sometime during the course of the day, it is known as intermittent fever. If the rise is quite high and sudden and the fall is equally rapid, the fever may be called as hectic fever. This type is usually seen in pyogenic infections. (Fig. 2.2 c)

If the temperature rises on every third day, the fever is called tertian and if it rises on every fourth day, it is known as quartan fever. Malarial infections are classic infections producing this type of temperature. (Fig. 2.2d, 2.2e)

(d) **Relapsing fever:** In this variety, the patient has pyrexia up to 40^0 C for a few days and it is followed by afebrile period of even up to one week. The pattern goes on repeating itself. (Fig. 2.2f)

Pel-Ebstein type of fever is a relapsing fever noted in some cases of Hodgkin's disease (in about 5 to 10% of patients). The fever lasts for about 3 to 10 days followed by afebrile period of the same duration. These cycles may repeat for a long period, even months, and may point towards the diagnosis. However, occasionally this type of fever may be persent in other infections also.

(e) **Low fever:** When height of temperature does not rise above 38^{0}C and occurs at any time of the day it is low fever. Common causes are tuberculosis, chronic infection anywhere in the body. (Fig. 2.2g)

Accompaniments of fever: Though most patients are aware that they have fever, some do not appreciate their bodily rise of temperature and may complain of bodyache and myalgia, which are the most common accompaniments of fever.

Other patients may have more specific symptoms, which can be attributed only to fever whatever may be its etiology.

(a) **Chills:** A true chill or rigor is described by the patient as a sensation of feeling intensely cold

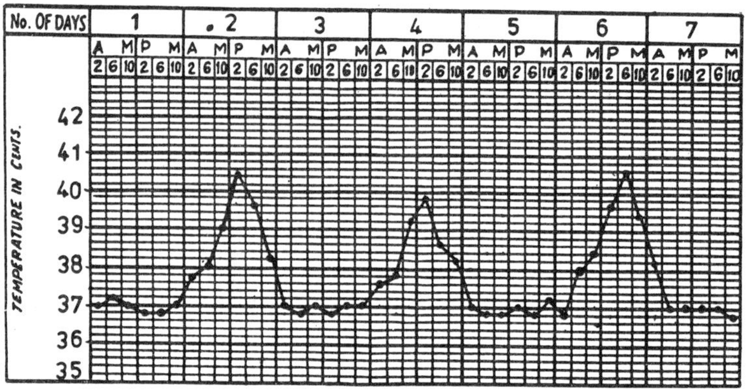

Fig. 2.2 d
Tertian fever

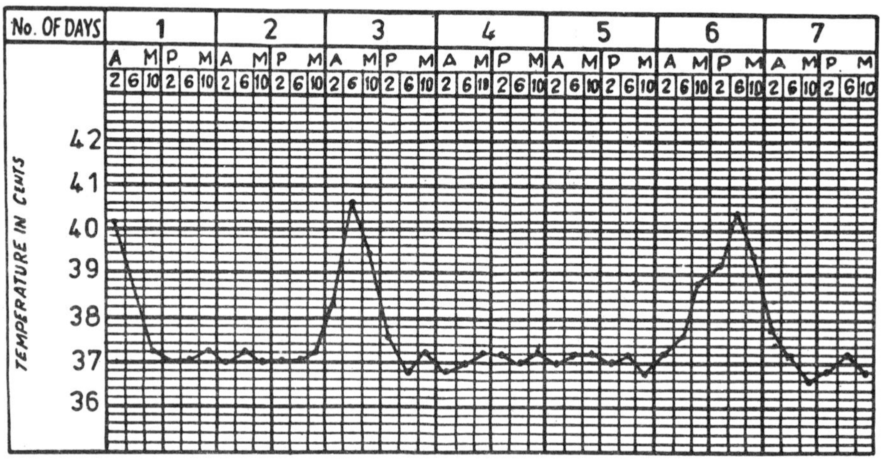

Fig. 2.2 e
Quartan fever

when he may demand blankets. It is accompanied by chattering of the teeth and intense shivering. It corresponds with the rise of body temperature.

They are always present in malarial fevers but can accompany any pyogenic infection.

Most of the patients who have temperature, have a sensation of cold or chill during its rise and this should be differentiated from a true rigor.

(b) **Tachycardia:** Fever is always associated with a rise in pulse rate. This rise is usually about 7 beats per minute for every 0.5^0 rise in temperature in adults. However in certain diseases like typhoid fever this rise in pulse rate is not appropriate to the rise in temperature and is known as relative bradycardia and is of diagnostic significance. This phenomenon is also observed in patients who have fever due to infections like meningitis (causing rise in intracranial pressure) and viral infections.

(c) **Sweating:** Sweating occurs in all patients

when the fever comes down. However, it is more marked in certain fevers like rheumatic or septic fever. Night sweats were supposed to be diagnostic of pulmonary tuberculosis though they can occur in any debilitating diseases. Continuous cold sweat occurs in very septic conditions and the temperature apparently does not seem too high. However rectal temperature should be recorded in such patients when it will usually be found to be very high. Profuse sweating occurs especially as temperature comes down by 'crisis' (suddenly due to normal or subnormal) when it comes down gradually it is by 'lysis'. (Fig. 2.2h and 2i)

(d) **Respiratory rate:** This is normally high in all fevers but is extremely high in respiratory infections like pneumonia or bronchiolitis in children.

(e) **Herpes labialis:** Small vesicles due to herpes simplex virus are formed on the lips during high fevers. Though at one time thought to be diagnostic of pneumococcal infections, they can occur during any high fever.

(f) **Delirium:** This can occur due to any infection. Usually this occurs when the temperature is high and is more common in chronic alcoholics or atherosclerotic individuals.

(g) **Febrile convulsion:** This is more common among small children and may be of great prognostic value. History of such convulsions during childhood is common in patients suffering from epilepsy.

Causes of fever: (a) Infections: bacterial, rickettsial, viral.

(b) Mechanical trauma causing tissue damage following fracture, operation.

(c) Neoplastic diseases: (i) Hypernephroma, (ii) hepatoma, (iii) pancreatic carcinomas.

(d) Diseases of the reticulo-endothelial systems: (i) Hodgkin's disease, (ii) lymphosarcomas, (iii) leukemias.

(e) Acute hemolytic crises.

(f) Vascular accidents: (i) Myocardial infarction, (ii) cerebrovascular accidents.

(g) Collagen disorders.

(h) Acute metabolic disorders like gout, porphyria.

(i) Heat pyrexias.

Mechanism of fever: Temperature of the body is maintained in its normal range by the temperature regulating centres located in the hypothalamus. It carries on its activity by controlling the heat gain

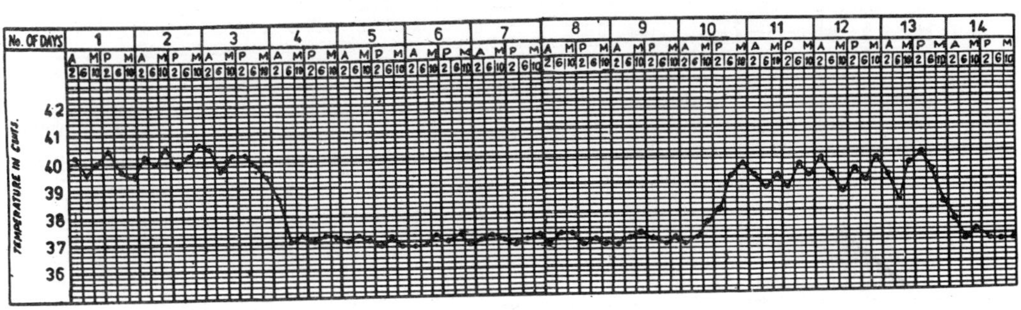

Fig. 2.2f
Relapsing fever

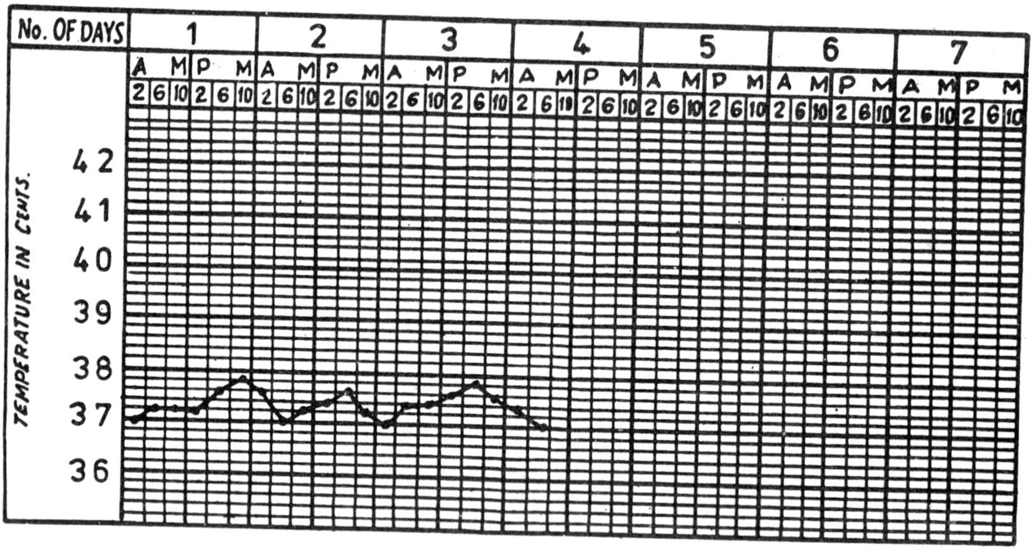

Fig. 2.2g
Low fever

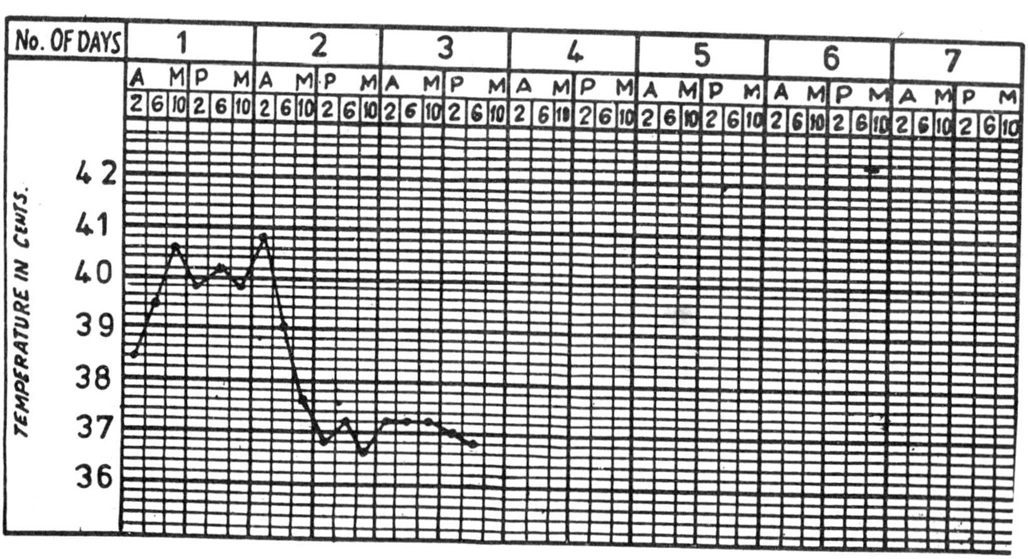

Fig. 2.2h
Hectic fever coming down by crisis

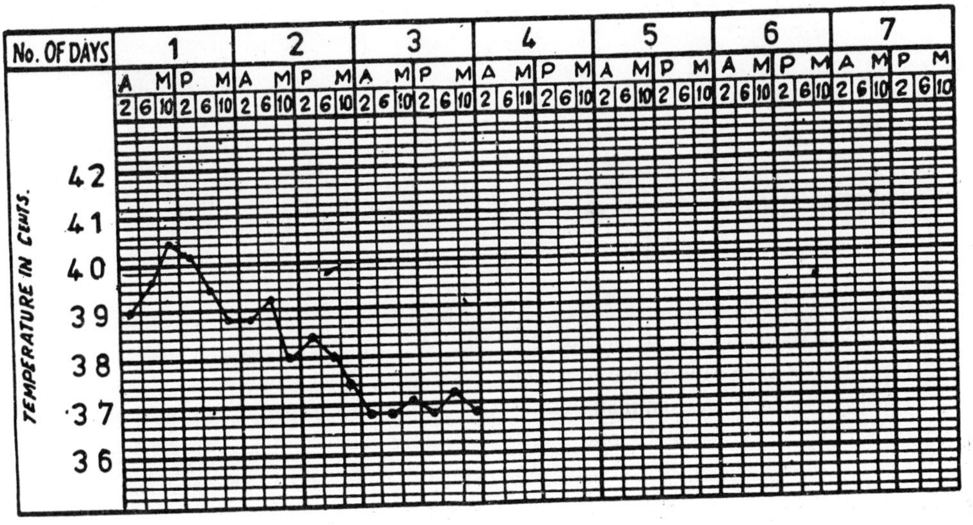

Fig. 2.2i
Fever coming down by crisis

or loss by controlling the vasomotor, pseudomotor and metabolic receptors.

In fever, the temperature regulating centre, which can be compared to a thermostat, is set at a higher level by the effect of pyrogens which are released by the invading organisms or by the tissues which undergo lysis due to trauma or inflammation.

Hence the thermostat which is thus set at a higher level increases the heat production in the body by shivering (muscular contraction) and by vasoconstriction (resulting in pallor). These changes give rise to the sensation of chill which is initially experienced by the patient. Conversely, when the fever comes down cutaneous vasodilatation and sweating occurs.

Section II: Alimentary System

3. Symptomatology and History Taking

A thorough history of any patient is extremely important, but more so in the case of one with the digestive system disorders. This is duc to many reasons. The physical signs on examination may be minimal or absent (as in the case of peptic ulcer) and the diagnosis may have to be suspected on history alone. Secondly, quite often the symptoms related to alimentary tract may be of systemic disorder (like diminished appetite and constipation), as in a case of myxodema. The patients who have psychogenic complaints presenting as alimentary disorders may be included in the same group and will have to be analysed carefully and accordingly. Lastly, the complaints may be minimal as compared to the physical signs.

As there is a wide variety of symptoms which the patients can present, it is convenient to discuss these symptoms according to the anatomical locations of the G.I. tract.

I. Symptoms related to Upper Alimentary Tract (mouth, tongue, oesophagus)

(1) Appetite:

(a) **Loss of appetite (Anorexia):** This is a common complaint which can be the result of any systemic disease or psychological upset and need not be primarily due to Gastro intestinal (G.I.) tract disease. Hence, fever due to any infection, cardiac failure, renal failure or myxodema may cause loss of appetite. Anxiety neurosis or especially depression also may cause the same complaint. It also may be an early symptom of megaloblastic anaemia.

Severe or complete loss of appetite, especially in an elderly person may be the earliest and for some time the only feature of gastric carcinoma. In hepato cellular damage, anorexia may be again the presenting symptom, but is usually associated with nausea and vomiting.

Anorexia nervosa is another syndrome affecting young females who have a total loss of appetite with loss of weight. In spite of this they are unusually active. Other features, of this syndrome are sub-normal temperature and low B.M.R.

(b) Excessive appetite : The alimentary affections which the patient complains of in this symptom are parasitic infections and sometimes malabsorption syndrome. However quite often it is a symptom of systemic disorders or it may be of psychological origin. Hyperthyroidism and diabetes mellitus are the two common systemic disorders leading to this complaint. Obesity due to compulsive cating may be of psychological origin.

(c) **Perverted appetite:** This is usually a symptom associated with either pregnancy or psychoneurosis.

(2) Taste:

Complete loss of taste is usually due to lesions of the facial or glossopharyngeal nerves. However, loss of taste is a common complaint of patients and is usually an interpretation of unpleasant taste in the mouth. This again can occur either due to systemic disorders, or G.I. disorders.

Chronic lung infections, renal failure and diabetes are diseases which commonly produce loss of taste. Drugs administered for various diseases (such as metronidazole for amoebiasis or phenformin for diabetes) can produce unpleasant taste in the mouth.

Any obstruction of G. I. tract like carcinoma of the oesophagus or stomach, a pharyngeal pouch or chronic gastritis can also produce this symptom. A sudden distaste for smoking (tobacco) is one of the earliest symptoms complained by patients who are affected by infective hepatitis.

(3) **Sore mouth:**

In this the patient complains of pain in the oral cavity which is aggravated by any irritant substance coming in contact with the mouth. Commonly this is due to ulcers in the mouth caused by a variety of disorders.

Aphthous ulceration is a common condition where there are multiple ulcers which come and go in crops. They start as minute vesicles which later on break down to form a white slough with a red rim. They are extremely painful and their exact cause is unknown. Acutely painful ulcers on tongue or in the oral cavity may be produced by sharp edges of caries teeth. These are traumatic ulcers.

Other causes of ulceration in the mouth are Vincent's angina and thrush (fungal infection by *Candida albicans*). Rarely the ulcerations may be spirochetal in origin. Local recurring ulcers in the mouth can be due to an ill fitting denture or sharp irregular teeth (traumatic ulcers). Angular stomatitis presents as linear cracks at the angle of the mouth and is usually due to riboflavin deficiency. Scurvy and blood dyscrasias can manifest as recurrent gingivitis. Rarely a hypertrophy of gums may indicate that the patient is being treated with dilantin sodium for epilepsy. Persistent ulcers in mouth may be due to agranulocytasis or local malignancy.

(4) **Sore tongue :**

The usual causes of a painful and sore tongue are either vitamin B complex (mainly vitamin B12) deficiency or iron deficiency. This variety of stomatitis presents as multiple red ulcers which are small in size and are centrally situated.

Malignant ulcers and leucoplakia usually do not cause pain in the earlier stages and they are usually situated on the lateral borders of the tongue.

(5) **Coated tongue :**

This could be due to a variety of reasons and is usually a source of anxiety to the patients.

Early morning coating of the tongue is usually present in people who breathe through their mouth at night.

Any febrile illness, where the amplitude of respiratory movements is increased, may cause coating on the tongue though it is commonly interpreted as a diagnostic sign of enteric infections. A black furred tongue is usually due to fungus infection following antibiotic therapy.

Large papillae and fissures which are normal anatomically, sometimes cause anxiety to the patients. These people should be reassured that there are no abnormalities in any way. Lastly, the coating of the tongue may be due to the faulty hygienic habits, like improper washing of the mouth after food.

(6) **Bad breath (halitosis):**

The smell of breath often can give a clue to diagnosis. Usually this is due to chronic infections in the upper respiratory tract or caries teeth and pyorrhoea. Rarely, stasis in a pharyngeal pouch, oesophagus or stomach (pyloric stenosis or carcinoma), may give rise to this symptom (as in achlasia cardia).

Bronchiactasis or lung abscess especially caused by *B. pyocyaneus* or *E. coli*, may cause this symptom much more frequently than G. I. disorders.

A musty breath (compared to the smell of a dead mouse) is present in patients with hepatic coma. The breath can be described as uriniferous in a case of uraemia while it has a peculiar sweet sickly odour in diabetic acidosis. Rarely, psychoneurotic patients persistently complain of bad breath which is not apparent on clinical examination. Alcohol, paraldehyde and organophosphorus emit peculiar smell and this may help to clinch the diagnosis.

(7) **Disorders of salivation**

(a) Excessive salivation is usually a result of

irritating painful lesions of the mouth or oral cavity. However, it is very distressing and persistent in oesophageal carcinoma.

Any condition which causes nausea is accompanied by reflex increased salivation. Parkinsonism and less commonly trigeminal neuralgia give rise to persistent increased salivation. Waterbrash is a particular form of increased salivation. Pregnancy and heavy metal poisoning may rarely cause this particular complaint.

(b) Decreased salivation or dryness of the mouth is commonly present in mouth breathers. Any condition causing dehydration will also cause the same compaint. Diabetes mellitus and fluid loss due to diarrhoea are the common causes of dehydration.

Any febrile illness where there is a combination of heavy sweating and increased respiratory movements also result in a dry tongue. Diseases of salivary gland or use of anti-cholinergic drugs which can decrease their secretion are rather uncommon but not rare causes of this complaint.

(8) Acid regurgitation

A complaint of bitter and sour fluid rising in the back of the mouth with local burning is commonly present in patients suffering from peptic ulcers. It is also complained of by patients who are suffering from hiatus hernia, oesophagitis or gastritis.

Heart burn is the term used when the irritation is felt retrosternally and is due to irritation of the oesophageal mucosa.

(9) Dysphagia

Dysphagia means difficulty in swallowing and is a symptom which must be taken seriously. However, when a patient complains of dysphagia, the following points should always be inquired into:

(1) How long is the patient suffering from this complaint?

(2) Whether it is of sudden onset or has it developed gradually?

(3) Is the difficulty more while swallowing solids or liquids? If for both, was it first noticed while swallowing solids and has it then progressed to liquids?

(4) Can the patient localise the site of obstruction? i.e., whether it is in the pharynx, midoesophagus or lower oesophageal area?

(5) Is it persistent or intermittent?

The common causes of dysphagia are as follows:

(A) **Upper or pharyngo-oesophageal,**

(1) **Intramural**

(a) Mucosa - Pharyngitis and tonsillitis Trauma
Sideropenia (iron deficiency anaemia)

(b) Muscular - Pharyngeal pouch
Myathenia gravis

(c) Neurological - Bulbar palsy
Globus hystericus

(2) Extrinsic pressure - Thyroid enlargement.
Retropharyngeal abscess.

(B) **Mid oesophageal**

(1) Intraluminal - Foreign body

(2) Intramural
- (a) Stricture
- (b) Carcinoma

(3) Extrinsic pressure
- (a) Mediastinal lymphadenopathy
- (b) Thyroid enlargement
- (c) Aortic aneurysm
- (d) Enlarged left atrium in case of mitral stenosis
- (e) Vascular ring

(C) **Lower oesophageal**

(1) Intraluminal - Foreign body

(2) Intramural
- (a) Mucosal - Peptic oesophagitis
Carcinoma oesophagus
Peptic ulcer in aberrant epithelium of lower end of oesophagus
- (b) Muscular - Spasm

Scleroderma
Diverticulum

(3) Extrinsic pressure
(a) Hiatus hernia
(b) Unfolding of aorta

The common causes of dysphagia which are encountered in practice are carcinoma of oesophagus, achalasia cardia, iron deficiency anaemia and peptic oesophagitis or oesophagitis caused by drugs and chemicals.

The patients who suffer from carcinoma, usually give history of a short duration. The symptoms are progressive without any let up and the initial difficulty is in swallowing of liquids. Usually the patient can localise the site quite accurately, though sometimes the patient complains of obstruction at the midsternal area in lower oesophageal obstruction. In advanced cases, the patients always complain of excessive salivation. Hiccoughs are commonly associated with carcinoma at lower end of oesophagus.

Patients who are suffering from achalasia cardia or cardiospasm, usually localise the hold up at the lower end of the oesophagus. Initially the difficulty may be periodic but later on becomes continuous.

A fair number of patients complain of difficulty more pronounced while swallowing liquids than solids.

Iron dificiency anaemia or sideropenia leading to dysphagia is very commonly in developing countries. This syndrome of dysphagia due to iron deficiency anaemia is known as Plummer-Vinson syndrome or Paterson-Kelly syndrome and almost exculsively affects women between the ages of 30-50 years. The difficulty in swallowing may be intermittent at first. It is usually localised to the pharyngo-oesophageal region and is associated with either atrophic changes of the oesophageal mucosa or by formation of a web distal to the level of cricoid cartilage.

Peptic oesophagitis leads usually to intermittent dysphagia, localised at the lower end of oesophagus and is usually associated with heartburn. It is sometimes aggravated by stooping which facilitates the regurgitation of the acid from the stomach into the oesophagus.

Globus hystericus is not really a difficulty in swallowing. Some patients complain of a lump like feeling in the upper oesophagus and describe it as causing a difficulty in swallowing. It is of psychogenic origin and careful analysis of symptoms will prove that it is not a genuine dysphagia.

Patients who have dysphagia due to oesophagitis caused by chemicals or drugs will give history of swallowing chemical like caustic soda, acids, etc. Swallowing of very hot liquids can also lead to oesophagitis.

II. Symptoms related to Lower Alimentary Tract and Abdominal Viscera

A basic knowledge of various symptoms related to the G. I. tract is essential while interpreting their clinical significance.

Symptoms are enumerated as follows :

A. Nausea and vomiting

Nausea means a feeling of imminent desire to vomit. It is usually associated with other vasomotor and autonomic disturbances which cause a fainting sensation, weakness, pallor and increased perspiration.

Vomiting means a forcible expulsion of the gastro-intestinal contents through the mouth (Retching is the term applied to the laboured respiratory movement which precede or accompany vomiting).

Whenever a patient complains of vomiting the following points should be noted :

(1) The time of onset of vomiting should always be noted. Early morning vomiting before breakfast is common in pregnancy or in toxic causes such as in uraemia. Chronic gastritis due to alcoholism also causes vomiting at this time.

Increased intracranial tension also causes early morning vomiting but this is characteristically not associated with nausea.

(2) Vomiting immediately after food is commonly of functional origin. However reflex vomiting also occurs immediately after food. So also loal causes of gastric irritation can produce this variety of

vomiting.

(3) Recurrent bouts of vomiting occurring two or four hours after food are usually due to pylorospasm caused by gastric or duodenal ulcer or duodenitis.

(4) Large amounts of vomitus brought out 12 to 48 hours after food is practically diagnostic of pyloric obstruction.

(5) Periodic episodes of vomiting preceded by unilateral headaches are common in migraine.

(6) Vomiting is often induced by the patients to relieve abdominal pain. This is common in patients suffering from gastric or duodenal ulcers.

Causes of vomiting

The vomiting centre and chemoreceptor trigger zone (CTZ) are situated in the medulla. Any stimulation of these areas by psychogenic, central or reflex nervous stimuli, toxins or alimentary tract irritation will cause vomiting.

Causes of vomiting

I. Psychogenic causes
   - (a) Emotional upsets
   - (b) Disgusting smells or sights
   - (c) Anorexia nervosa

II. Central causes
   - (a) Increased intracranial tension
   - (b) Concussion

III. Reflex causes
   - (a) Migraine
   - (b) Labyrinthine disorder
   - (c) Tabetic crises

IV. Metabolic
   - (a) Pregnancy
   - (b) Uraemia
   - (c) Liver cell failure
   - (d) Drugs like digitalis, anti-inflammatory drugs, etc.

V. Alimentary tract irritation
   - (a) Pharyngeal irritation
   - (b) Oesophageal irritation or obstruction.

VI. Gastric Causes
   - (a) Gastritis
   - (b) Gastric ulcers
   - (c) Carcinoma of stomach
   - (d) Allergy of food
   - (e) Reflex disturbances of stomach, due to diseases like gall bladder, appendix, etc.
   - (f) Pyloric obstruction

VII. Intestinal obstruction and parasitic infestation.

VIII. Others:
   - (a) Acute myocardial infarction
   - (b) Acute renal colic.
   - (c) Acute biliary colic

Character of vomitus:

The naked eye examination of vomitus can give information of much value. It should always be examined whenever possible and the following points should be noted.

(a) **Quantity:** Large quantities of vomitus are characteristically seen in pyloric obstruction. Small quantities are seen when the vomiting is due to oesophagitis or gastritis.

(b) **Odour:** Gastric acid gives a characteristic sour odour to the vomitus and signifies pyloric obstruction and its absence may signify either vomiting proximal to the stomach (achalasia cardia or pharyngeal pouch) or presence of achylia gastrica. A fecal odour to the vomitus signifies intestinal obstruction or it may rarely be due to gastrocolic fistula. Carcinoma of the stomach causing partial obstruction also gives rise to a peculiar foul vomitus.

(c) **Colour:** Bright red appearance of vomiting means presence of blood (hematemesis) and its causes are discussed later on.

Coffee ground — dark brown coloured vomiting is due to the presence of blood in the vomitus which has remained in the stomach for some length of time. It is commonly seen in toxic conditions like uraemia or cerebral haemorrhage, or as a terminal event in unconscious patient.

Presence of bile imparts a yellow or green colour to the vomitus. It is commonly present but its excess may signify intestinal obstruction distal to second part of duodenum. It is absent in vomiting due to pyloric obstruction.

(d) **Constituents:** Mucus: Mucus is present very commonly and it appears like a white jelly like substance. Excessive amount of mucus may denote gastric stasis or malignancy.

Foods: Presence of food which is eaten more than 8 to 12 hours ago usually signifies pyloric obstruction. Repeated vomiting of retained food may occur in achalasia cardia or hour glass stomach.

Pus : This is a very rare constituent and its presence signifies either a rupture of extrinsic abscess in the stomach or suppurative gastritis.

Foreign bodies: Vomiting of round worm is common when there is a heavy infestation of intestine by these parasites.

Gall stones may be vomited rarely when there is a cholecystogastric or cholecystoduodenal fistula.

B. **Heartburn**

Heartburn (pyrosis) is a sensation of heat or burning which is felt retrosternally and is usually attributed to reflux of acid from the stomach into the oesophagus. It may be present even in cases of achalasia cardia, where there is no acid in the stomach and probably the real cause for this phenomenon is abnormal motility or neuromuscular activity of the lower end of the oesophagus.

The common causes of heartburn are hiatus hernia, peptic oesophagitis, peptic ulcers and faulty eating habits.

C. **Aerophagy and belching**

Aerophagy is defined as swallowing of air. Physiological swallowing of air is impossible. The action really is a sucking in of air. Persons who suffer from aerophagy relax the superior sphincter of the oesophagus and air is sucked into the oesophagus due to the negative pressure in the oesophagus. Some amount of this air goes into the stomach and increases the size of the gastric bubble.

Belching is the release of air into the oesophagus from the gastric fundal air bubble. This action is sudden and involuntary.

(Aerophagy and belching occur commonly as a reflex action due to discomfort, in either chest or abdomen. Cardiac ischemia, hiatus hernia, gall stones and a peptic ulcer are common examples of such a condition.)

D. **Hiccups**

Hiccup is a sound produced by spasmodic contraction of the diaphragm with adduction of the vocal cords. This is usually produced by impulses arising from structures supplied by the phrenic or vagus nerves. These afferent impulses are passed through the phrenic nerve.

Common causes of hiccups are :

1. Reflex origin in hypersensitive subjects (Temperature change, hot or cold food, etc.)
2. Irritation of phrenic nerve –
   a. Phrenic nerve neuritis
   b. Pressure due to oesophageal tumours, diphragmatic hernia, pericarditis.
   c. Irritation due to influenza, bronchitis, asthma.
3. Dilatation of the stomach
4. Carcinoma of the stomach
5. Hepatic and splenic diseases irritating the diaphragm
6. Following abdominal surgery
7. Toxic conditions like uraemia or febrile illness.
8. Central irritation due to brain tumour, apoplexy, encephalitis or meningitis.
9. Epidemic hiccup.

E. **Abdominal pain**

Pain in the abdomen is an extremely common symptom. Due to the wide variations in its presentation that is its localisation, character, radiation, etc., and secondly due to the fact that it can be produced not only by affection of the abdominal viscera but also due to disease of the spine, the abdominal musculature, the nervous system or thoracic diseases, a discussion as to its mode of production is presented first. Abdominal pain of organic origin is produced in the following three ways:

I. Visceral pain

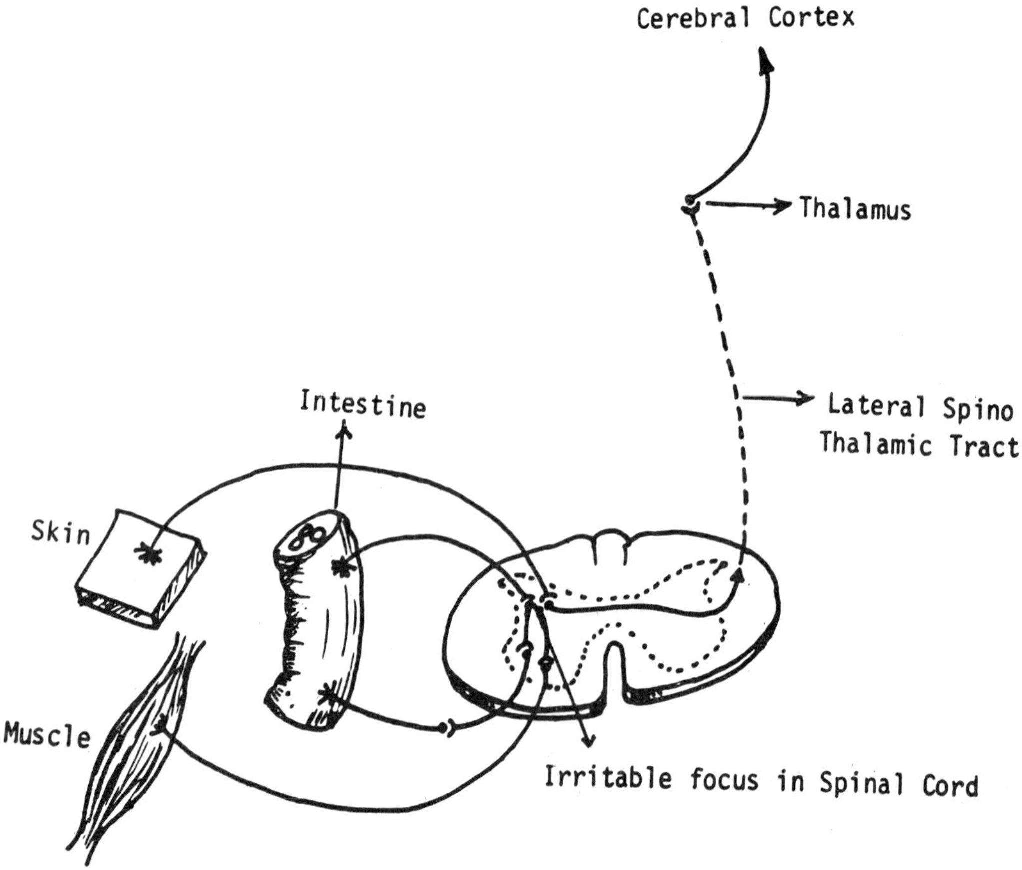

Fig. 3.1

To illustrate Mackenzie's theory of referred pain. Impulses from a viscus are received by spinal cord and they start an irritable focus in spinal cord. Due to the irritable focus, neighbouring neurons also get involved and increase the tone of muscles innervated by same segments.

II. Referred pain

III. Due to peritoneocutaneous reflex

I. Visceral pain

This is produced by a stimulus acting upon sensory nerve endings in the viscus. The stimulus is usually either distension or contraction of the viscus. These impulses travel via afferent visceral fibres which accompany the sympathetic nervous system and then travel to posterior root ganglia via the white rami communicants. They enter the posterior horn of the spinal cord along with the somatic neurones.

True visceral pain is thus produced by stimuli travelling through these nerves and the cerebrospinal nerves do not participate in its production.

True visceral pain is felt as a deep situated pain, and is described commonly as an ache. It can be mild to severe in intensity and is usually colicky in nature. It is diffuse an vaguely localised to the middle of the abdomen. However, it can be localised in a general way to that portion of the abdomen which corresponds segmentally to the location of the stimulated viscus.

It is most commonly and classically seen in

obstruction of viscera such as intestines, stomach and bile ducts. The pain threshold is reduced when an organ is inflamed and then it can be precipitated by small irritations (example acidic irritation of a peptic ulcer).

II. Referred pain

The second mechanism which comes into play when the visceral pain fibres are stimulated is the referred pain. (Fig. 3.1)

It is usually produced by inflammatory or neoplastic diseases rather than by diseases producing alteration in motility. Its character is sharp, cutting in nature and it is well localised and is superficial. It is usually felt more laterally than visceral pain (which is usually felt in the midline) and usually radiates over a fixed pathway.

III. Pain felt due to peritoneocutaneous reflex (Morley's reflex)

In this type of pain, the sympathetic fibres do not participate. The parietal peritoneum is supplied directly by cerebrospinal (somatic) nerve endings. The stimulation of these nerve endings cause pain which is felt along the somatic distribution of the same sensory nerve.This type of pain is again produced by inflammation of the viscera rather than any changes in its functions. It is very often associated with spasm (rigidity) of the abdominal muscles and is responsible for the phenomenon of guarding.

(All these types of pathways may be used on the presentation of an inflammation of a hollow viscus).

Psychological factors

Pain is a subjective sensation which is felt by the patient and hence the patient's sensitivity to pain plays a great part in its interpretation. The intensity of pain which is felt by the patient may vary. Some people may be intolerant to even minor pains, while others can tolerate even a severe pain stoically.

Analysis of pain

Whenever a patient complains of pain it is necessary to ask him a fairly detailed questionnaire. The following points which are known as Ryle's ten questions should be asked in a systematic way.

1. Situations (including depth from surface);
2. Localisation;
3. Character;
4. Severity;
5. Duration;
6. Frequency;
7. Special times of occurrence;
8. Paths of reference and radiation of pain;
9. Aggravating factors;
10. Relieving factors.

(1 & 2) **Situation and localisation:**

Where is the pain situated?

Can the patient localise in which abdominal quadrant it is the worst?

Is it possible for him to exactly point towards the area by his own finger?

Is it in midline and cannot be localised properly?

Can the patient describe whether it is superficial or felt as a deep situated pain?

(3 & 4) **Character and severity:**

How does the patient describe it?

Is is described as griping, colicky, stabbing or sharp cutting pain?

Does it come in waves or is it a dull constant ache? Is the patient tossing and turning around in bed without finding a comfortable position? (as happens in colicky pain).

Or is he afraid to move as that increases the pain? (as happens in peritoneal irritation especially perforation).

5. **Duration:**

How long ago did the pain start?

Is it constant since then or has it been waxing and waning?

Did the pain start suddenly or was it of gradual onset?

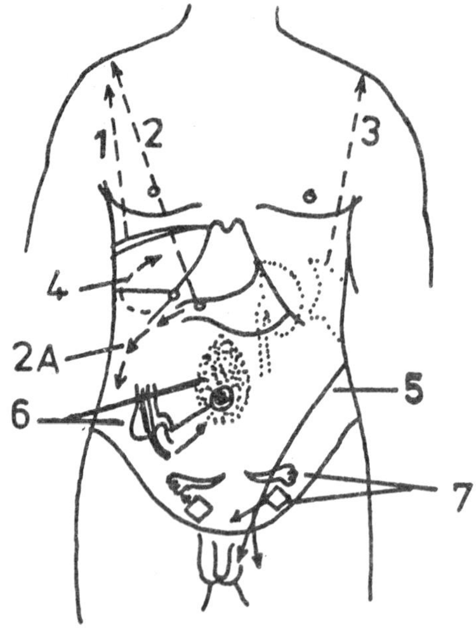

Fig. 3.2 — Sites where the referred pain from various organs is felt.

1. Pain due to perforation of appendix or typhoid ulcer is referred to right shoulder.
2. Pain of peptic ulcer perforation is referred to right shoulder.

2A. Pain of peptic ulcer perforation may also travel along paracolic gutter and be referred to iliac fossa.

3. Splenic pain is referred to left shoulder.
4. Biliary colic radiates posteriorly to inferior angle of scapula.
5. Renal colic is referred to groin, testis and inner side of thigh.
6. Appendicular colic or pain is first felt at umbilicus and then in epigastrium and later at right iliac fossa.
7. Pain due to fallopian tube (salphingitis) is referred to hypogastrium.

6. **Frequency:**

If the patient is suffering from the pain for some length of time, then whether it is present practically every day or does he have any pain-free intervals of weeks or days in between?

Or whether the attacks of pain come intermittently without any apparent reason, last for some time and then disappear completely?

7. **Particular time of occurrence:**

Does the pain come on at any particular time of day or night?

Does the patient have to wake up in the early hours of the morning due to the pain?

8. **Paths of referred pain and radiation of pain (sites):** — Fig. 3.2

9. **Aggravating factors:**

What is its time relation to hunger and food?

That is whether the patient feels the pain more when he is hungry, or after food?

Does any particular type of food bring about the pain?

If so, whether it is tasty food, chillies or spices, alcohol or only a specific dietary item which causes the pain?

10. **Relieving factors:**

Does anything relieve the pain?

Description of certain common 'pains'

1. **Duodenal ulcer:** The pain of duodenal ulcer in its typical form presents a fairly constant clinical picture. The pain is steady, growing, burning or hunger like discomfort, which is situated high up in the epigastrium slightly to the right of the mid-line. It is localised to a small area and usually does not radiate. Only when the ulcer penetrates and adheres to the pancreas, the pain is described as a dull boring pain at the back. The pain usually develops 2 to 3 hours after meals and is immediately relieved after food or alkalies. Hence the patient usually attributes it to hunger and hence it is also known as 'hunger pain'. The pain sometimes awakens the patient from sleep in the early hours of the morning and thus the patient usually forms a habit of eating a few biscuits or drinking a glass of milk, at this time to relieve this pain.

The pain of duodenal ulcer exhibits what can be termed as periodicity. The symptoms appear and last for a few days and then disappear for an interval of few weeks or even months without any apparent reason.

Exacerbation of these symptoms tends to last longer and the pain-free intervals become shorter, so that subsequently after a few years the pain may be a fairly constant feature. No exact explanation of this phenomenon is known but it is a classic feature in the history of a patient suffering from duodenal ulcer.

2. **Gastric ulcer:** The pain of gastric ulcer is also felt in the epigastrium but more to the left of the mid-line.

The pain is again described as burning or aching but may be atypical and the patient may describe it as a sensation of discomfort or bloating. The pain is fairly well localised and though initially there is a relief from pain after eating, an acute bout of pain is precipitated about half an hour after food. Hence the patient of gastric ulcer correlates the pain with the act of eating and hence is afraid to eat properly with a resultant loss of weight. The pain of gastric ulcer is relieved by alkalies.

There is usually no nocturnal pain and the nonperiodicity of pain as experienced by patient having duodenal ulcer.

Pain of gastritis or gastric ulcer is often caused by anti-inflammatory drugs, psychological tensions and irregular food habits.

3. **Intestinal colic:** Pain of intestinal colic can be divided roughly as that due to small intestinal colic and that due to large intestinal colic.

Small intestinal colic usually presents as a characteristic colicky pain which is usually periumbilical or supraumbilical. The localisation of this pain may be poor. Initially it is very severe and each bout increases in severity reaching crescendo and then after sustaining at this highest level for a few minutes subsides fairly quickly. These bouts go on recurring until in severe obstruction the muscular tone of the smooth muscle subsides and the pain loses this intermittent nature and may remain as a dull ache. Constipation is a fairly common accompaniment of this sort of pain. Vomiting is usually a late phenomenon.

Large intestinal colics are not so typical and may be localised to the areas where there is pathological involvement.

4. **Appendicular:** In its characteristic form, this condition produces a very typical picture. Pain is the first symptom and it usually starts around the umbilicus but can be located in the epigastrium. The intensity may vary from mild to severe. It is usually followed by nausea and vomiting. This is an important diagnostic point. If the nausea and vomiting precede the abdominal pain, the disease process is more likely to be an infection such as gastroenteritis.

The reason why the pain of appendicular inflammation or irritation is localised to the umbilical area is that the sensory innervation of the appendix corresponds to the tenth spinal segment and hence the pain initially is referred to that area.

After a few hours, the pain shifts to the right iliac fossa as the peritoneum covering the apendix is inflamed. This is accompanied by local tenderness, guarding and rebound tenderness (peritoneo-cutaneous reflex, Morley's reflex). This is usually accompanied by fever of a moderate degree and leucocytosis. Sudden sensation of appendicular pain is usually of severe prognosis as it indicates either perforation or gangrene of the appendix.

The appendicular pain is usually accompanied by constipation but in some cases diarrhoea may occur, especially with pelvic appendicitis with local peri-appendicular abscess formation. A coated tongue with foetor oris (foul breath) is a very common sign seen along with acute appendicitis.

5. **Perforation** (of peptic ulcer, appendix or typhoid ulcer): The pain of peritoneal irritation or inflammation is usually of a very severe intensity and always begins fairly suddenly. It is initially located directly over the inflamed area and the intensity is dependent upon the type and amount of the irritating substance as well as the rate at which the substance is poured into the peritoneal cavity as a result of perforation. Hence a small quantity of acidic gastric juice from a perforated peptic ulcer or pancreatic juice containing its digestive enzymes give rise to a

severe peritoneal irritation as compared to that produced by a slow leak of blood or urine or bile.

The pain of perforative peritonitis is aggravated by changes in tension of the peritoneum. Hence the patient suffering from this condition lies still in bed and avoids all movements as compared to the patient with colicky pain who is usually tossing and turning in bed to find out a favourable position which will relieve the pain. This pain is always accompanied by a board-like rigidity (can be compared to the feel of a wooden board, hence the name). It is due to spasm of the abdominal muscles and in the initial phases, the muscles overlying the pathological viscera demonstrate it. Later on the rigidity becomes generalised as the peritonitis spreads over the whole of the peritoneum.

6. **Biliary colic:** The pain of biliary colic is produced by either distention or inflammation of gall bladder, or both. It can also be caused by spasm of cystic duct or common bile duct. Distention of the gall bladder is caused by the obstruction of the ducts due to gall stones. The pain starts abruptly and increases to its maximum pitch fairly suddenly. It remains at this level for a fairly long period lasting for hours at a time and the attack subsides as rapidly as it starts.

The pain is felt in the epigastrium and it radiates along the costal margin to the right hypochondrium and the lower angle of the right scapula. It may also radiate to the right shoulder and rarely to the left hypochondrium. Radiation to right lumbar region is also noted fairly commonly. The pain is accompanied by local guarding and tenderness. A sensation of soreness persists over the area of acute pain for a number of days following the acute attack of colic. Severe restlessness is a common symptom.

7. **Pain due to acute pancreatitis:** Pain produced by this condition is acute, very severe and continuous. Though generalised, the pain is localised in the upper abdomen and slightly to the left. It radiates to the back. In severe attacks, the pain is accompanied by shock, tachycardia, pallor and cyanosis. Small frequent vomiting of bilestained fluid is a usual accompaniment. Rigidity of the abdominal muscles is not marked and this point may serve to distinguish it from acute perforation.

8. **Hepatic pain:** The pain is felt in the right hypochondrium and is due to stretching of the hepatic capsule either by inflammation or congestion. Pain is severe, constant in nature and is aggravated by deep breathing and coughing as these actions produce a movement of the diaphragm which irritate the hepatic capsule.

9. **Renal colic:** This presents as a typical attack of sudden severe pain which starts either at the back in the lumbar region or at the side of the abdomen on one side, and then radiates down the abdomen up to the testis or groin on the same side. The onset is fairly sudden and the pain goes on waxing and waning, but lasts for few hours. It is associated with vomiting and difficulty or frequency of micturition and occasionally fever (if the colic is due to renal infection). Severe restlessness is associated.

F. Hematemesis and melena

Hematemesis means vomiting of blood and melena means passage of dark black stools, which are best described as tarry.

Whenever a patient complains of these symptoms certain points should be remembered. Inquiry of the patient should be conducted to determine the duration and the severity of the bleeding. Severity can be determined not only by the amount of blood vomited but also to a certain extent by the associated symptoms. A loss of blood up to 500 ml in the bowels usually does not produce any associated symptoms, but any loss above this amount certainly produces symptoms of diminution of blood volume. The cause of hematemesis and melena also has to be found out and questioning the patient regarding the common causes of GI bleeding should follow.

Frank bleeding — red blood per rectum usually points towards bleeding from the lower intestines — i.e., from jejunum downwards. Sometimes a massive bleeding from stomach and duodenum can produce frank bleeding per rectum.

Black stools resembling melena may be produced following oral iron therapy. Rarely bismuth or charcoal ingestion may colour the stools black.

The following line of questioning should be followed to evaluate the patient's complaint of hematemesis and melena:

1. How many hours ago was the onset of hematemesis?

2. What was roughly the quantity of blood vomited? (It is always better to ask the patient in terms of how many cupfuls he has vomited rather than in terms of ounces).

3. What was the colour of the vomited blood?

Red colour will indicated that the vomiting of blood was immediately after bleeding in the stomach. Dark red or black colour indicates that the vomiting of blood has taken place some time after the bleeding and the acid gastric juice has converted the haemoglobin into haematin. Coffee ground colour vomiting indicates that the blood has remained in the stomach for a fairly long time before being vomited.

4. Is there any associated melena or is there melena without hematemesis?

(Hematemesis usually produces melena when the bleeding is even of moderate quantity. Bleeding from the stomach and duodenum gives rise to both hematemesis and melena but bleeding from jejunum downwards produces only melena.

Minimum amount of blood required to produce melena is about 50 to 100 ml and the bleeding should be rapid. Any bleeding which is slower than this or less in quantity may not manifest clinically as frank melena and can be detected only microscopically as occult blood. After a single large bout of gastric bleeding, melena may persist for as long as two or three days and occult blood may be found in the stools for as long as a week).

5. Does the patient complain of any giddiness especially when standing or in a sitting position? Or was the bleeding associated with sweating, palpitations, syncope and a sensation of sinking?

These questions will help to establish the severity of the bleeding. A severe gastrointestinal haemorrhage is associated with all the other clinical features of shock while a mild bleeding, will produce no associated symptoms or only mild giddiness.

6. Does the patient give a history of any upper abdominal pain relieved by food, a few months or even years before the onset of hematemesis?

A typical history suggestive of peptic ulcer may be obtained but even a vague history of epigastric distress on and off may suggest the same diagnosis.

7. Is there any history of chronic alcoholism or jaundice in the past?

This would suggest that the cause of the bleeding is cirrhosis of liver, which gives rise to oesophageal varices.

8. Or did the bleeding follow ingestion of any drug like aspirin or alcohol?

Acute gastritis following aspirin is a very common cause of GI bleeding. However, aspirin or sometimes cortisone may precipitate bleeding from a chronic peptic ulcer.

9. If there is no history of any abdominal pain or drug ingestion, the patient should be asked the following questions:

Is there any cough either acute or chronic or is there any history of recent upper respiratory tract infection or surgery?

Rarely hematemesis may be due to vomiting of blood which is swallowed from respiratory tract lesions and the patient may not complain of any haemoptysis.

10. Does the patient give a history of fever for about a week preceding melena?

Typhoid infection can give rise to melena especially in the second week of its course.

Differentiation between hematemesis and hemoptysis is given in Table 3.1

G. Distention of abdomen

A sensation of distention for which fullness, bloating gaseous discomfort or any number of other synonyms are used is an extremely common symptom complained of by the patient.

Table 3.1

Hematemesis	Hemoptysis
1. With vomiting	1. With cough
2. Altered or coffee coloured blood	2. Frank red blood
3. Clots may be passed with frank blood	3. Fresh frothy
4. With food	4. Without food
5. Gastrointestinal symptoms present	5. Respiratory symptoms present
6. Vomitus not stained for following days	6. Sputum is tinged pink for following 2-3 days
7. Acidic	7. Alkaline
8. Associated with melena	8. Usually melena absent unless blood is swallowed

Distention being a subjective symptom, the first point to be remembered is that it can be of a functional origin in which case it will not be accompanied by any clinical signs.

Organic distention of the abdomen can be either generalised or localised. A generalised abdominal distention has classically been described as being caused by fat, facces, fluid, foetus or flatus. A localised distention is due to disease of the underlying viscera.

The following line of questioning should be adopted to analyse this complaint :

1. Is the distention generalised or localised?

2. Has the onset been fairly sudden or is it gradual?

3. Is there history of incessent vomiting or/ and loose motions. Such symptoms lead to hypokalemia and distension.

Gradual onset may be noticed by the patient as an increasing tightness of his clothes and a sensation of heaviness of the abdomen.

Sudden abdominal distension can be caused by either intestinal obstruction or sudden onset of ascites following portal vein thrombosis. Acute peritonitis following infection or perforation may have distension as its main symptom along with acute pain, whenever hypokalemia leads to generalised abdominal distension. There is severe asthenia and patient lies flaccid with cold limbs.

Gradual distension of abdomen is usually due to insidious formation of ascites. The common causes of this condition are cirrhosis of liver and tuberculous peritonitis. A gradually progressive abdominal tumour like ovarian cyst may also be present.

3. Is there any history pointing towards chronic hepatic disease like alcoholism, jaundice or hematemesis?

This will point towards cirrhosis of liver as the cause of ascites.

4. Is there any history of fever especially low grade fever in the evening or is there any associated history suggestive of pulmonary tuberculosis?

Tuberculosis of the abdominal peritoneum is a very common cause of ascites and may be the cause of a rapid increase in the ascites in cirrhosis of liver, as it very often supervenes as a secondary complication in this condition. Ascites with severe cachexia indicates malignancy.

5. Is there any dyspnea or orthopnea associated with the ascites?

A massive ascites will cause these complaints as the diaphragm is pushed upwards due to the pressure of the fluid resulting in reduced vital capacity of the lungs.

However, ascites can be caused by cardiac failure and here the dyspnea will usually precede the ascites.

6. Is there any edema of the feet or swelling of the face associated with the distension?

Appearance of edema of legs following that of distension points towards abdominal diseases as the cause of distension while appearance of edema of legs first and then distension later will point towards cardiac lesions as the cause of the distension.

Edema of face, distension of abdomen and edema of feet can be the effect of generalised hypoproteinemia. However if edema of face, especially predominant in early morning is the most prominent feature of the history, the cause is likely to be a renal disease. Rarely appearance of edema of face and ascites without any edema of feet may be clinical feature of constrictive pericarditis.

7. Is there any change in bowel habits or any

fairly noticeable loss of weight before the appearance of abdominal distension?

This may point towards an adbominal malignancy as the cause of ascites causing the distension.

If the distension is localised, the line of questioning to be adopted should be as follows :

(1) What is the exact situation of the swelling in relation to the abdominal quadrants?

(2) For how long has the patient noticed the swelling?

(3) Is it gradually increasing in size or stable since its appearance?

(4) Does the patient feel that the swelling moves from one place to another?

(5) Is there any pain associated with it?

(6) Is it associated with systemic symptoms like fever, weakness, etc.?

(7) Has the patient lost weight rapidly since its appearance or prior to it?

H. **Localised swelling:**

Though any organ in the abdomen can be affected in such a way as to give rise to a localised swelling, the common organs which give rise to localised swellings are the liver, spleen, stomach, colon — especially the ileocecal region and the kidneys.

Liver enlargement is noticed very often by the patient as a swelling in the right hypochondrium and one of the most common causes is congestion of the liver due to congestive cardiac failure. Hepatoma and hepatitis due to viral and amoebic infection also give rise to hepatic swelling.

Spleen can be enlarged to a very large size and a dragging sensation in the left hypochondrium is usually associated with this swelling.

Tumours of the stomach can present first as localised swelling in the epigastrium. However much more commonly pyloric obstruction caused either by peptic ulcer or malignancy produces obstruction of the stomach when the patient classically complains of a lump in the upper abdomen which movers from left to right side. This is due to the violent peristaltic movements of the stomach, which become particularly prominent after food.

Renal lumps may first be noticed as unilateral swellings. They may have no other associated symptoms but if the swelling is due to obstructive hydronephrosis due to stone, renal colic is usually present with it. Similarly, if there is an infective element in the obstruction, fever with rigors is usually added to the symptomatology. Very rarely polycystic kidneys may present as gradually increasing bilateral renal lumps.

The ileocecal region is commonly affected by disease process and a lump may be the presenting complaint. Common causes of such a lump are ileocecal tuberculosis, appendicular abscess, colonic malignancy or rarely amoeboma (typhlitis).

I. **Diarrhoea and dysentery**

Diarrhoea can be defined as frequent evacuation of unformed abnormal stools. Dysentery can be defined as diarrhoea with the presence of blood and / or mucus in the stools.

A detailed history is a must when the patient complains of these conditions as it may point towards the causative lesion or give an approximate idea about the nature of investigations to be done in such a case.

(1) How long does the patient have this diarrhoea? i.e., is it an acute or a chronic diarrhoea?

(2) What is the approximate number of stools passed in 24 hours?

(3) What is the consistency?

Is it completely watery or is it semi-liquid or semi-solid?

(4) Is there any particular time of the day when it is worst or is there any relation to food?

(5) Did it start after ingestion of any food which could have been contaminated?

(6) Is there presence of mucus and blood?

(7) If present, are the stools accompanied by blood and mucus or does the patient pass only blood and mucus as a motion?

This may differentiate between amoebic and bacillary dysentery. In amoebic dysentery, the stools are made up of fecal matter with blood and mucus, while in bacillary dysentery, the stools may contain only blood or mucus.

(8) What is the quantity and nature of stools?

Large frothy stools may point towards steatorrhoea and also giardiasis.

(9) Are the stools extremely foul smelling?

A severe infection especially causing acute diarrhoea gives rise to a very foul smell.

(10) Is there any urgency and tenesmus along with the diarrhoea?

Involvement of rectum (proctitis) usually gives rise to these two symptoms. Sometimes there may be so much urgency that patient may soil the clothes.

(11) Is there any history of alternating constipation and diarrhoea? This may indicate a tuberculous infection of the small intestines.

(12) Is there any associated fever along with the diarrhoea?

J. Constipation

Constipation is a term used by patients in many ways. It is most commonly used to describe diminishing frequency of bowel habits, but may also be used to describe passing of hard stools or difficulty in defecation.

(1) What is the duration of constipation?

(2) How was the onset?

If it started suddenly with an initial history of bleeding per rectum, thorough investigation should be conducted to exclude malignancy of the lower intestinal tract.

(3) Is it alternating with diarrhoea?

(4) Is there any abdominal distension and vomiting associated with it?

(5) Is the constipation habitual and of long duration?

A complete history of dietetic habits and sedentary habits should be examined. Rarely a true constipation may present as spurious diarrhoea. This is due to irritation of the colon by the hard inspissated fecal masses.

K. Change of bowel habits

If a person above forty years of age complains of change of habits of recent origin, he should be investigated for malignancy of large bowel.

L. Jaundice

Jaundice is a yellow discolouration of the skin and mucus membranes due to excessive accumulation of bilirubin in the blood. An increased production of bilirubin due to excessive and abnormal destruction of the red blood cells, a defective metabolism of bilirubin in the liver, or an obstruction in the passage of bilirubin in the bile ducts, are the three modes of production of jaundice. These types are known as hemolytic, hepatocellular and obstructive jaundice, respectively.

The history of a patient should be elicited to differentiate between these three types.

(1) How was the onset?

Was it sudden, subacute or very insidious so that the patient has difficulty in recollecting the exact time when it first started?

(2) Was there any fever, nausea and vomiting at the onset?

This is a typical feature at the onset of hepatocellular jaundice. An aversion to tobacco in smokers is also present at the onset of hepatocellular jaundice.

(3) Was there any pain in the abdomen suggestive of gall bladder colic? Or is there any continuous dull boring pain in the upper abdomen suggestive of carcinoma of the head of pancreas?

A transient dull pain in the right hypochondrium may indicate infective hepatitis.

(4) Is the jaundice gradually progressive?

Or is there any intermittent waxing or waning in its intensity?

Obstructive jaundice due to carcinoma of the head of pancreas will give rise to a steadily progressive jaundice while that caused by gall stones may be intermittent.

(5) What is the colour of the urine and stools?

In obstructive jaundice, the urine will become progressively yellow or reddish and the stools will remain acholic (white) once they become so.

In hepatocellular jaundice, the stools will turn white after a few days and a return of yellow colour to the stools will usually herald a recovery.

In hemolytic jaundice, both urine and stools will be excessively yellow in colour.

(6) Is there any associated itching of the skin?

Though classically presumed to be a symptom of pointing towards an obstructive pathology as the cause, it is also present in patients who have a cholestatic type of affection in viral hepatitis.

(7) Are there any previous incidences of jaundice in the past?

Hemolytic jaundice and Serum B hepatitis usually recur and may be associated with incidences of fever at the onset.

(8) Is there any history of any progressive loss of weight with severe loss of appetite?

Malignancy causing an obstruction of the bile ducts or secondary deposits in the liver may result in this particular complaint.

(9) Is there any history of previous blood transfusions or drugs?

Blood transfusions may give rise to serum hepatitis. Incubation period may be as long as 6 months after the transfusion.

Drugs may cause jaundice by direct hepatotoxicity (as chloroquine, etc) or they may cause an allergic response in the biliary canaliculi, resulting in cholestatic type of jaundice (chlorpromazine).

PAST AND PERSONAL HISTORY

This should be elicited according to the nature of the complaints and will depend upon the presenting complaint and the probable diagnosis arrived at after taking the history.

Details of these evaluations will be discussed along with the discussion of common diseases affecting the G.I. system which follows after the description of examination.

4. Alimentary System — Clinical Examination

Examination can be carried out as

I. General

II. Systemic

I. **General Examination:** In examination of alimentary system important points to be noted in general examination are :-

1. State of consciousness
2. Change of behaviour

Appearance : Whether the patient is in acute pain and doubled up, or whether the patient is restless because of acute pain (acute renal or biliary or intestinal colic)?

Face

Eyes : Sunken - dehydration

Pallor - anaemia cirrhosis

Icterus - cirrhosis and other causes of jaundice

Hypertelorism with mongoloid face- hemolytic anaemia.

Mouth : 1. Pale - bleeding gums in leukaemia

2. Pallor of lips - in leukaemia and severe anaemia

3. Sore tongue - stomatitis in multiple vitamin deficiencies

- ulcers on tongue
- halitosis
- foctor hepaticus

coated tongue - Enteric fever

Parotid : Enlargement in cirrhosis and in malnutrition

Skin : Spider naevi

edema of feet

distribution of body hair

gynaecomastia

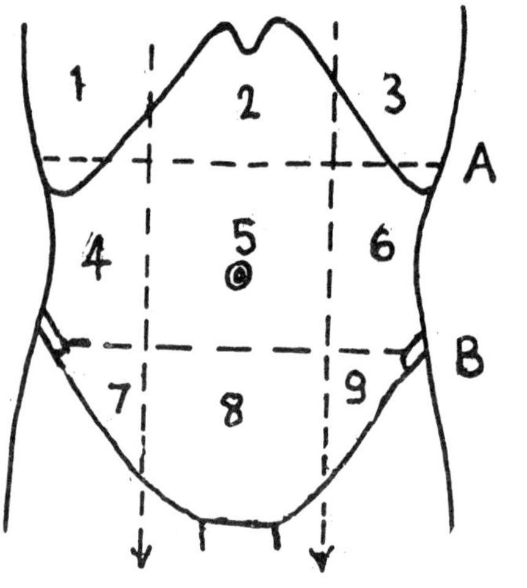

Fig. 4.1

Vertical lines pass through mid inguinal points — (mid point between symphysis pubis and anterior superior iliac spine)

1. Right hypochondrium
2. Epigastrium
3. Left hypochondrium
4. Right lumbar
5. Umbilical
6. Left lumbar
7. Right iliac fossa
8. Hypogastrium
9. Left iliac fossa

A. This line passes at the tip of the 10th costal cartilage.

B. This line passes through anterior superior iliac spines.

Systemic Examination

The routine of inspepction, palpation, percussion and auscultation should be followed when examining the alimentary system.

The patient should be examined in a good light, preferably in a recumbent posture with a pillow below the head to relax the abdomen. The bed should be firm to prevent undue sagging of the abdomen.

Anatomical landmarks

For convenience of description and localisation of the abdominal organs, the abdomen is arbitrarily divided into 9 regions.

This is done by drawing of imaginery lines over the abdomen as shown in figure (Fig. 4.1).

The vertical lines are drawn vertically upwards from points between the anterior superior iliac spines and symphysis pubis. The upper horizontal line is drawn joining the tenth costal cartilage (i.e., the lowest level of the costal margins) and the lower horizontal line is drawn joining the two anterior superior iliac spines.

The areas or the regions thus mapped out are from right to left:

1. Upper abdomen: right hypochondrium, epigastrium and left hypochondrium
2. Middle portion of the abdomen: right lumbar, umbilical and left lumbar
3. Lower abdomen: right iliac, hypogastrium and left iliac.

These zones provide easy reference points in relation to which the various abnormalities found on examination can be described.

Inspection : The inspection should follow in a systematic manner and the points to be noted are as follows :

1. Shape or contour of the abdomen,
2. Skin over the abdomen including umbilicus,
3. Abdominal wall,
4. Abnormal swellings,
5. Visible peristalsis,
6. Veins,
7. Arteries,
8. Hernial sites.

1. Shape or contour of the abdomen: A normal abdomen varies so much in contour from person to person that there can be no fixed norm for its description.

However, roughly the varieties which are seen in normal person can be described as follows :

i. Flat abdomen — usually seen in young persons where the thorax and the abdomen are at the same level.

ii. Protruberent due to accumulation of fat.

iii. Scaphoid abdomen is seen in thin persons or in persons with chronic malnourishment. Here the anterior abdominal wall is sunken and sometimes the lumbar spine can be seen as causing a bulge in the abdominal wall.

A symmetrical bulging of the abdomen is caused by various disease processes.

A distended abdomen should be observed to note whether the bulging is more laterally (i.e., in the flanks) or it is in an anteroposterior direction. Bulging which is more in the flanks is usually due to accumulation of fluid in the abdomen. However, obesity, pregnancy or a large ovarian cyst sometimes gives a similar distension. Bulging in an anteroposterior diameter can be produced by gaseous distension. But the most common cause of this condition is intestinal obstruction.

2. Skin over the abdominal wall including umbilicus

The skin over the abdominal wall should be observed for presence of previous scars of operation. Old or recent branding marks and marks produced by application of lecches may point towards the site of the underlying disease processes.

Lineae albicantes (linea alba) are produced by prolonged stretching of the abdomen and are evidence of previous pregnancies abdominal tumours or ascites.

Striae gravidarum is the term used to describe these lines when they are the result of previous pregnancies. Linea nigra is the term used to describe the black line produced by deposition of melanin in the midline and is also seen in females who have had multiple pregnancies.

Red linear striae are evidence of either Cushing's syndrome or prolonged therapy with steroids.

Repeated application of fomentations by hot water bottles can produce a diffuse mottled discolouration.

Abdominal skin appears to be smooth, shining and stretched when there is abdominal distension due to a pathological cause. In such cases, the umbilicus is either transversely stretched or everted. In extreme cases of ascites, it may protrude out as an umbilical herniation. Obese persons with large abdomens may show umbilicus deeper than normal.

The abdominal skin may show presence of multiple small nodules which are evidence of widespread hematogenous metastasis. However, these are rarely the result of an abdominal malignancy.

In extreme dehydration, the skin of the abdominal wall can be used as a guideline. It can be wrinkled by pinching and these wrinkles do not disappear when they are due to dehydration. However, in old people this sign is not reliable. Any marks of tapping done or liver biopsy should be looked for if patient has already been treated in the recent past.

3. **Abdominal wall**

Abdominal wall should be observed first for its movements. In males, the respiratory movements are abdominothoracic while in females, they are thoraco-abdominal. In both sexes the movements should be equal and smooth.

Complete absence of movements with respiration is indicative of generalised peritonitis, while in localised peritonitis only the portion of the wall over the inflamed organ will show the restricted movements.

The next point to be observed is the position of the recti muscles. They may be separated to a slight extent or there may be a wide gap between the two. The patient should be asked to lift up his head from the pillow to make the gap between the two recti prominent. In its mildest form, there is a small epigastric herniation of mesenteric fat which could be the cause of the pain. Wide diverication (separation) of recti is common in patients who have long-standing ascites. (Pl. 4.1)

4. **Abnormal swellings**

Any enlargement of the abdominal viscera due to new growths, inflammation or congestion may give rise to abnormal swellings.

Enlargement of liver and spleen are common causes of visible swellings in right and left hypochondrium respectively, and usually these swellings can be seen to move up or down with respiration. (Pls. 4.2 a, b & c)

Enlargement of the gall bladder, kidney or a tumour of the stomach, pancreas or colon can be seen as visible swellings. An ovarian cyst in a female can cause a lump in either iliac fossa. A distended bladder or a pregnant uterus causes a swelling which is rounded and is arising from the pelvis in the mid-line.

5. **Visible peristalsis**

Normal peristaltic movements are seen commonly in thin individuals or in females, who have lost the tone of the abdominal muscles due to repeated pregnancies.

Whenever, peristalsis is visible, the exact site and the direction in which the peristaltic wave is seen to progress should be carefully noted.

Gastric peristalsis is seen when there is pyloric obstruction. The peristaltic waves are seen in the epigastrium preceding from left to right side.

Large intestinal obstruction can also produce peristaltic wave in the epigastrium and here the wave is seen passing from right to left.

Small intestinal obstruction gives rise to visible peristalsis in the umbilical and surrounding region and here the peristalsis shows a typical 'step ladder' pattern.

All these peristaltic movements are seen better if the abdomen is observed transversely. Gastric peristalsis in pyloric obstruction can be made more prominent if the patient drinks a glass of water. Any cold stimulus like a spray of ethyl chloride to the abdomen also stimulates the underlying peristalsis.

6. **Veins**

Distended abdominal veins are usually produced either by obstruction to the inferior vena cava or portal vein. Patient should be in an upright position when the flow is examined.

Few small veins are seen infrequently over normal abdomen. Normal direction of the blood flow in the abdominal veins is from above downwards in the lower half of the abdomen and below upwards in upper half of abdomen.

In inferior vena cava obstruction, the direction of blood flow is always from below upwards in lower half of abdomen. In superior vena cava obstruction, flow is in above downward direction in upper half of abdomen.

In the portal vein obstruction, the direction of blood flow in the abnormally dilated veins is always from the umbilicus in a radial fashion. 'Caput medusae' or the markedly engorged veins radiation from the umbilicus are occasionally seen clinically.

The direction of the blood flow should be tested by selecting a vein with no side branches and compressing it with one finger of either hand held near each other. The fingers are then drawn apart so that the vein collapses under them. The presssure of these fingers is released in turn and the side from which the vein fills up is determined. (Fig. 4.2)

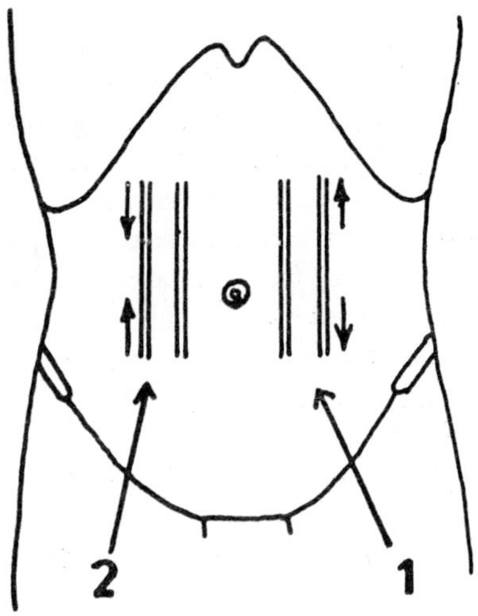

Fig. 4.2

Diagramatic representation of direction of blood flow through superficial abdominal veins : -

1. Normal	—	Flow is below upwards, above the level of umbilical and above downwards below the level of umbilicus.
2. Abnormal	—	in inferior or superior vena cava obstruction direction is reversed. (see Text)

7. **Arteries**

Normal aortic pulsations are seen in very thin individuals and children.

Any hyperdynamic circulatory state like thyrotoxicosis or aortic regurgitation also will produce visible pulsations of the abdominal aorta.

Aneurysm of the aorta gives rise to a pulsatile swelling in the epigastrium and a tumour of the abdominal organs in this area will also transmit pulsations from the aorta in the same area. Clinically, the pulsations due to aortic aneurysm will be obvious while those due to the other condition will not be so. Moreover, the pulsations due to abdominal aortic aneurysm will persist in the knee chest position while those due to transmission through a lump will disappear.

Hepatic pulsations are seen in the case of tricuspid incompetence or due to a hepatic hemangioma. Hypertrophic right ventricle will transmit its pulsations to the epigastrium directly resulting in visible epigastric pulsations.

8. **Hernial sites**

Inguinal rings should always be observed especially with the patient in standing position. Palpation of the rings should also be done simultaneously to determine the presence or absence of small bubonoceles.

PALPATION:

Palpation, which is the most important part of the abdominal examination, should be carried out with the patient comfortably lying down on his back. The legs should be drawn up and a pillow should be placed below the head to ensure that the abdominal muscles are relaxed properly. Only while palpating the lower abdomen, the patient should be asked to extend his legs. For ensuring that the abdominal muscles are properly relaxed, the patient should be asked to breathe in and out through his mouth.

The palpating hand should not be cold and before starting, the examiner should take care to warm his hands by rubbing them together.

Some patients are abnormally ticklish and even the most gentle touch of the examiner's hand will tickle them. A bed sheet should be interposed between the palpating hand and the patient's abdomen to avoid this as much as posible.

Methods of palpation : Superficial and deep palpation are the two common methods of palpation followed routinely. However, bimanual palpation or ballottment is used to palpate the kidneys while a method known as 'dipping' is followed in presence of ascites.

1. **Superficial palpation:** Gentle light palpation should be done initially to elicit minimum degree of tenderness or guarding.

The feel of the normal abdominal wall is soft and yielding and there is no guarding or rigidity. In very obese individuals, the presence of excessive fat in the abdominal wall may cause a feel of generalised increased resistance while there will be an unusual laxity or lack of resistance in females who have had repeated pregnancies or in those patients who are suffering from a severe cachectic illness.

The palpation should always be carried out from an area which is normal and not from the area where the patient is complaining of pain. This will prevent initial pain to the patient which will result in a generalised abdominal resistance because of apprehension.

The initial light palpation may give the information regarding an underlying tumour or an enlarged solid organ, similarly a distended urinary bladder can be detected more easily on gentle palpation.

2. **Deep palpation:** This should follow superficial palpation if there is no area of marked guarding or rigidity anywhere.

This method is used for palpating deep seated abdominal organs or any deep seated tenderness. However, disease of abdominal wall can also give rise to tenderness during deep palpation. This should be excluded by asking the patient to lift his head from the pillow and making the abdominal wall tense. The tense abdominal muscles will cause more pain if the disease is superficial.

3. **Bimanual palpation :** This precedure is followed routinely for palpation of the kidneys and retroperitoneal mass if present.

One hand of the examiner is kept in the loin posteriorly and the other arm is placed over the anterior aspect of the abdomen. The posterior hand pushes the kidney forward and if enlarged, it is felt by the hand placed over the abdominal wall. Normally, the lower pole of the right kidney may be palpable in a thin person.

4. **Dipping :** This method is followed to feel the abdominal viscera in presence of ascites. Due to the presence of a tense ascites the enlargement of the abdominal viscera may not be felt by the routine method of palpation. The examiner should keep his hand flat on the abdomen and the fingers then should be suddenly pushed in the abdomen by flexing them at the metacarpophalangeal joints. This will displace the fluid over the viscera (like spleen or liver) and the enlarged organ is palpated easily.

Abnormal findings on palpation

1. **Muscle guarding or rigidity:** In this condition, the resistance offered by the abdominal musculature is increased. There may be a

generalised peritonitis.

Localised guarding and rigidity is due to inflammation of abdominal organs causing local peritonitis. For example, an inflamed appendix will give rise to guarding and tenderness in right iliac fossa or a perforated peptic ulcer in the initial stages will cause only epigastric tenderness and rigidity.

2. **Tenderness:** This usually signifies an inflammation of the underlying abdominal organ. The patient will complain of pain when the palpating hand presses on the inflamed organ.

Rebound tenderness is elicited as follows. Deep pressure of a constant nature is applied to an abdominal area for some time and then the pressure is suddenly withdrawn. When a deep seated abdominal organ is inflamed, the patient will complain of sudden severe pain which is known as rebound tenderness.

Palpation of abdominal viscera

After routine palpation, the various abdominal viscera should be palpated and their abnormalities if any should be noted as follows:

LIVER:

Normally the edge of the liver may be palpable during deep inspiration. However, the method to be followed when looking for any enlarged liver is as follows:

The palpation should start as low as the right iliac fossa and then the examiner should proceed towards the right costal margin. This procedure should be followed so that a marked enlargement of the liver should not be missed. The patient should be asked to take a deep breath when palpating in this manner, so that the edge of the liver which moves up and down with respiration can be easily felt. The left lobe of the liver is palpable in the epigastrium and should be checked for its enlargement.

If the liver is palpable, the following points should be noted.

1. **The size of the enlarged liver :** Ideally this should be measured and expressed in terms of centimeters below the costal margin in midline, in mid-clavicular line and in mid-axillary line. But in usual clinical practice, it is expressed in terms of finger breadths below the costal margin.

A grossly enlarged liver is seen in congestive cardiac failure, malignant deposits, blood dyscrasias and amoebic abscesses. A moderately enlarged liver is seen in alcoholic hepatitis, fatty degeneration and obstructive hepatitis in cirrhosis and infective hepatitis. In infective hepatitis and anaemia it may only be slightly enlarged.

2. **Surface of the liver:** This should be palpated to find out whether it is smooth or irregular. Smooth surface of the enlarged liver is encountered when the enlargement is due to congestive cardiac failure, hepatitis and amyloidosis.

A finely granular surface points towards portal cirrhosis while irregular large nodules if not very hard will indicate post-hepatitic cirrhosis.

Secondary deposits in the liver will be felt as hard irregular nodes over the surface of the liver. Sometimes, there may be a characteristic depression in their centre which is known as umbilication.

3. **Edge of the liver :** This should be palpated to determine its consistency, regularity and to note whether it is rounded or sharp.

A fatty liver has a soft rounded edge while that enlarged due to congestive cardiac failure has a firm regular edge. Edge of a cirrhotic liver is also sharp. A liver enlarged due to carcinomatosis has a hard irregular margin.

4. **Tenderness :** Tenderness over the liver indicates the presence of inflammatory lesions like viral or amoebic hepatitis. However, liver which is enlarged due to congestive cardiac failure is also markedly tender, especially in its acute stage. Even a grossly enlarged liver due to malignant disease or cirrhosis, is non-tender.

5. **Consistency:** A very hard liver usually

indicates a malignant disease. A firm consistency is found in cirrhosis of the liver and in hepatic enlargement due to chronic congestive cardiac failure. Liver enlarged due to fatty infiltration is soft in consistency.

6. **Movements with respiration:** Amoebic abscess of the liver causes restricted or absent movements of the liver with respiration.

7. **Pulsations over the liver:** Pulsations of the enlarged liver are usually due to tricuspid incompetence. Very rarely hemangiomatous tumours of the liver may cause a pulsatile swelling of the liver.

Whenever a liver is found to be enlarged on palpation, the location of its upper margin should be checked by percussing its upper border. If the upper margin is below the 6th space in mid-clavicular line it is much likely to be due to push from thoracic cavity because of emphysema, etc.

8. Bruit over liver may be heard in malignancy of liver.

SPLEEN:

Normally the spleen is not palpable even on deep inspiration. It has to enlarge at least thrice its normal size to be palpable.

For palpation of the spleen, the examiner should start the palpation in right iliac fossa (so as not to miss a grossly enlarged spleen) and should proceed towards the left costal margin. The patient should be asked to breathe in and out deeply so that the lower portion of the spleen can be felt more easily.

The spleen can also be palpated bimanually. The left hand of the examiner should be kept posteriorly over the left lumbar region and exert a pressure forwards. The right hand should be kept over the abdomen anteriorly in the left hypochondrium. The patient is asked to take a deep breath and the spleen is felt by the hand anteriorly. Care should be taken not to exert a heavy pressure by the hand placed anteriorly, as the spleen hugs the anterior abdominal wall during its descent. The inability to feel a palpable spleen is due to the mistake of palpating too deeply.

The following points should be noted if the spleen is palpable:

1. **Size:** This should be described as enlargement in centimeters or finger breadths below the costal margin. A massive enlargement is seen in Malarial, chronic mycloid leukaemias and kala azar.

In portal hypertension and anaemia (hemolytic or iron deficiency) or leukaemia, a moderate enlargement is seen while minimal enlargement is caused by anaemias or toxic conditions like typhoid fever or infective endocarditis or even tuberculosis.

2. **Consistency:** Infections or septicemic conditions usually cause a soft enlarged spleen.

Spleen in portal hypertension and blood dyscrasias is firm, while that due to a long-standing malarial infection may be hard.

3. **Edge:** The characteristic notch in the anterior margin should always be looked for, to confirm that the organ enlarged is spleen itself.

4. **Movements with respiration:** Spleen moves freely upwards and downwards with respiration and the movement is medially directed. This differentiates it from the enlarged left lobe of liver and kidney which moves directly downwards during inspiration.

Whenever spleen is palpable, its upper margin should be checked by percussion. Normally, the upper level of dullness is encountered in the eighth intercostal space in the mid-axillary line while percussing from above downwards.

An enlarged spleen has to be sometimes differentiated from an enlarged left kidney, as seen in Table 4.1.

The most important points are the free movements on respiration and the presence of a notch in the anterior margin. The other points are variable and not reliable for clinical differentiation.

Table 4.1

Spleen	Kidney
1. Usually causes a superficial swelling	1. Swelling usually deep seated
2. Moves very well with respiration and the movement is directed medially	2. Moves with respiration and movement is directed downwards
3. Characteristic notch in the anterior margin	3. No notch felt
4. Fingers cannot be insinuated between spleen and costal margin	4. Fingers can be insinuated between the two
5. No band of resonance on the enlarged surface	5. Vertical band of colonic resonance on the anterior surface
6. Fingers can be insinuated between the mass and the posterior spinal muscle	6. No space between the mass and these muscles
7. Tenth rib is dull on percussion posteriorly	7. Tenth rib is not dull on percussion posteriorly

GALL BLADDER:

Normal gall bladder is never palpable and it can be felt only when enlarged. When enlarged it is felt typically as a pear shaped swelling beneath the costal margin on the right side and it moves up and down with respiration. Sometimes, the enlargement can be very large in which case the swelling can extend up to the right lumbar region.

If the gall bladder is enlarged when the patient has jaundice, the obstruction to the gall bladder is usually outside the bile duct, such as carcinoma of the head of pancreas. Cholecystitis causes a fibrosis of the gall bladder and the thickened walls of the gall bladder are unable to distend. This phenomenon is known as Courveisier's Law.

The swelling of the gall bladder is usually associated with tenderness. Murphy's sign is eliciting this tenderness by keeping the fingers below the right costal margin at the 9th intercostal cartilage and asking the patient to take a deep breath. If the sign is positive, there is a sudden catch in the breathing process due to the tender gall bladder coming in contact with the palpating hand.

KIDNEYS:

The best method of palpating the kidneys is bimanual palpation. One hand of the examiner is placed posteriorly in the lumbar region and the kidney is pushed forwards. The other hand is kept over the anterior aspect and pressed down. The patient is asked to take a deep breath and if the kidney is enlarged it is felt easily. In normal circumstances, only the lower pole of the right kidney may be palpable especially in thin individuals.

If the kidney is enlarged, then its approximate size, surface, consistency should be noted. At the same time, tenderness should be looked for.

ABDOMINAL LUMPS:

After palpating these organs, the examiner should look for any abnormal swelling or lump. Of course, if there is a huge or an obvious lump, it will be noticed by the examiner as soon as the palpation begins.

The following points should be noted whenever a lump is felt in the abdomen.

(i) **Anatomical location:** This should be described in relation to the abdominal divisions (i.e. epigastric region-lumbar region, etc.). A large tumour may occupy more than two or three of these regions and they should be described as such.

The importance of this is that the anatomical localisation will give a clue as to which organ may be affected giving rise to the lump.

It should also be determined whether the lump is intra-abdominal or is in the abdominal wall. This can be done by asking the patient to raise his head from the bed. A tumour in the abdominal wall will become more prominent by this procedure.

(ii) **Shape and size:** The shape should be described as oval, rounded or enlarged and its approximate dimensions should be described. It should also be noted whether all the borders of the lump can be defined. When a lump is arising from pelvic cavity, its lower margin cannot be reached.

(iii) **Surface:** The surface should be checked to see whether it is smooth, nodular or irregularly nodular. A cirrhotic liver will present a nodular surface, while a malignant liver will have a hard irregularity and nodular surface.

(iv) **Consistency:** A very hard consistency is usually due to a malignant swelling but a very tense cystic swelling of an organ may give rise to the same feeling.

Liver when enlarged will have a varying consistency depending on the cause of enlargement. An inflamed liver is usually soft, a cirrhotic liver is firm, while hepatic enlargement due to malignancy is usually hard.

(v) **Mobility of the lump and relation to respiratory movements:** The mobility of the lump should be looked for by attempting to push it gently in various directions. A floating kidney is very freely mobile. Colonic and intestinal lumps as well as gall bladder swellings, can also be mobile if they have not developed adhesions to the surrounding structures. Colonic lumps are less mobile. Lumps in connection with small bowel are mobile in direction at right angles to the attachment of mesentery. Lumps which have peduncle and which arise from retroperitoneal structures are quite mobile. (Fig. 4.3)

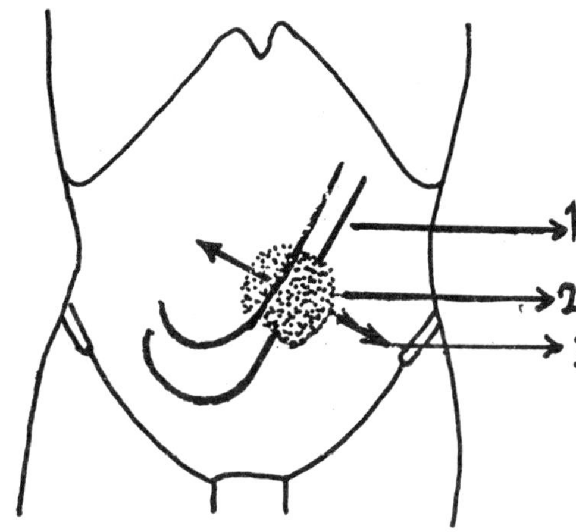

Fig. 4.3
Lumps in connection with small bowel

1. Attachment of mesentery
2. Lump in abdomen in relation to the mesentery and small bowel
3. Direction of mobility of lump is perpendicular to the attachment of mesentery

Usually upper abdominal swellings connected with liver, spleen, stomach and to a certain extent renal lumps move freely up and down with respiration. However, this also can be restricted or absent if there are adhesions due to inflammation.

(vi) **Tenderness:** Usually lumps due to inflammation or congestion are tender. However, any rapidly growing tumour can also give rise to tenderness due to stretching of the surrounding structures. Malignant lumps are usually painless.

(vii) **Pulsations:** The lumps should be checked for presence or absence of pulsations. If present, an attempt should be made to check whether these are due to pulsations of tumour itself or whether they are transmitted to the lump from the abdominal aorta. The pulsations will be expansile when they are due to primary pulsations of the tumour (like those produced by an aneurysm of the abdominal aorta). The transmitted pulsation will disappear especially if the patient is asked to assume the knee chest position, so that the tumour separates from the abdominal aorta.

Fluid in the peritoneal cavity (ascites)

Whenever there is fluid in the abdominal cavity there is a generalised increase of resistance to palpation. However, this is variable and depends upon the amount of fluid in the abdomen.

Usually palpation and percussion have to be combined to determine the presence of fluid. However, the presence of fluid thrill is seen by the palpatory method.

Technique of eliciting fluid thrill

For eliciting the fluid thrill, the examiner should tap the abdomen in one flank and palpate the other flank. In presence of ascites, the wave generated by tapping the abdomen is easily left by the other hand. However, the fat present in the abdominal wall especially in obese people can easily transmit this wave. This should be avoided by asking either the patient or an assistant to hold his hand firmly in the midline of the patient's abdominal wall. This will stop the wave from being transmitted through the abdominal wall. About 1 litre of fluid in abdominal cavity is necessary to give positive fluid thrill.

Mesenteric inflammation

A characteristic doughy feel (a feeling of increased resistance which can be compared to the dough prepared prior to making chapatis) is imparted to the abdomen when there is a tuberculous inflammation of the peritoneum including the mesentery. This doughy feeling disappears when and if there is ascites due to the inflammation.

Percussion

Normal abdomen has a characteristic tympanitic note on percussion. Liver dullness and Traube's semilunar space which is tympanitic are the normal variations in this tympanitic note.

As a rule a mere tympanitic note is of less significance than a dull note. The presence of gases in the hallow viscera may cause an exagerated note. However, in presence of intestinal obstruction, this will be very much more marked.

Obliteration of the normal liver dullness can have an important clinical value when the abdomen is distended. This points towards perforation as the cause of abdominal distention. The gas released in the peritoneal cavity rises below the diaphragm causing this obliteration.

However, this should always be confirmed by sonography or radiological investigations.

Dullness on percussion

Enlargement of any solid viscera or a mass will cause an abnormal dullness over that particular area.

However, the dullness produced by presence of fluid is very typical and the following points should be looked for when the presence of free fluid in the abdomen is suspected.

(a) **Horse shoe shaped dullness :** As the free fluid in the abdomen settles in the flanks and lower regions of the abdomen, the intestines float to the anterior abdominal wall (when the patient is lying supine). This is the basis of this sign.

To elicit this, the examiner should start percussing in the epigastrium and not anywhere else. For in a very tense ascites, this may be the only region which is tympanitic. From this tympanitic area, the percussion should proceed in all directions systematically in a radial fashion. As soon as the dullness is encountered in a paricular direction that point should be marked. Finally, if any imaginery line is drawn (or with the help of a skin pencil) it will be seen that it resembles a horse shoe with its open end pointing towards the epigastrium. (Fig. 4.4)

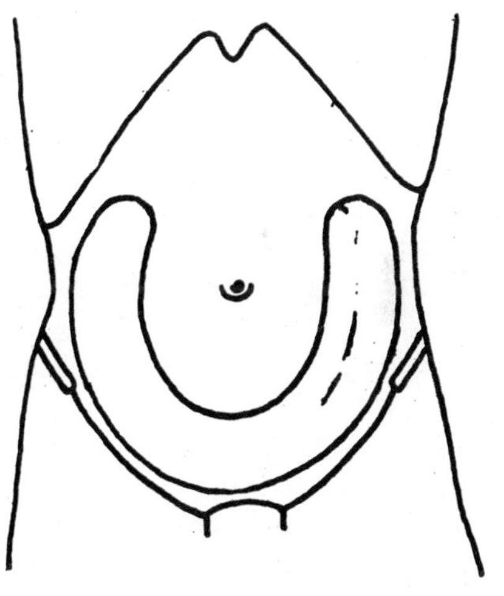

Fig 4.4

To show horse shoe shaped dullness in case of ascites

(b) **Shifting dullness :** The anatomical reason for this sign is also the same, i.e., the gas filled intestines float on the surface of the free fluid in the peritoneal cavity. About 750 ml fluid should be present in abdominal cavity to get shifting dullness.

The percussion should again start in the epigastrium or a point in the midine which is tympanitic and then proceed towards the flanks. The lateral border of the abdomen is dull. The finger over the abdominal wall should be kept in position and the patient should be asked to turn in such a way that the flank which is being percussed is now uppermost. After waiting for a short while (so that the intestines can float upwards in this new position) the percussion over the finger which is kept in position is repeated. The area which was previously dull will now be tympanitic. The examiner should now percuss the original area in the midline which was tympanitic at first. This will now be found to be dull thus proving that the dullness has shifted from one place to the other.

(c) **Percussion of the umbilical area in knee chest position (Puddle's sign):** When there is a suspicion that there may be a minimum amount of fluid in the abdomen the patient is asked to assume the knee chest position and the umbilical area is percussed from below. This will be dull if there is fluid which will of course gravitate towards this area which is now the lowest in the abdominal cavity.

To get positive Puddle's sign, about 500 ml fluid should be present in abdominal cavity.

Auscultation: On routine auscultation of the abdomen, peristaltic sounds are heard which can vary from person to person and to a certain extent depend upon the state of the intestines (whether empty or full of food contents). Certain people have occasional loud rumblings which are audible even without the aid of stethoscope.

Absent peristaltic sounds: The absence of peristaltic sound is of ominous clinical significance and has more place in surgical diagnosis.

A rigid abdomen with absent peristaltic sounds will indicate the presene of perforation. Similarly, immediately after abdominal surgery, peristaltic sounds are absent and their return indicates a very important step in recovery.

Paralytic ileus which may follow an intestinal obstruction or necrotising enterocolitis, may also be associated with toxic conditions. It causes feeble or absent peristaltic sounds. Hypokalemia is another condition leading to diminished peristalsis.

Exaggerated peristaltic sounds: Pathological increase in these sounds is heard when there is a subacute intestinal obstruction. Similarly, in diarrhoeas and dysentery, the peristaltic sounds are increased because of increased intestinal motility.

Splash: A loud splash can be produced by shaking the patient and auscultating over the epigastrium when there is a pyloric obstruction. However, some normal persons also exhibit this splash after food.

Murmurs: An abdominal bruit may be heard either in the epigastrium or the lateral sides of the abdomen at the level in patients who have renal artery stenosis. Care should be taken not to press the chest piece too firmly in the epigastrium as otherwise an artificial systolic murmur may be produced by compressing the abdominal aorta. Bruit over right hypochondrium indicates malignancy in the liver.

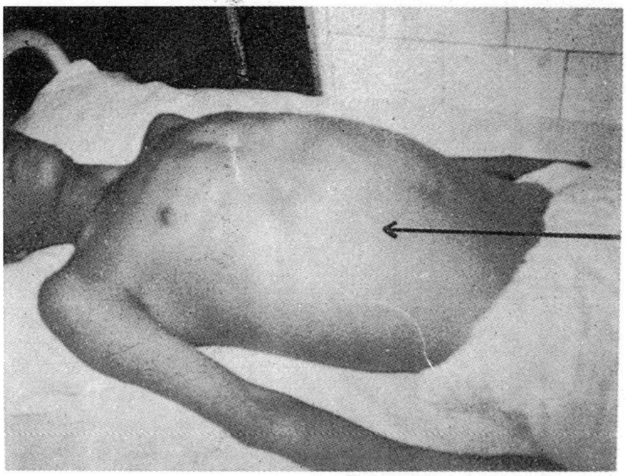

a

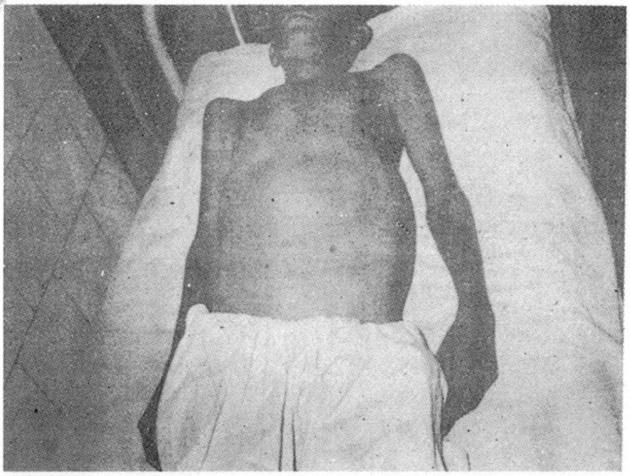

b

c

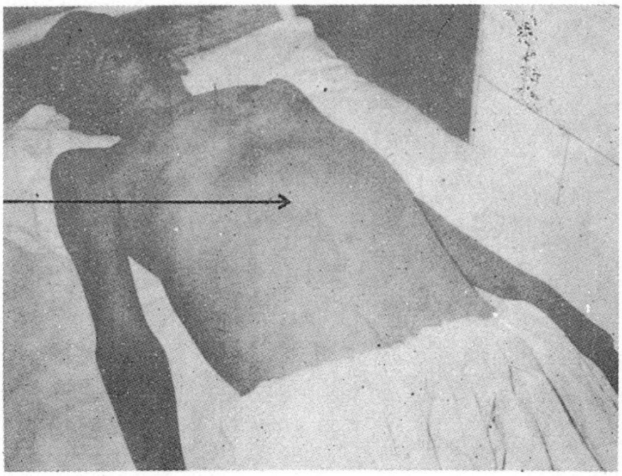

P1. 4.2 a, b and c Mass in abdomen in left hypochondrium

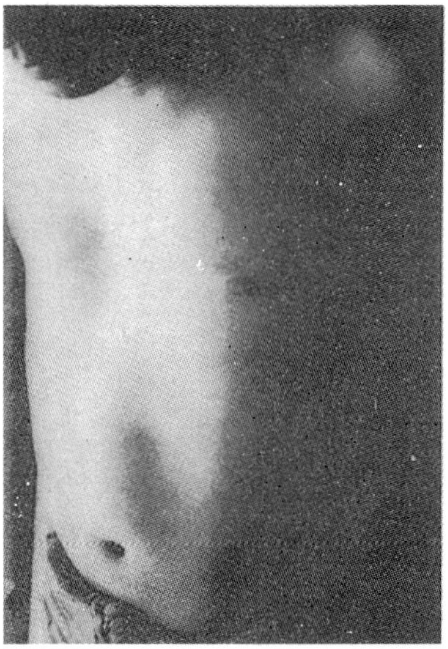

Pl. 4.1 Diverication of recti.

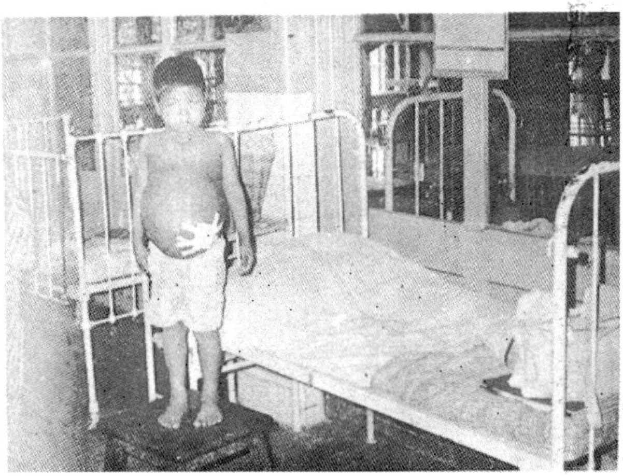

Pl. 5.1 Ascites. Note generalised distension of abdomen.
Note swollen face of a case of nephrotic syndrome

5. Alimentary System: Common Disorders Encountered

HEPATOMEGALY

Hepatomegaly means an increase in the size of liver.

Etiology:

1. Due to parenchymal diseases

i) Hepatitis - Viral: acute or chronic active variety.
Amoebic : amoebic hepatitis and amoebic abscess.

Malaria
Kala azar
Tuberculosis : especially miliary tuberculosis
Drug induced hepatitis : like that due to carbon tetrachloride, isoniazid, paracetamol, chlorpropamazine, etc.
Schistosomiasis
Weil's disease
Syphilis
Actinomycosis

ii) Cirrhosis: Laennec's cirrhosis (alcoholic)
Postnecrotic following hepatitis B virus infection
Biliary
Wilson's disease
Hemachromatosis

iii) Infiltrations : Fatty degeneration (alcoholic or toxic)
Glycogen storage disorders
Amyloidosis
Leukaemic deposits
Wilson's disease
Hemachromatosis

iv) Space occupying lesions : Metastatic deposits
Primary hepatoma
Angioma
Solitary or multiple cysts (hydatid)
Pyaemic abscess or amoebic abscess.
Gumma of liver

v) Hemopoietic disorders: Multiple myeloma
Hemolytic anaemia, Leukaemia.

vi) Congenital hyperbilirubinemias like : Crigler-Najjar syndrome
- Dubin-Johnson's syndrome

II. Due to hepatobiliary causes

i) Biliary obstruction due to gall stones, tumour or stricture of bile ducts.
ii) Cholangitis.

III. Vascular

i) Congestive cardiac failure
ii) Cardiac cirrhosis
iii) Constrictive pericarditis
iv) Budd-Chiari syndrome (hepatic vein thrombosis)
v) Portal vein thrombosis

Symptoms:

If onset is associated with loss of appetite, nausea, vomiting and fever and aversion to smoking, it is most likely to be viral hepatitis.

Histroy of Colicky pain in (R) hypochondrium without fever and onset of jaundice usually means gall stone causing obstruction. Similar colicky pain with high fever is likely to be due to cholangitis. High fever with rigors and with severe continuous pain in (R) hypochondrium suggests amoebic hepatitis.

Gradual loss of appetite, no definite onset but continuous deterioration of health usually points to cirrhosis or hepatoma.

Loss of appetite and rapid cachexia is usually seen in either secondary or primary carcinomas of liver. If the patient complains of jaundice it will be either due to infective, obstructive or haemolytic etiology. In infective etiology, urine colour will be yellow from the onset but the stools become white or acholic after sometime. The first sign of recovery will be return of colour of the stools.

In obstructive variety if the obstruction is due to gall stones the urine will be yellow and the stools will be acholic but there can be remissions in this history. However, if the obstruction is permanent, the stools will remain acholic.

In the haemolytic variety, the patient will complain of both urine and stools to be high coloured.

In quite a few patients with hepatomegaly the symptoms due to hepatic enlargement will be absent or negligible as compared to the other symptomatology of the disease, i.e., in chronic congestive cardiac failure, constrictive pericarditis, leukaemias, amyloidosis or multiple myeloma.

Rarely there will be absolutely no symptoms as when the hepatomegaly is due to old malarial or kala azar infection and the patient may complain of heaviness or lump in right hypochondrium.

Past history:

Previous H./o. biliary colics

H/o. receiving injections or undergoing laboratory tests where blood had to be collected.

H/o. infective hepatitis (post-necrotic cirrhosis).

H/o. fever with rigors in the past (malarial).

H/o. haematemesis and melena (portal hypertension).

H/o. exertional dyspnoea or other cardiac symptoms.

H/o. chronic sepsis (amyloidosis).

H/o. operations on the biliary tract may suggest a residual stone or stricture. Anaesthetics used during the surgery may cause fatty degeneration.

Personal history:

Socio-economic:

H/o. poor nourishment — predisposes to portal cirrhosis

Personal habits:

H/o. alcoholism:

H/o. drug ingestion — as a habit
— for diseases
— for psychiatric illness e.g., chlorpromazinc.

H/o. occupations bringing the patient in contact with rats as in sewer cleaners (Weil's disease)

H/o. loss of appetite.

H/o. loss of sexual libido

H/o. reduction in frequency of shaving

H/o. loss of axillary, chest and pubic hair

Family history:

H/o. jaundice in many members of the family suggests haemolytic jaundice or congenital hyperbilirubinemias.

H/o. splenectomy in relatives may point to haemolytic anaemias.

Signs

General examinations:

Poorly nourished in cirrhosis, chronic alcoholism, malignancy of the liver. (Cachexia can be especially prominent in the extremities in these conditions.)

Nails: Pale, revealing anaemia;

Clubbing is present in cirrhosis or malignancy.

Pulse and B.P.: May be of collapsing character in hepatocellular failure.

Skin examinations: Pinpoint haemorrhages of purpura or ecchymosis due to prothrombin deficiency may be seen. Scratch marks on the skin usually indicate obstructive or cholestatic lesions. Palmar erythemia-Liver palms and spider naevi are common in hepatocellular failure of cirrhosis.

Slaty colour of the skin suggests hemochromatosis, xanthoma on the extensor surface of tendons of wrists and ankles or on eyelids may indicate cholestatic jaundice.

Other features on general examinations:
Bilateral parotid swelling
Dupuytren's contracture.
Loss of axillary and pubic hair
Spider naevi
Gynaccomastia
Testicular atrophy
Eyes-Kayser-Fleischer ring in cornea in Wilsons disease.
Foetor hepaticus-hepatocellular failure.

Jaundice: — Mild yellow colour (lemon yellow) is due to haemolytic jaundice.
— Deeper yellow or orange means infective hepatitis.
— Greenish yellow colour suggests chronic obstructive jaundice.

Other systems:
C.V.S. — Soft systolic murmur
— Cirrhosis of liver
— Anaemia

RS — Lung signs — Tuberculosis
— malignancy

CNS — Change of consciousness
— incoherent speech — hepatocellular failure
— flapping tremors — hepatocellular failure
— choreiform movements — Wilson's disease

Examinations of alimentary system

Palpation of liver: Massive enlargement of the liver is felt in malignancy of the liver where only one or two large hard masses may be palpable or liver may be hard with multiple nodules on the surface.

Moderate enlargement of the liver is also felt in post-necrotic cirrhosis where the liver is multinodular and firm in consistency. Smooth uniform enlargement of the liver is felt in fatty infiltration. Hepatic enlargement due to cirrhosis is smaller as compared to the above causes and the surface is finely nodular.

Tender enlarged liver is present in amoebic abscess or hepatitis and congestive cardiac failure.

Palpable spleen: Palpable spleen should always be looked for along with hepatomegaly. Spleen is always palpable when hepatomegaly is due to cirrhosis, malaria or kala azar infections, leukaemias and reticulosis, amyloidosis.

It may be palbable when hepatomegaly is due to congestive cardiac failure, Budd-Chiari syndrome or in hemolytic anaemias. It is also palpable in diseases like Gaucher's disease and Niemann Pick's disease.

Ascites : Presence of massive ascites and splenomegaly when the liver is enlarged is due to portal hypertension caused by cirrhosis of liver.

In congestive cardiac failure, ascites may be present but with massive edema of feet. The only exception to this is constrictive pericarditis which causes hepatomegaly with minimal ascites and no edema of feet. Ascites without splenomegaly is found when the peritoneum is also involved by malignancy involving the liver.

Investigations :

Blood count : Anaemia normochromic in cirrhosis or in myeloid metaplasia.
Hypochromic microcytic following bleeding in cirrhosis of liver.
Abnormal WBC in leukaemias
Low WBC count and low platelet count in hypersplenism.

Urine : May show presence of bile salts or bile pigments or increased urobilinogen in hemolytic anaemia.

Stools : Presence of occult blood
Acholic in obstructive lesions
Excessive stercobilinogen in hemolytic condition.

Liver function tests:

Serum proteins — $\frac{\text{albumin}}{\text{globulin}}$ ratio

SGOT-PT (Transaminases)

— S.bilirubin — Total
Direct
Indirect

— Alkaline phosphatase

— Prothrombin time

— Cassoni's test - for hydatid cyst

— For hepatoma :

1. Alpha feto proteins
2. Serum aldolase
3. Serum nucleotidase
4. Blood sugar

— Liver biopsy - if cause is in liver itself

Ultrasound : For any cold areas and to see gall bladder and kidneys and also for ascites and local collection of fluids.

X-ray chest and abdomen — for evidence of tuberculosis

— evidence of malignancy

— gall stones

— liver enlargement

SPLENOMEGALY

Etiology:

I. Infective:

a. Bacterial: Infective endocarditis, enteric fever, septicemias, syphilis, miliary tuberculosis.

b. Viral: Infective hepatitis, infectious mononucleosis

c. Protozoal: Malaria, kala azar, trypanosomiasis

d. Fungal: Histoplasmosis

e. Parasitic: Echinococcus, bilharziasis

II. Congestive: (due to obstruction to hepatic venous blood flow)

Obstruction above the liver	a. Congestive cardiac failure b. Constructive pericarditis c. Budd Chiary syndrome
Obstruction inside the hepatic parenchyma	d. Cirrhosis of liver e. Schistosomiasis f. Congenital hepatic fibrosis
Obstruction below the liver	g. Portal vein thrombosis

III. Blood diseases:

Leukaemias, hemolytic anaemias, polycythemia vera anaemias-iron deficiency and megaloblastic, idiopathic thrombocytopenic purpura.

IV. Lipoid storage disorders:

Gaucher's disease, Neiman Pick's disease.

V. Neoplastic diseases:

Hemangiomas, sarcomas, lymphomas, Hodgkin's disease, lymphosarcomas, primary and secondary malignancy.

VI. Collagen disorders:

Systemic lupus erythematosus, Felty's syndrome.

VII. Miscellaneous

Amyloidosis, hematoma of the spleen, sarcoidosis.

Causes of splenomegaly: Can be classified on clinical basis (depending on size of spleen).

1. Massive enlargement of spleen (extending up to left iliac fossa).

— Chronic myeloid leukaemia

— Malaria

— Kala azar

2. Moderately enlarged spleen (spleen enlarged midway between umbilicus and left costal margin)

— Anaemia — hemolytic
— iron deficiency
— megaloblastic

— cirrhosis — leading to portal hypertension

— leukaemia

— purpura

— tuberculosis (miliary or abdominal)

— Septicemia

3. Just palpable spleen:
   1. Infective endocarditis;
   2. Tuberculosis;
   3. Toxaemia and septicemia;
   4. Anaemia;
   5. Idopathic thrombocytopenic purpura;
   6. Enteric fever
   7. Rheumatoid arthritis (Still's disease);
   8. Lymphoma

Symptoms:

1. Patient may have no symptoms except a dragging sensation in the left hypochondrium due to massive splenomegaly.

2. H/o. fever with rigors in malaria or kala azar infections.

H/o. irregular or hectic fever for a long period in bacterial endocarditis, brucellosis, tuberculosis.

H/o. relapsing type of fever in Hodgkin's disease.

H/o. high fever of short duration in typhoid or septicemic infections.

3. H/o. pallor with severe generalised weakness in leukaemias, hemolytic anaemias.

4. H/o. hemorrhagic purpuric spots or bleeding from the gums in leukaemias or purpura or infective endocarditis.

5. H/o. bone pains in Gaucher's diseases, leukaemias or metastatic deposits

6. H/o. lymphadenopathy in Hodgkin's disease and tuberculosis.

Past history:

H/o. jaundice in the past — in cirrhosis of liver

H/o. hematemesis or melena — in congestive splenomegaly

H/o. fever with rigors in the past — in malaria

H/o. ingestion of drugs in purpura

H/o. pulmonary tuberculosis

H/o. viral infection in recent past for purpura

H/o. open heart surgery in past — Infective endocarditis

Personal history:

H/o. chronic alcoholism leading to cirrhosis of liver

H/o. diet in malnutrition

H/o. sudden loss of weight over a short period

Family history:

H/o. lipoid storage disorders

H/o. hemolytic anaemias

Signs

General examinations:

Facies:

Pallor of the face : due to anaemia
Suffused face : due to polycythemia vera
Disky pigmentation : due to hemolytic anaemia hemochromatosis
Mongoloid facies : hemolytic anaemia

Sclera:

Presence of icterus : due to hemolytic anaemia
Pinguecula : due to Gaucher's disease

Cornea : Kayser Fleischer rings due to copper deposition in Wilson's disease

Gums :

Bleeding and pale : leukaemias purpura

Lymphadenopathy generalised : Glands usually discrete and not matted. May be enlarged markedly. Consistency may be rubbery. (Hodgkin's disease, lymphatic leukaemias, lymphosarcoma)

Nails :

Pallor due to anaemia
Splinter hemorrhages and Clubbing — due to infective endocarditis

Skin : Petechie and ecchymosis due to leukaemias
Spider naevi : due to cirrhosis of liver
Osler's nodes : in infective endocarditis

Pigmentation of face and limbs Grey brown pigmentation mainly on the flexor and medial aspects of upper arms — Kala azar.

Bony tenderness:
Over the sternum and pelvic bones : In leukaemias, Gaucher's disease Amyloidosis
Edema of feet : Congestive cardiac failure and cirrhosis of liver.

Fever:
Hodgkins , Kala azar,
Leukaemias , Malaria, Tuberculosis,
Septicemia , Infective endocarditis.

Systemic examinations:

1. Pulse : Tachycardia — bounding pulse — Anaemia
2. Blood Pressure : High pulse pressure — Cirrhosis
3. R.S. : Signs of tuberculosis
4. C.V.S. : Enlarged heart (infective endocarditis)
   — pressure of old rheumatic valvular lesion like MS or MI or AS - AI (infective endocarditis)
   — Congenital heart disease
   — PDA—VSD—Fallot's tetralogy, etc. (for infective endocarditis).
5. C.N.S. : Embolic phenomena manifesting as hemiplegia (in infective endocarditis)
6. A.S. : Inspection : Caput medusae — in portal hypertension fullness left hypochondrium

Palpable Spleen : Diagnosed by following features:
- lump in left hypochondrium
- firm
- moving with respiration
- notch on anterior border felt
- no band of resonance
- fingers cannot be insinuated in between lump and left costal margin
- dullness continuous with that over 10th rib posteriorly
- tenderness over spleen
- splenic infarcts

(Note that spleen has to enlarge 3 times its size to be palpable clinically).

Liver : enlarged nodular in cirrhosis
enlarged — in hemolytic anaemia
iron deficiency anaemia
tuberculosis
lipoid storage diseases

Lump in abdomen — glandular mass in case of leukaemia or Hodgkins or lymphosarcoma

Investigations

1. BLOOD COUNT:

RBC : A — Increased in polycythemia vera
B — Reduced in anaemias, leukaemias, hemolytic anaemias
C — Reticulocytosis in hemolytic anaemias
D — Spherocytosis in hereditary spherocytosis

WBC : Leucocytosis with normal cytology in pyogenic infections. Leucocytosis with abnormal cytology in leukaemias.

Platelets : Thrombocytopenia : in leukaemias and purpuras
Increased platelet count in polycythemia vera

Smear for parasites : Malarial parasites may be seen especially during rigors

Blood culture : Presence of *Streptococcal viridans* and other organisms confirming subacute infective endocarditis.

Specific blood investigations :

ESR — Raised in leukaemias and malignant conditions

Serum bilirubin increased in hemolytic anaemias in infective hepatitis rarely in cirrhosis.

Flocculation tests : in kala azar

Paul bunnel : for infectious mononucleosis

Coombs test — hemolytic anaemia

Abnormal haemoglobin studies for hemolytic anaemia

L.E. cell phenomenon : S.L.E.

Serum iron and copper : for hemochromatosis and Wilson's disease

Serum proteins : Cirrhosis of liver : multiple myeloma

Ultra Sound : in size of spleen and for splenic infarcts.

CIRRHOSIS OF LIVER

I. **Definition :** It is atypical regenerative fibrosis of liver due to varied etiological factors, characterised by change in architecture of liver and pseudolobule formation.

II. **Causes :**

1. Infections — Viral hepatitis (B)
2. Alcohol
3. Metabolic — Wilson's disease
   Hemochromatosis
   Galactosaemia
   Congenital tyrosinosis
4. Biliary — Intrahepatic causes
   Extrahepatic causes
5. Hepatic vein obstruction —
   V.O.D. (Veno occlusive disease)
   — Budd-Chiari syndrome obstruction to hepatic veins
   — C.C.F.— cardiac cirrhosis
6. Toxic — Chemicals
   Isoniazid
   Drugs Methyl dopa
   Methotrexate

III. **Types** —Micronodular — granular — alcoholic (Lannec's)
—Macronodular
—Mixed

IV. **Predisposing factors** — Malnutrition
— Infections like
— Schiztosomiasis
— Granuloma

V. **Symptoms:**

H/o. distension or abdomen — in pancreatitis;
H/o. attacks of dyspepsia ;
H/o. steatorrhoea - anorexia - pancreatitis;
H/o. weight loss;
H/o. jaundice;
H/o. dragging sensation in right hypochondrium;
H/o. gradual distension of abdomen — especially flanks;
H/o. swelling of legs;
H/o. hematemesis or melena and epistaxis;

VI. **Past H/o. alcoholism;**
infective hepatitis;
attacks of biliary colic;
persistent jaundice;
dyspnoea on exertion;
drug ingestion;

VII. **Personal history**

Diet

Occupation— people working in

i. Factories dealing with toxic chemicals
ii. Coal tar industries

Alcoholism
i. Executives in companies and mill workers;
ii. Changed bowel habits — steatorrhea— because of pancreatic deficiency caused by pancreatic calcification because of alcoholism.
iii. Changes in colour of stool.

VIII. Clinical examination

General examination : Poor nutrition;
Foctor hepaticus;
Jaundice;
Clubbing;
Pallor;
Collapsing pulse;
Edema of feet and/or face;
Haemorrhagic spots and patches;
Palmar erythema;
Loss of sexual hair;
Testicular atrophy;
Parotid enlargement;
Spider naevi;
Gynaecomastia.

Alimentary system : Distension;
— Abdomen wall — prominent and with distended veins;
— Caput medusae;
— Hernial orifices.

Palpitation : — enlarged liver;
— enlarged spleen;
— fluid thrill.

Percussion : — shifting dullness,
— horse shoe shaped dullness

C.V.S. — Enlarged heart; } in case of cardiac cirrhosis
— Signs of CCF

(Mechanism of Ascites in Cirrhosis of Liver)

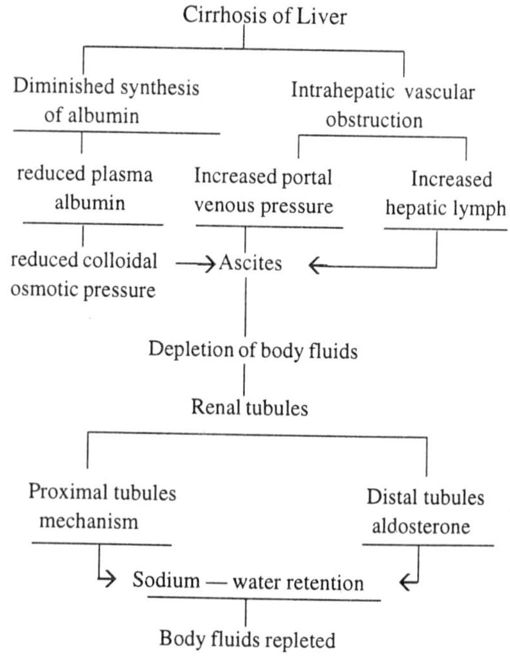

C.N.S. — Change in mental disposition
— Flapping tremors
— Stupor
— Choreiform movements

Investigations : CBC - for anaemia;
Urine for bilirubin;
Blood- alkaline phosphatase;
SGOT-PT;
Electrophoresis of proteins;
Sodium, potassium, chloride
Serum copper and iron
Serum bilirubin
Serum Ammonia for hepatocellular failure

Immunological states :
i. Mitochondrial antinuclear antibodies;
ii. Australia antigen;
iii. Alpha-1 fetoprotein;

Ba. swallow-Oesophagoscopy for oesophageal varices

Liver — Biopsy;
Scan;
Ultrasound examination for confirmation of diagonis :

Prognosis judges as follows :

- —alcoholic cirrhosis, if patient abstains, prognosis better.
- —If decompensation follows any acute cause like alcohol or hemorrhage or infection — progress may be better if & because the precipitating cause is correctable.

Prognosis is bad : If decompensation is gradual

- —Persistent jaundice;
- —CNS manifestations are present and persistent;
- —Ascites — especially if resistant to diuretic therapy;
- —Shrunken liver;
- —Persistent hypoprothrombinaemia;
- —Serum albumin less than 2.5 gm%.

ASCITES

Ascites can be defined as presence of fluid in the peritoneal cavity.

Fluid which accumulates in the peritoneal cavity can either be transudate or exudate.

Causes of transudate:

1. Congestive cardiac failure;
2. Hypoproteinemia;
   a. Cirrhosis of liver;
   b. Renal causes - nephrotic syndrome;
   c. Nutritional; hypoalbuminemia.
3. Polyserositis;
4. Associated with ovarian tumour (Meig's syndrome).

Causes of exudate:

1. Infections : Tuberculosis, pyogenic bacterial infections;
2. Neoplasms : Secondary metastasis involving the peritoneum or direct spread firm abdominal viscera including ovaries. Rarely primary mesothelioma of the peritoneum.
3. Chylous : Lymphatic obstruction due to filariasis, tuberculosis, trauma or tumour.
4. Rarely due to collagen disorders, eosinophilic peritonitis or Crohn's disease.

Symptoms:

1. Gradual accumulation of fluid may remain unnoticed until it reaches a significant amount.

2. Increase in the size of abdomen which is noticed by the patient.

3. Dyspnea and orthopnoea due to accumulation of large quantity of fluid in abdomen.

4. If there is edema of other parts of the body, their relation to the onset of ascites should be asked for.

i. Edema of feet following ascites is due to cirrhosis of liver.

ii. Edema of feet before the onset of ascites is due to congestive cardiac failure.

iii. Edema of face which is more in the morning and preceding ascites is due to nephrotic syndrome or renal pathology.

iv. If the ascites is a part of a generalised anasarca and if the patient is unable to tell the sequence of events as above, it could be due to hypoproteinemia of nutirtional origin.

5. Sudden development of ascites may occur in cirrhotic patients or in patients who have borderline levels of serum albumin, when sudden loss of proteins occurs in form of haemorrhage or severe diarrhoea. Portal vein thrombosis may also lead to sudden development of ascites.

Past history:

H/o. hematemesis and melena (due to portal hypertension);

H/o. infective hepatitis;

H/o. exertional dyspnoea or rheumatic fever;

H/o. renal colic with hematuria/pyuria or burning micturition, oliguria.

Personal history:

Socioeconomic :

H/o. poor nourishment causing cirrhosis of liver.

Personal :

H/o. alcoholism;

H/o. loss of appetite (either due to cirrhosis of liver or due to presence of abdominal malignancy)

H/o. change in bowel habits (due to colonic malignancy)

H/o menstrual periods (menorrhagia or amenorrhoea due to ovarian tumours)

Signs:

General examinations:

I. Build and nutrition: Poorly nourished in cirrhosis; chronic alcoholism; Abdominal malignancy.

Pot belly and thin limbs (due to wasting of muscles) leads to 'Spider man'. (Pl.5.1)

II. Edema of face or generalised may mask the undernourished state in renal diseases or in hypoproteinemic condition.

Examination of neck:

i. J.V.P. raised if ascites is due to congestive cardiac failure.

ii. Presence of matted cervical glands point towards tubercle as the etiological factor.

iii. Supraclavicular (Virchow's) glands are indicative of gastric malignancy.

III. Nails:

i. Pallor due to anemia;

ii. Clubbing due to cirrhosis of liver.

IV. Skin

Spider naevi

Pallor-anaemia

Circumoral pigmentation, Pigmentation of skin } Multiple vitamin deficiency

V. Pulse and blood pressure and heart:

i Corresponding changes if there is any cardiac disease causing C.C.F.

ii. Collapsing in nature due to cirrhosis of liver.

iii. Apex beat — shifted upwards to outwards because diaphragm is raised.

VI. Endocrine changes like palmar erythema, spider naevi, loss of axillary and pubic hair, etc. point towards cirrhosis as the cause of ascites.

VII. Edema of feet:

(i) Always present when the ascite is due to C.C.F.

(ii) Usually present but may be absent in conditions like cirrhosis of liver or in peritoneal diseases causing ascites.

(iii) Present as a part of generalised anasarca in hypoproteinemia and nephrotic syndrome.

Abdomen

Inspection — appearance — fullness in flanks
— protuberant abdomen
— Prominent veins
— Umbilicus transverse or everted — hernia may be present
— Caput medusae
— Scrotal edema may be present

Palpation : (1) Visible lump
(2) Girth— to be measured at umbilicus in sitting position
(3) Flow in veins
(4) Liver enlargement
(5) Spleen enlargement

Percussion : Horse shoe shape dullness
Shifting dullness
Confirmation of upper border of liver

Ascultations : Peristalsis
Bruit over abdomen — usually indicates primary or secondary malignancy of liver.

Investigations

1) X-ray chest

2) C.B.C.
3) E.S.R.
4) Blood urea
5) Serum proteins — albumin
— globulin
6) Serum electrolytes — Na
— K
— Cl
7) Urine — albuminuria massive in nephrotic syndrome.
8) Sonography

Ascitic fluid:

Transudate: Sp. gr. less than 1015
Proteins less than 2 gms
Cells few endothelial
No clot formation

Exudate: T. B. peritonitis: Sp. gr. more than 1015
Proteins more than 3 gms%
Cells + lymphocytes

Malignancy: Sp. gr. more than 1015
Haemorrhagic
Clot formation
Proteins more than 3 gm%

Liver Biopsy:

Management: Treatment of the cause
Salt free diet;
Proteins — ½ gm/kg
— Diuretics.

6. Alimentary System: Common Diagnostic and/or Therapeutic Procedures

Most common ones are: Ascitic Tapping and Liver Biopsy.

Ascitic tapping

Indications :

Diagnostic : to determine the nature of fluid

Therapeutic : — Increasing distension leading to discomfort.
— Sudden increase in girth of abdomen.

Procedure : Consent, premedication as in case of pleural tapping. Patient should empty the bladder, and should be seated at the edge of the cot with feet hanging from sides. Area should be cleaned with antiseptics.

Site — either in midline-midway between umbilicus and pubic symphysis or on one side at the lateral border of rectus — Midway between umbilicus and anterior superior iliac spine.

Local infiltration with lignocaine should be done and No. 18-20 needle is inserted through the infiltrated area and few ml. of fluid withdrawn with help of syringe. Thereafter, syringe should be disconnected and fluid should be allowed to flow drop by drop till patient feels comfortable.

Complications : (1) Hepatic coma in case of cirrhosis;
(2) Introduction of infection;
(3) Injury to intestine;
(4) Injury to bladder;
(5) Puncture of ovarian cyst.

Liver Biopsy

Indications — Diagnostic and prognostic

Contraindications — Bleeding tendencies and prolonged prothrombin time.

Precautions : (1) Consent of the patient or the parents in case the patient is minor.
(2) Bleeding time, clotting time and prothrombin time should be done and should be within normal range.
(3) Blood should be grouped and cross matched, in case any severe blood loss occurs or is anticipated.

Premedications:

(1) Inj. diazepam 5-10 mg. should be given i.m. to sedate the patient.
(2) Inj. pethidine should be used with caution when chronic liver disease is suspected.
(3) Inj. atropine.

Procedure:

(1) Patient should be reassured.
(2) Patient should be in semi-reclined position at 45^0.
(3) Percuss the liver and set the area of liver dullness which remains dull even in inspiration.
(4) Site chosen should be in anterior or mid-axillary line.
(5) Local anaesthetic (xylocaine) should be used up to capsule of liver. It should be given along upper border of rib.

Vim silverman needle

(a) Introduce the trocar with cannula.
(b) Remove the trocar.
(c) Insert the prongs.
(d) Keep prongs in and slide the cannula over the prongs.
(e) Twist the cannula and prongs through 180^0 and withdraw swiftly.
(f) Put the piece of liver into a bottle of saline and transfer it to solution of formalin.
(g) Apply benzoin seal.

Menghini's needle

(a) Syringe with 3-4 ml normal saline and needle is taken.
(b) Enter the liver, inject the saline 1 ml in the capsule of the liver while entering.
(c) Thereafter exert constant negative pressure on the syringe and withdraw.
(d) Transfer the piece of liver in saline as stated above.

Post-procedure order

(a) Nil by mouth for 4-6 hours.
(b) Let the patient lie on right lateral position
(c) Half hourly TPR and BP
(d) Watch for bleeding
(e) Take abdominal girt half hourly
(f) Watch for distension

Advantages of the second procedure (with Menghini's needle) are that chances of bleeding are minimal. The only drawback is that failure rate is high.

Section III: Respiratory System (R.S.)

7. Symptomatology and History Taking

Many diseases of the Respiratory System (R.S.) cause anatomical and physiological disturbances, but all of them indicate a relatively small group of symptoms. These are enlisted below and then the method of analysing them follows.

The symptoms relating directly to the respiratory system affection are:

A Cough;
B Expectoration;
C Hemoptysis;
D Dyspnea;
E Chest pain;
F Upper respiratory tract symptoms;
G Wheeze and stridor.

In addition to these, patients with respiratory system affection may complain of the following constitutional symptoms :

A. Fever;
B Sweating;
C Anorexia;
D Weakness;
E Loss of weight.

Symptoms directly related to respiratory system affection

A Cough:

Cough can be described as a violent expiratory blast which occurs against partially closed glottis. It is a protective mechanism which guards against the entry of foreign substances into the tracheobronchial tree and also relieves the broncho-pulmonary secretions. Usually, it is caused by irritation of the respiratory mucous membrane which through the 'cough centre' in

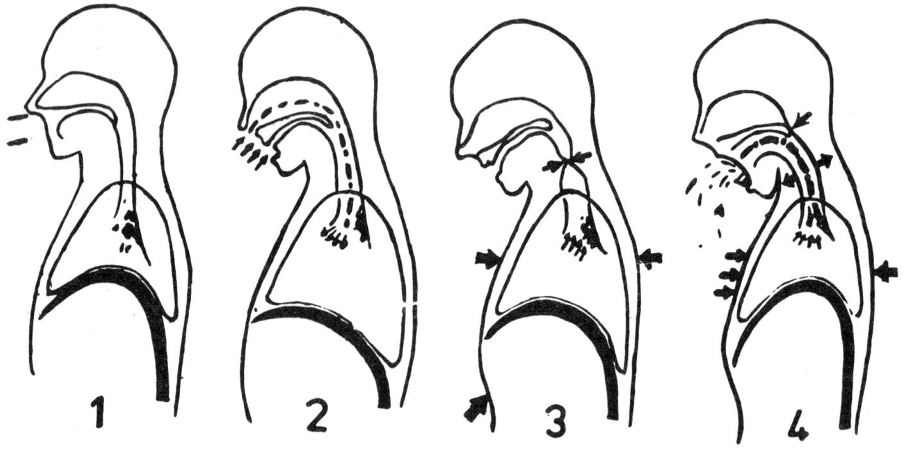

Fig. 7.1
Mechanism of cough

1. Stage of irritation. 2. Stage of inspiration. 3. Stage of rise in pressure, i.e., raising of diaphragm and rise in intrathoracic and intra-abdominal pressure. 4. Stage of expulsion.

the medulla produces the cough reflex.

It can also be produced voluntarily.

The act of coughing can be divided in four phases (Fig. 7.1).

(i) 1st phase is the initial irritation.

(ii) 2nd phase is a deep inspiration.

(iii) 3rd phase is the stage when the glottis is tightly closed and the expiratory intercostal and abdominal muscles contract tightly producing a rise in the intra-thoracic and intra-abdominal pressures.

(iv) 4th phase is the stage when the intra-thoracic pressure rises to a very high level, the glottis opens slightly and the intra-thoracic pressure falls. Hence the intra-abdominal pressure becomes higher than the intrathoracic pressure resulting in pushing up the diaphragm. This produces a violent explosive movement of air from the lower to the upper respiratory tract.

During this phase, as soon as the glottis opens, the palate closes off the nasopharynx and hence any material which is expectorated enters the mouth and is then thrown out.

The following inquiry should be carried out when *cough* is the presenting symptom :

i) **Duration and onset of the complaint:**
How long has the cough been present?
If it is of a long duration it will signify a chronic respiratory allergy or infection. Cough of short duration with a sudden onset may signify, a foreign body, an acute irritation, an infection, or acute allergic phenomenon.

ii) **Types of cough :**

a) Is the cough dry or productive? Dry cough is usually associated with upper respiratory tract infection or irritation and early stages of pulmonary tuberculosis. A harsh irritating dry cough usually signifies an irritation of trachea. When the trachea is compressed from outside (as in case of mediastinal mass) it may produce a harsh brassy cough which has also been described as a 'gander cough'. A loud cough may be present in hysterical patients to draw attention from others. A productive cough signifies free fluid or exudate in the respiratory tract and occurs in chronic bronchitis, bronchiectasis and lung abscess.

b) Whether the cough is paroxysmal? i.e., Does it start suddenly and continues as repeated bouts and stop fairly abruptly? Usually a paroxysmal cough is spasmodic in nature and may be associated with wheezing.
The common causes of this type of cough are bronchial asthma or asthmatic bronchitis, eosinophilic bronchitis, whooping cough, foreign body and left ventricular failure causing pulmonary edema. In children, miliary tuberculosis and acute bronchiolitis can produce this symptom. Paroxysmal cough is usually more at night.

c) Is the cough of short duration and is it associated with pain?
A short cough is common in upper respiratory infections. In pleural inflammation, the cough is short and there may be sudden partial voluntary suppression to avoid the pain produced by the cough.

iii) **Factors influencing the production of cough:**
Whether the cough is present at a particular time or whether any change of posture starts or increases the bout of cough?

a) **Time :** Cough which is worse in the early morning on getting up and usually associated with expectoration is a classic feature of bronchiectasis. Cough which wakes up the patient in the early hours of the morning and which is associated with dyspnea may be produced by either bronchial asthma or left ventricular failure.
Chronic upper respiratory infections especially, chronic sinusitis with postnasal discharge can also produce cough when the patient goes to bed. Paroxysmal cough is usually nocturnal because tracheo-laryngo bronchitis is more at night.

b) **Posture :** Change of posture producing cough with expectoration is usually present in lung abscess or bronchiectasis. Dry brassy cough occurring in supine posture shows compression of trachea and main bronchi due to mediastinal mass.

B. **Expectoration :** i.e., phlegm brought out by bout of cough.

1. Is the expectoration large in amount or scanty?
   If large in amount can the patient roughly assess the quantity?
   A large quantity of sputum is produced by patients suffering from bronchiectasis or lung abscess. As much as 300 to 450 cc of sputum (2 to 3 cupfuls) can be expectorated in 24 hours. Sputum produced by a bronchiectatic patient separates into three layers if it is collected in a conical flask. The top layer is mucoid, the middle layer is mucopurulent and the lower-most layer is purulent. The sputum produced by a patient suffering from lung abscess separates into 2 layers when collected similarly. The top layer is mucoid while the bottom layer is purulent.
2. What is the appearance of the sputum?
   Mucoid sputum is clear white and sticky and is usually scanty. It is usually produced due to chronic bronchitis and upper respiratory infections. If it is very sticky, it can be coughed up as casts of the bronchi, especially in patient suffering from bronchial asthma. Laennec's pearls are small sago-like round particles of very thick sticky sputum. Mucopurulent sputum usually indicates active bacterial infection. It appears sticky, creamy yellow and gelatinous and has gelatinous consistency. Yellowish or purulent sputum is usually seen in bronchiectasis or lung abscess.It indicates the presence of an active infection in the lung.
   A typical rusty brown sputum is characteristic of pneumonia. Prune juice or red current jelly appearance of sputum is suggestive of bronchial carcinoma. An anchovy sauce like sputum is produced when an amoebic liver abscess ruptures into the lung.
   Pink, frothy sputum is characteristic of pulmonary edema. A greenish coloured sputum (usually foul smelling) is seen when there is an infection of the lung parenchyma due to gangrene of the lung. It may contain disintegrated lung tissue. Rarely black sputum may be produced by patients suffering from anthracosis.
3. Does the sputum have an offensive odour?
   A very foul smell of the sputum indicates lung abscess or rarely gangrene of the lung. In cases of bronchopleural fistula and bronchiectasis, the sputum may be very foul smelling.

C. **Hemoptysis:**

Hemoptysis means expectoration or spitting out blood.

The most common confusion occurs when the patient is not sure whether he has a genuine hemoptysis or whether he has vomited the blood.

Blood which is coughed up is always bright red and frothy due to admixture with air. The sputum may be stained bright red in colour for a few days after the initial bout. It is usually alkaline in reaction. Blood which is vomited may be bright red but is more commonly dark red or brown. It is not frothy and the reaction is acidic in nature.

The following inquiry should be carried out when the patient complains of hemoptysis :

1. Was it sudden like a bolt from the blue? This can happen as a presenting symptom of pulmonary tuberculosis.
2. Or is it associated with long standing cough? Pulmonary tuberculosis, malignancy, bronchiectasis or lung abscess can give rise to this type of hemoptysis.
3. What is the quantity? Is it massive or is it only blood tinged sputum?
   A large or massive hemoptysis can occur

in patients suffering from pulmonary tuberculosis, bronchiectasis or rarely lung abscess. Mitral stenosis can also give rise to severe degree of hemoptysis.

Causes of Hemoptysis:

(i) Respiratory : Children — Whooping cough
- Eosinophilic bronchitis
- Bronchiectasis
- Lung abscess

Young adult:
- Pulmonary tuberculosis
- Bronchiectasis
- Lung abscess
- Pneumonia
- Bronchitis

Above 40-50 years : (middle aged and above)
- Bronchiectasis
- Bronchial adenoma and carcinoma
- Secondaries in lung from elsewhere
- Other causes as in young adult

(ii) Cardiac :
- Mitral stenosis
- Pulmonary embolism
- Acute pulmonary edema due to left sided failure
- Aortic aneurysm
- Arteriovenous malformation
- Primary pulmonary hypertension
- Rarely systemic hypertension

(iii) Miscellaneous (General causes)
- Bleeding disorders like purpura, etc.
- Anticoagulant therapy
- Local bleeding from respiratory tract, e.g. after instrumentation like bronchoscopy.
- Haemorrhagic fever especially septicemia
- After tonsillectomy
- Pulmonary mycoses

The points differentiating hemoptysis from haemetemesis are discussed under haemetemesis in alimentary system. (section II)

Blood tinged sputum may occur in bronchitis or tuberculosis. However, it can be associated with any disease causing violent or persistent cough.

D. **Dyspnea:**

Dyspnea may be defined as consciousness or awareness of breathing difficulty.

Dyspnea due to respiratory system involvement may be due to emphysema, infection, fibrosis or infection of the lung parenchyma, obstruction to the trachea or bronchi or when there is either fluid or air in the pleural cavities. It is also a presenting symptom in foreign body, bronchial asthma, and miliary tuberculosis; and acute bronchiolitis in children.

The following points should be looked into when analysing respiratory dyspnea :

1. How was the onset?

   A very rapid onset will indicate spontaneous pneumothorax, pulmonary infarction, foreign body causing a collapse of the lung or edema of the glottis or larynx. A diphtheritic membrane obstructing the larynx is common cause of dyspnea in children.

   In cases of pleural effusion, dyspnea can develop over a period of a few days. When the effusion becomes massive, or in case of empyema, dyspnea can occur suddenly.

2. Is the dyspnea paroxysmal?

   Bronchial asthma will give rise to its own classic picture of paroxysmal dyspnea.

3. Is the dyspnea practically continuous or worsens on exertion?

   In emphysema, interstitial fibrosis, chronic obstructive pulmonary disease (C.O.P.D.) and in any other chronic lung disorders, dyspnea is a permanent feature. Initially, the dyspnea may be present when the patient is at rest and in very severe cases may make the patient orthopneic.

4. Is it precipitated by exposure to any allergen or change in weather?
   An allergic response to any particular object may cause a violent spasm of the bronchi resulting in dyspnea.
5. Is it associated with chest pain or fever?
   A pleuritic pain may result in dyspnea as the patient is unable to take a deep breath and has to take repeated short breaths.
   Dyspnea associated with fever indicates an infective process like pneumonia, empyema or hydropneumothorax and pyopneumothorax.

E. **Chest pain :**

Pain in chest due to respiratory disease is usually due to involvement of the pleura. Lung tissue (parenchyma) is insensitive and hence even a fairly advanced disease in the lungs which does not involve the pleura, does not give rise to any pain. Rarely a deep seated pulmonary neoplasm may give rise to deep aching pain.

If the patient complains of chest pain the following points should be looked into:

What is the exact site of the pain?

When did the pain start and was its onset sudden or gradual?

Is there any radiation of the pain from behind forwards and which regions are affected?

Is the character dull or is it cutting, sharp or burning in nature?

Is it affected by coughing, deep breathing or sneezing?

Are there any relieving factors?

Pleural pain is produced by irritation of the parietal pleura. The visceral layer has no pain endings and hence it is insensitive to pain. The pain due to pleural inflammation is referred along the corresponding intercostal nerve and hence its site varies. However, it is usually sudden in onset and is described as a sharp cutting pain or stitch like pain radiating from behind forwards and aggravated by coughing, deep breathing and sneezing. (These manoeuvres increase the intrathoracic negative pressure producing an increased pull or tension on the parietal pleura and aggravate the pain). If the respiratory movements on the affected side are dampened by the patient lying down on the affected side, the pleural pain is relieved to some extent.

As the pleural pain is referred along the intercostal nerves, the radiation of this pain may be felt over sites away from the thorax. Hence, pleural infalmmation which involves the areas supplied by 8 to 12 thoracic segments of the spinal cord will cause pain, which is referred to the abdomen.

Diaphragmatic pleura is supplied by phrenic nerve in its central portion and by the fifth and sixth intercostal nerve in its peripheral portions. Hence, the involvement of the central portion will cause pain which is referred to the superior ridge of the trapezious muscle on the same side. The involvement of the peripheral portion will cause pain referred along with fifth and sixth thoracic segments.

Apical pleurisy usually presents as a dull pain in the apical areas of the lungs. The pain is not affected by respiratory movements as there is minimal expansion of these areas during respiration.

F. **Upper respiratory tract symptoms:**

The following questions should be asked to elucidate the history :

i. Is there any history of recurrent colds or sore throat?

ii. Is there any hoarseness of voice? Hoarseness may be of recent origin in case of laryingitis but elderly patients with persistent hoarseness should be submitted for laryngoscopy to rule out malignancy of larynx. Hoarseness can also be because of paralysis of recurrent laryngeal nerve due to tuberculosis or malignant mediastinal mass.

iii. Does the patient complain of pain or pricking sensation in throat?

iv. Is there any history of any operation on the upper respiratory tract recently?

G. **Wheeze and stridor:**

Wheeze : Musical sound produced mainly

on expiration (as the bronchi become narrower and shorter in expiration) which is present in patients with air-ways obstruction like asthma or chronic and acute bronchitis.

Stridor: Musical noise (louder) caused by obstruction in the trachea or larynx. Usually inspiratory because of the more rapid air flow during inspiration. May occur with neoplastic or inflammatory conditions.

Constitutional symptoms usually associated with respiratory disease:

A. **Fever:**

Fever or elevation of body temperature is associated with respiratory disease whenever there is infection or degeneration of tissues. With infections like sinusitis or tracheo-bronchitis fever is of short duration (a few days) and does not follow any specific pattern. A low grade fever with evening rise of temperature is characteristic of tubercle infection either of the lung parenchyma or pleura. A similar low rise but not necessarily confined to evenings may be present in patients suffering from malignant disease of the lungs. Pleurisy with effusion may give rise to high irregular or continuous fever. A high intermittent fever associated with chills indicates either a lung abscess or severely infected bronchiectasis or infected hydropneumothorax. A high continuous temperature may indicate a pneumonic process affecting the lung parenchyma and empyema. This fever can also be of the hectic variety.

B. **Sweating:**

This is caused by sympathetic overactivity, and though associated with fever, it may be out of proportion to the degree of fever.

Sometimes drenching night sweats may occur in pulmonary tuberculosis. The explanation of this phenomenon is unknown.

C. D & E. **Anorexia, Weakness, and Loss of Weight:**

They are usually present in patients suffering from chronic respiratory disease.

Weakness and loss of weight are present when the total expenditure of energy is greater than that derived from the food intake. This imbalance occurs whenever the total metabolism of the body is increased either due to fever or due to increased consumption by the overacting respiratory muscles. In addition to this factor there may be an excessive loss of protein due to infection causing a large amount of sputum. Malignancy or tissue destruction also affects the metabolism in a similar way.

8. Respiratory System — Clinical Examination

EXAMINATION OF THE RESPIRATORY SYSTEM

Before proceeding with the examination of the chest following points in general examination should be observed : (1) Clubbing of nails; (2) build of the body; (3) obvious weight loss; and (4) obvious tachypnea. These are discussed in general examination earlier.

It is essential to know the boundaries of the thoracic contents. Hence a brief description of the important landmarks is given below:

Surface Anatomy: (refer Fig. 8.1 a & b)

A. **Important lines:** These are conventional topographic lines which demarcate the various areas of the chest wall and are 'drawn' in anatomical position.

i. Midclavicular line: This runs vertically downwards from the middle of the clavicle over the anterior chest wall up to the lower costal margin.

ii. Anterior axillary line : A vertical line parallel to the midclavicular line which runs through the anterior fold of the axilla.

iii. Posterior axillary : A similar line through the posterior axillary fold.

iv. Mid-axillary line : A vertical line parallel to the above lines running down over the lateral chest wall through the middle of the axilla (apex of axilla).

v. Midscapular line: A vertical line through the middle tip of the inferior angle of the scapula to the renal angle. The arm should be hanging

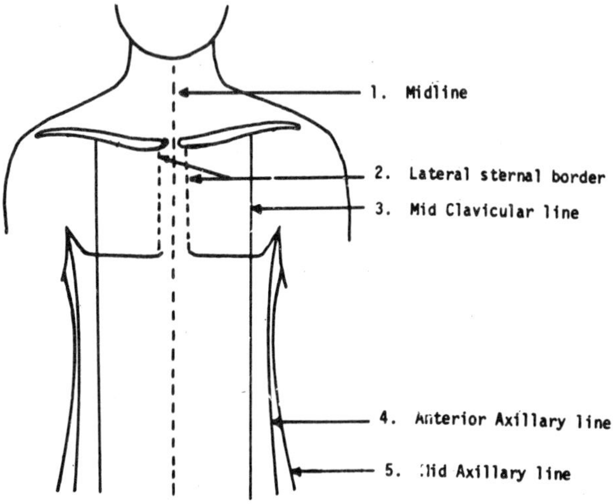

Fig. 8.1 a
Lines on anterior wall of chest.

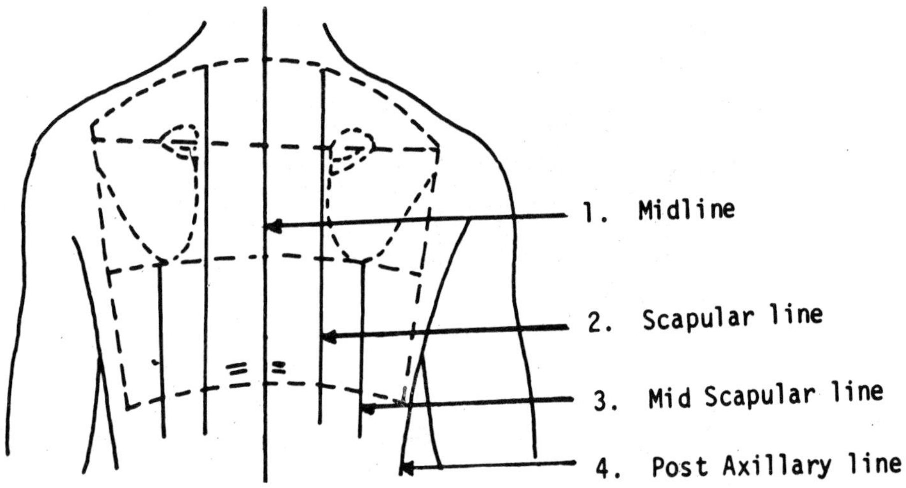

Fig. 8.1 b
Lines on posterior wall of chest.

down by the side when this line is drawn.

vi. Scapular line — A vertical line along the most medial border of scapula.

B. **Landmarks on the posterior chest wall:** (Pl 8.1)

i. The spinous process of seventh cervical vertebra : This is easily seen and felt when the patient is in erect position with head bent slightly forward. It is the first very prominent spinous process felt if spinous processes are palpated from C_1 downwards.

ii. The 1st thoracic spinous process : This is most prominent and it is immediately below the spinous process of the seventh cervical vertebra.

iii. The IIIrd thoracic spinous process : When the patient is sitting or standing upright with his arm by his side, this process lies at the level of the root of the spine of the scapula.

iv. The VIIth thoracic spinous process : In the same position as above the VIIth thoracic spinous process lies at the level of the inferior angle of the scapula.

C. **Landmarks on the anterior chest wall :**

The sternal angle or the angle of Louis.

This marks the junction of the manubrium of the sternum with its body. The second costal cartilage is attached at this junction and hence the 2nd intercostal space can be easily marked below it.

The bifurcation of the trachea lies at this level and so also at the upper level where the lung borders meet anteriorly. It also indicates the upper level of the atria.

i) **Surface markings of the pleura and the lungs:** (Fig. 8.2)

The hilum of the lungs corresponds to an area, which is roughly rectangular in shape and is situated posteriorly between the vertebral borders of the scapula and the spine at the level of fourth, fifth and sixth vertebrae.

The apices of the lungs lie in the root of the neck on either side and they are closely covered by pleura. They occupy an area which can be demarcated by a line drawn from the

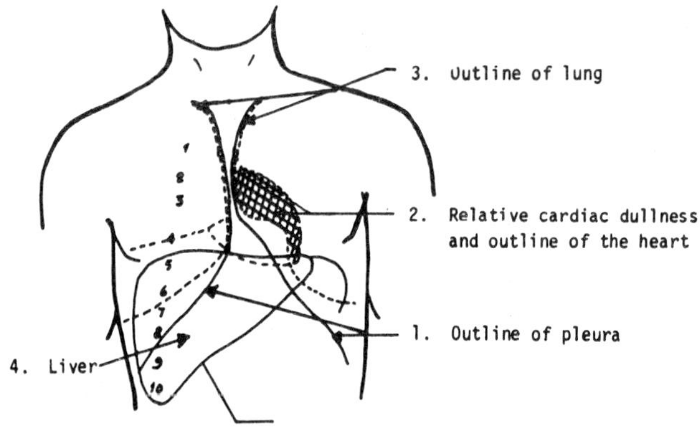

Fig. 8.2

Outlines of pleura, lung, heart and liver. Note their interrelationship.

sternoclavicular junction which curves upwards to about one inch above the calvicle and then descends to join the inferior border of the clavicle at the junction of its lateral and middle thirds.

The anterior border of the pleura on the right side corresponds to a line drawn from the right sternoclavicular joint to the centre of the angle of Louis and then vertically down the sternum up to the xiphisternum. The anterior border of the right lung also exactly corresponds to this line.

The anterior border of pleura on the left side corresponds to a line drawn from the left sternoclavicular joint to the centre of the angle of Louis. This when goes down vertically up to the level of fourth costal cartilage it turns laterally to the left sternal border and runs downwards to the VIIth costal cartilage on left side. However, the left anterior border of the lung does not correspond to this line. It follows this line up to the fourth left costal cartilage and then follows a line which runs lateral along the left fourth costal cartilage to a point about 2 cms from the left sternal border. From there it curves downwards and ends at the sixth costal cartilage about 2.5 cms from the sternal border.

Examination of the respiratory system should follow the usual system of :

1. Inspection;
2. Palpation;
3. Percussion;
4. Auscultation.

Inspection of the chest :

This is the most important part of the examination of the respiratory system and the examiner may be able to locate the nature and the site of the disease during this procedure.

It should always be carried out in adequate light, and the chest should be observed from :

a. The front (may be best observed when examined from the foot-end of the bed).

b. The back (preferably with the patient in siting up position).

c. From the sides.

d. From above downwards over the shoulders of the patient to observe the apical regions.

It will not be possible to follow this procedure in a severely ill patient. In these cases, he should be turned from side to side and the back should be observed.

The following points should be noted on inspection of the chest.

A. The size and the shape of the chest.

B. Deformities of the chest.

C. Respiratory movements.

D. Different types of breathing.
E. Position of the apex beat and trachea.
F. Presence of collateral veins.

A. The size and shape of the chest:

The normal characteristics vary with the build of the individual. The chest is broad, short and deepset in the sthenic individual and long, flat or narrow in the asthenic individual.

It is bilaterally symmetrical and oval or elliptical in shape and the anteroposterior diameter is slightly smaller than the transverse diameter (Ratio is 5 : 7).

The intercostal spaces are broader in front than they are behind and there is a depression in the sternum which is most prominent at this lower end. The sub-costal angle is normally about 70^0 to 110^0 (average about 90^0). This angle is more acute in males than in females.

B. Deformities of the chest:

These must be looked for carefully as certain diseases of the lungs can produce characteristic changes in the contour of the thorax. So also any abnormality of the thoracic walls due to disease processes can produce abnormal signs in the chest.

Deformities of the chest can be either symmetrical or asymmetrical.

Symmetrical deformities:

1. Funnel chest: (Cobbler's deformity, pectus excavatum)

In its most typical form, the body of the sternum is curved backwards and it forms a deep depression on the anterior wall. This depression has its centre at the xiphisternal junction. The chest cage hence becomes narrower and longer due to this deformity. (Plate 8.2) In mild forms, there may be only a prominent hollowing at the lower end of the sternum. It usually produces no symptoms and is usually hereditary.

In very rare severe cases there may be symptoms like dyspnea and palpitations due to displacement of the heart or lungs. Dysphagia has been reported due to compression and kinking of the esophagus.

2. **Pigeon breast:**

This is a protrusion deformity of the anterior chest wall. Both the sternum and the costal cartilages are protruding anteriorly and hence the resemblance to that of a pigeon's breast is seen.

Sometimes the whole body of the sternum is protruded anteriorly and then it can also be called a 'keel' breast.

3. **Rachitic chest:**

There are various types of deformities produced due to childhood rickets. They occur due to the fact that the soft bones (affected by the rachitic process) yield to the stress produced by the respiratory muscles and diaphragm (costal attachment of diaphragm is at costochondral junction).

a: **Harrison's grooves** (lower 6 ribs)

Harrison, an English physician, first described these grooves over a century ago. They are horizontal depressions on the thoracic wall and they correspond to the attachments of the diaphragm. They extend laterally from the sixth and seventh costal cartilage downwards from the xiphoid process and produce an appearance of transverse constriction of the thorax. (Pl. 8.3)

b. **Rickety rosary:**

The costochondral junctions, especially of the lower 6 ribs remain enlarged due to rickets in childhood. This is due to the enlargement of the metaphyseal end of the ribs which are involved in the rachitic process. (Pl 8.4)

The appearance is that of a row of beads which is nearer the sternum at the upper end and then goes out laterally to the lower end (rarely a similar rosary may be seen in advanced cases of scurvy called scorbutic beading or rosary).

c. **Longitudinal grooves:**

These may be seen in either side of the sternum and are produced by the softened ribs being pulled in due to the negative pressure in the chest.

d. **Other deformities due to rickets:**

Rarely pigeon breast deformity or a funnel shaped depression of the lower sternal end may be produced due to rickets.

4. **Barrel chest:**

This is produced due to emphysema. The word emphysema is derived from the Greek word meaning over inflation and the lungs are fixed in a position of over inflation. Hence the thoracic cage reflects these changes.

The thorax becomes barrel like, the anteroposterior diameter becoming more or less equal to the transverse diameter. The ribs are horizontal and appear fixed in a position of deep or mid inspiration. The intercostal spaces are widened. The lower ribs flare upwards. The angle of Louis becomes more promient and the subcostal angle is wide. (Pl. 8.5) The upper thoracic spine becomes kyphotic. The respiratory excursions of the thorax are minimal and they are mainly abdominal. The accessory muscles of the respiration are prominent and hypertrophied. (Pl 8.6)

5. **Flat chest:**

A thoracic cage which is narrow and long due to reduced anteroposterior diameter is known as flat chest. (Pl. 8.7). The sternum is nearer to the vertebral column and in advanced cases the scapula appears to be winged. It is then also known as alar chest.

Asymmetrical deformities:

Most often these are caused by deformities of the vertebral column. However, disease of the chest and lungs may cause unilateral deformities which may be generalised or localised.

1. **Scoliosis:**

This is commonest deformity of the thoracic spine and it causes a lateral curvature of the spine, which is usually associated with some rotation of the vertebrae in their longitudinal axis. There is compensatory curvature below scoliosis. (Pl. 8.8)

Due to this, the thoracic cage assumes a typical

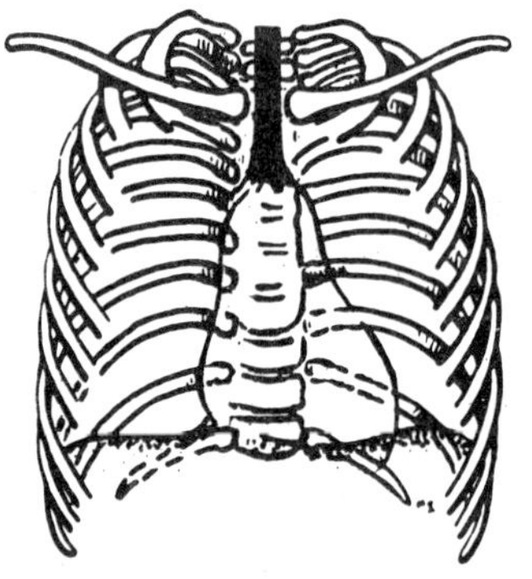

1

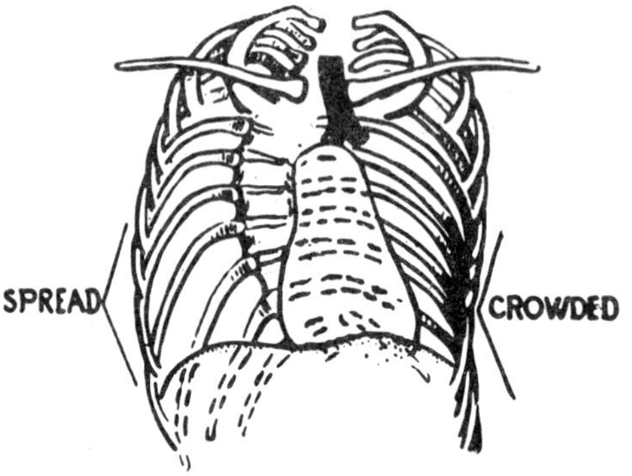

2

Fig. 8.3

1. Normal contour of chest. Note the normal widening of spaces.
2. Contour of the chest in kyphoscoliosis. Note the widening of spaces on the side of scoliosis and crowding of ribs and narrowing of spaces on the other side.

appearance. On the side of the convexity the ribs ar separated widely and are angulated at their posterior aspects due to the rotation of the vertebrae.

For some unknown reasons, scoliosis is more commonly seen on right side. This causes bulging of the posterior aspects of the ribs on the convex side. On the concave side the ribs are crowded together and as their articulation with the vertebrae are rotated, the anterior aspect of the rib cage becomes bulging on that side. The lung gets compressed on the side where the ribs are crowded.

2. **Kyphosis:**

This is a fairly acute angular curvature of the thoracic spine with a posterior convexity.

This causes a hump in the spine. The ribs tend to crowd together and hence the anterior portion of the chest and the sternum bulge forward mimicking a pigeon breast deformity. (Pl. 8.8)

3. **Kyphoscoliosis:**

This is a combination of the above two deformities. It can cause a severe displacement of the thoracic viscera. Externally it can produce a combination of the deformities described above. (Fig. 8.3)

Unilateral generalised deformity of the thoracic cage:

These can be manifested either as bulging or retraction.

a. Unilateral bulging of the chest can be produced either by pneumothorax or pleural effusion.

b. Unilateral retraction can be produced by either collapse of the lung or fibrosis of pulmonary tissue or pleura. (Pl. 8.9)

Local deformities of the thoracic cage:

Any local pathology of the underlying organs which results in swelling may cause a localised bulging. Hence encysted effusions or local disease of the ribs, etc., can produce this abnormality.

Localised retraction is most commonly associated with pulmonary tuberculosis and is observed in the supraclavicular and infraclavicular regions. Such retraction in infraclavicular regions may lead to depression of shoulder on the same side. A pleural fibrosis can also cause a retraction of the chest wall mostly in the lower aspect of the chest.

C. Respiratory movements:

They should be first checked for the rate and amplitude as a whole and also equality of movements on both sides.

I. Respiratory movements as a whole:

Normal rate in an adult is about 18 to 20 respirations per minute. It is affected by psychological and physical factors. In disease processes the rate as well as rhythm of the respiration can be affected.

The amplitude of chest movements has no absolute standard and hence varies from individual to individual. Shallow or deep breathing can be determined only by clinical experience.

Usually, a rapid rate is associated with movements of the accessory muscles of respiration.

Deep and rapid breathing (tachypnea) is indicative of acidosis.

A decreased rate of respiration may be associated with morphine or barbiturate poisoning. Rarely, it may be seen in patients suffering from myxoedema.

II. Equality of movements on both sides of the chest:

This should be carefully checked. An inspection from the foot-end of the bed is very helpful to check this. Not only attention should be paid to the movements as a whole, but very particularly the onset of movements on both sides should be checked. Very often the only evidence of abnormal movements is delay in the start of the movements on one side (The lag of movement on one side).

It should be remembered that whenever there is an inequality of movements, the side which moves less is the side affected by the disease process. The common causes of restriction of movements on one side are pulmonary infections like tuberculosis or pneumonia or pleural disease like effusion or pneumothorax.

Any local retractions of the chest wall should be checked. A slight indrawing of the lower intercostal spaces during inspiration is normal. A bilateral marked retraction of the intercostal spaces occurs in conditions like bronchial asthma and sometimes in emphysema and in conditions where there is an obstruction to the respiratory passages. The respiratory distress leads to strong contraction of the diaphragm. The strong pull of the diaphragm causes retration of intercostal spaces. An unilateral retraction over a localised area suggests either collapse or fibrosis of the lungs or pleura. Sub-costal retraction and intercostal retraction show distressed breathing.

D. Types of breathing:

Following are the different types:

1. **Cheyne Stokes breathing:** (Fig. 8.4)

This is a characteristic type of breathing in which a period of apnea is followed by gradual increase in the rate and amplitude of respiratory movements which reach a peak and then again gradually subside to the apneic phase. This type of breathing is indicative of central respiratory **failure.**

2. **Biots breathing: (Fig. 8.5)**

In this, two or three inspiratory movements are superimposed upon one another before the expiratory movement. There are periods of apnea

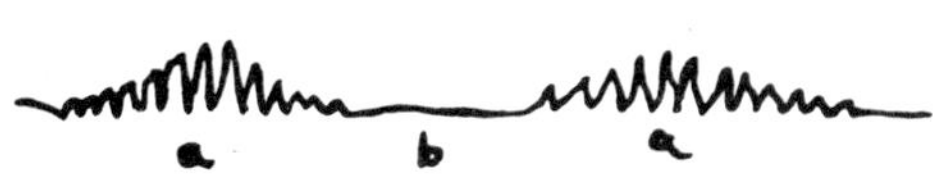

Fig. 8.4
Cheyne Stokes breathing.

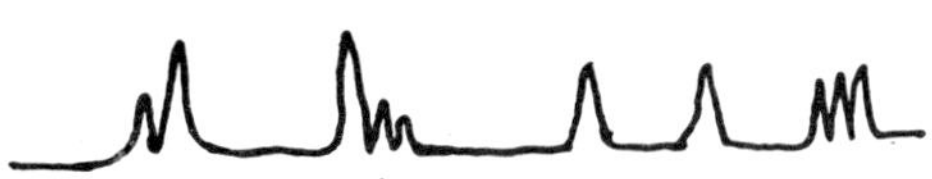

Fig. 8.5
Biot's breathing.

in between several periods of shallow or deep inspiration. This type of breathing is indicative of advanced central respiratory failure.

3. **Kussmaul breathing:**

This is seen classically in patients suffering from diabetic acidosis. The respirations are very deep in amplitude and expiratory phases are prolonged. The respirations have a sighing character.

4. Prolongation of the expiratory phase is classically seen in bronchial asthma and leads to prolonged wheeze associated with expiratory phase.

E. Position of the apex impulse and trachea:

It is very important to determine the exact position of the apex impulse and trachea as they provide important clues to the underlying disease processes.

However, as the positions of these can be determined very easily and more correctly on palpaltion, the discussion of their normal position and variations will be deferred until then. The sternomastoid muscle on the side to which the trachea is deviated may be prominent and this sign is designated as Trail's sign or sternomastoid sign.

F. **Presence of collateral veins:**

Their presence over the front of the chest wall usually means obstruction of the superior vena cava. The cause of the obstruction is usually mediastinal mass — neoplastic in nature.

Sometimes small veins are seen along the lateral chest walls in emphysema.

PALPATION

Palpation of the respiratory system is done to record the following points:

1. To confirm the findings regarding movements of the chest wall as seen during inspection.
2. To confirm or determine the position of the apex beat and the trachea.
3. Examine the tactile vocal fremitus. (TVF)

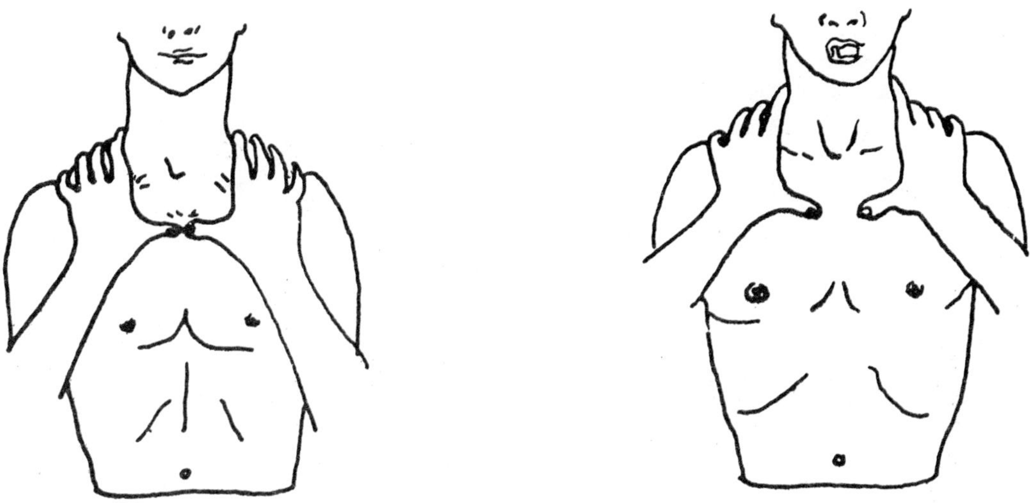

a. Before inspiration . b. After inspiration.

Fig. 8.6
Examination of movements of upper lobes.

4. To note the presence of any other findings detected on palpation.

1. **To confirm the respiratory movements:**

A reduced distensibility of a portion of a lung is noted by diminished movements of the overlying portion of the chest wall. Hence when diminished movement of a portion of the chest is confirmed, it means that some disease process is involving the underlying pleura or lung.

a. **Movements of upper lobes: (Fig. 8.6)**

The anterior chest wall overlying the upper lobes moves forward during inspiration because the anterior ends of the first four ribs are elevated. This is examined as follows : The palms of both hands are kept symmetrically over the anterior chest wall and the fingers overlie both the trapezii. The skin of the front of the chest is then stretched by dragging the palms of both hands until they lie in the infraclavicular areas. The thumbs are made to meet each other end to end and the hands are allowed to follow the stretched skin. The hands will move upward and laterally when the chest expands and the tip of the thumbs will be separated. If both the upper lobes are healthy, the movements of thumbs will be equidistant from midline and if they are not, the thumb on the affected side will traverse over a shorter distance.

b. **Movements of the middle lobe of the right lung or the lingular segment of the left upper lobe: (Fig. 8.7 a, b)**

These underlie the corresponding fifth and sixth ribs and are expanded when these ribs are elevated by the respiratory muscles. The expansion takes place both in an anteroposterior and lateral direction. However, it is mainly the lateral movement which is checked by the following method. Both hands are kept in the axillae as shown, with the fingers outstretched and the palms are laid flat against the chest wall. The skin is then stretched medially until both the thumbs meet in the midsternal line. During inspiration the thumbs move away from each other and should move over an equal distance if the underlying lungs are healthy.

To check the movements of the apices, the palms of the hands are kept over the apices from behind.

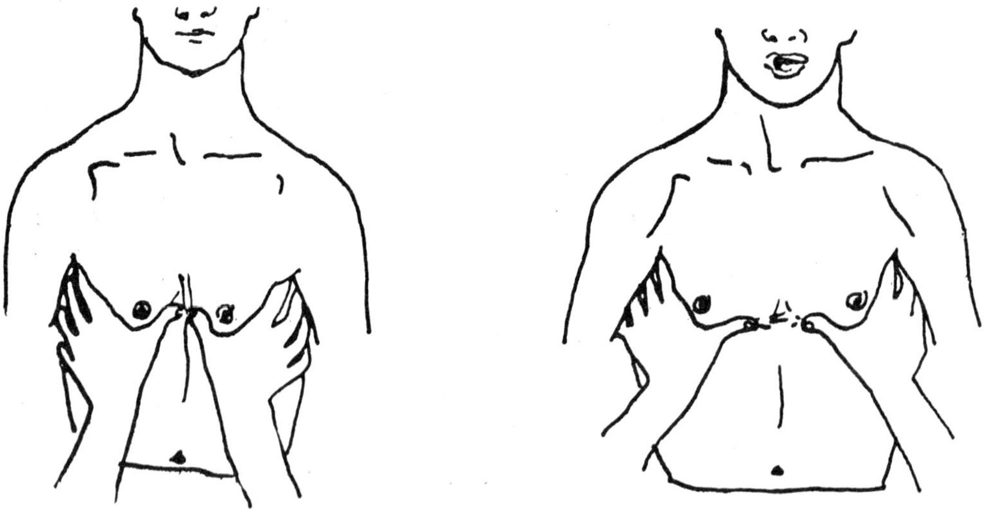

a. Before inspiration.

b. After inspiration.

Fig. 8.7
Examination of movements of middle lobe (R) and lingula (L).

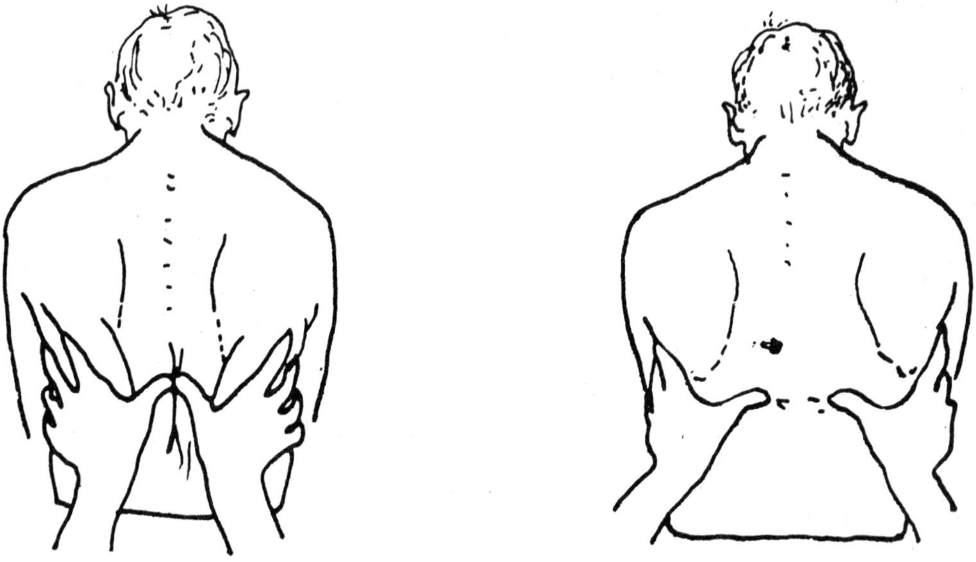

a. Before inspiration.

b. After inspiration.

Fig. 8.8
Examination of movements of lower lobes.

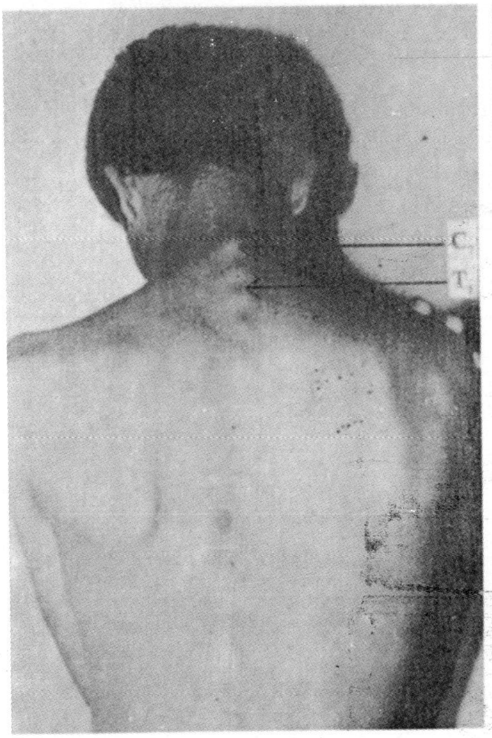

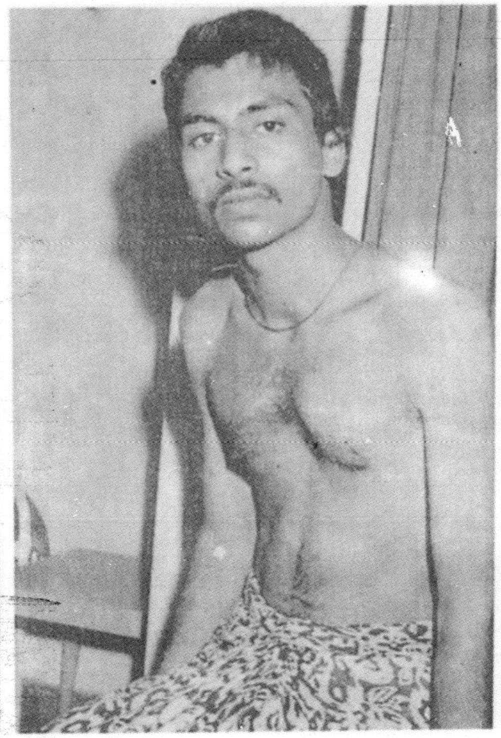

Pl. 8.1 To show cervical and dorsal spine to identify the spinous processes.

Pl. 8.2 Pectus excavatum---Cobbler's chest

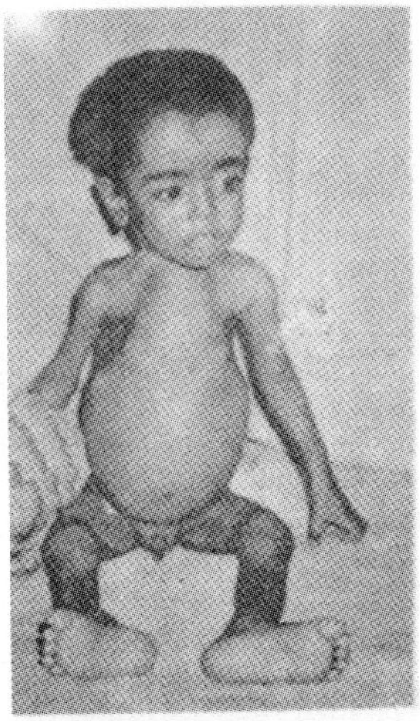

Pl. 8.3 Harrison's grooves. Note bilateral Harrison's grooves producing violin shaped chest- Cause - advanced rickets.

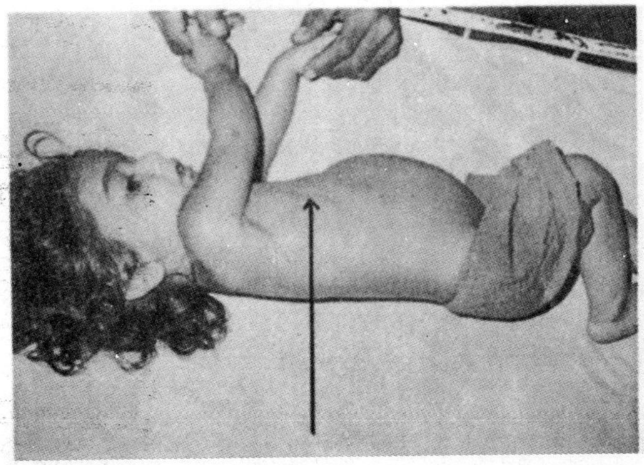

Pl. 8.4 Rickety rosary

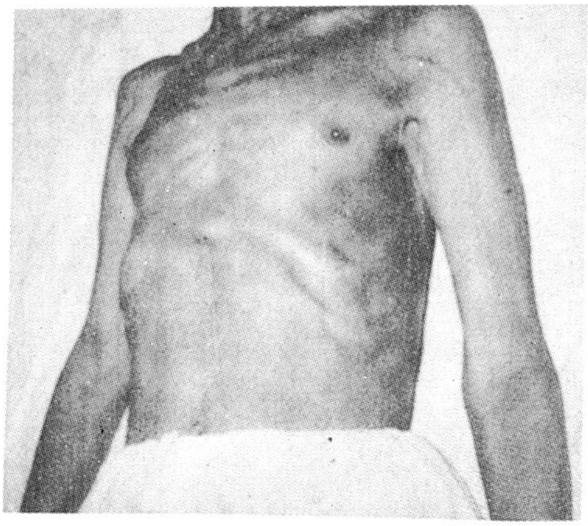

Pl. 8.5 Wide subcostal angle

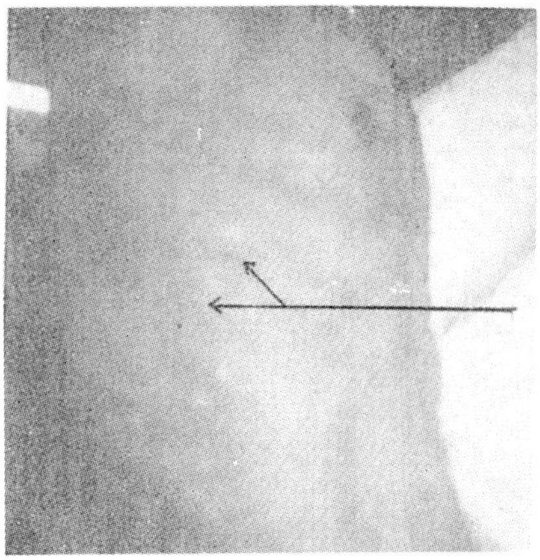

Pl.8.6 Emphysema with intercostal recession

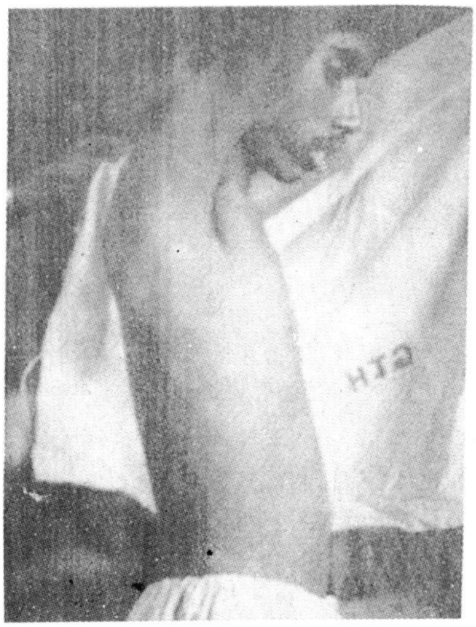

Pl. 8.7 Flat chest

Pl.8.8 Flat chest on right side. Note the retraction in supra and infraclavicular fossae on (R) side

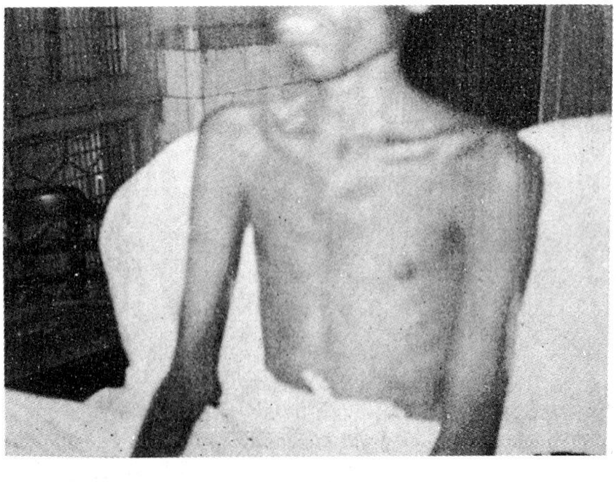

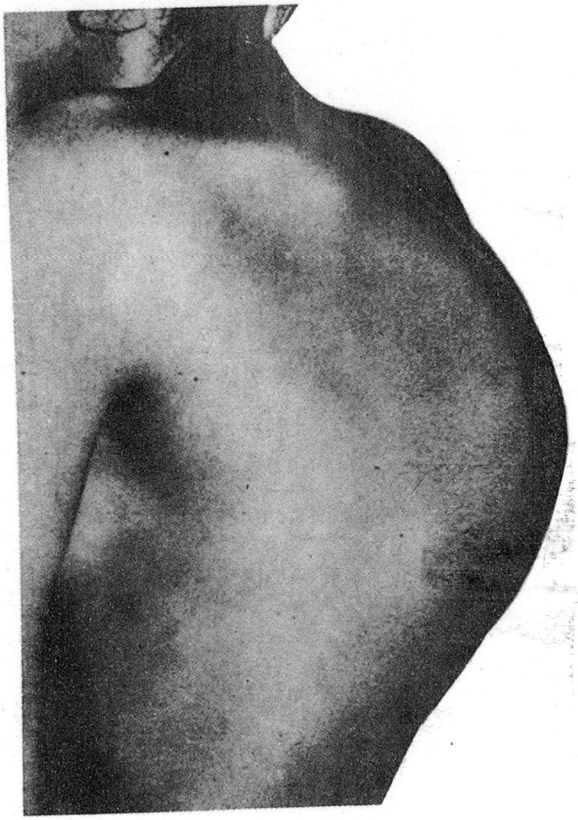

Kyphoscoliosis.

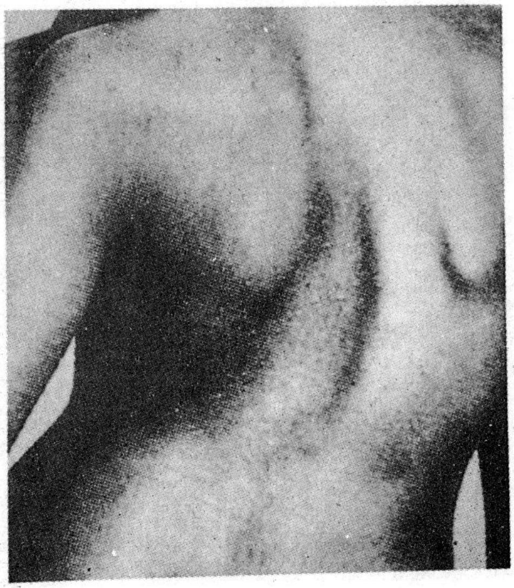

Scoliosis.

Pl. 8.9 Scoliosis and Kyphoscoliosis.

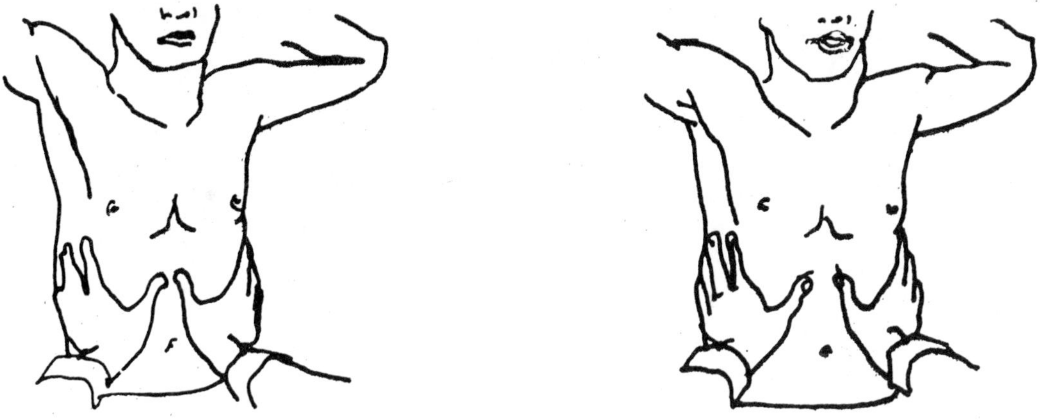

a. Before inspiration. b. After inspiration.

Fig. 8.9
Examination of movements of diaphragm.

The patient should preferably be sitting up with head bent forwards. The thumbs should meet each other in the centre, in the midline posteriorly. The expansion of these regions is noted when the patient takes a deep breath.

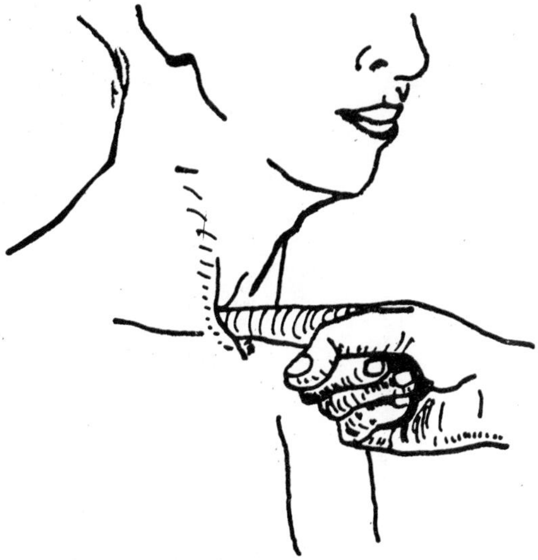

Fig. 8.10
Confirmation of position of trachea on palpation. Note that the neck should be still more extended than what is shown in the figure.

c. **Movements of the lower lobes:** (Fig.8.8 a, b)

The palms are kept over the posterior aspect of the chest wall, and the fingers curve below the scapular margins. The thumbs are made to meet in the centre and the movements tested as described above.

d. **Movements of the diaphragm:** (Fig. 8.9 a,b)

The patient should be asked to lie down in a supine position and the examiner's hands are placed lightly over the lower ribs as shown in figure. Both thumbs are placed along the costal margins and their tips should meet in the centre near the xiphoid process. The thumbs should follow the movements of the costal margins. If the diaphragmatic pull is normal, the angle at the xiphoid process increases equally on both the sides.

2. To confirm or determine the position of the apex beat and the trachea:

The position of the apex beat is first noted on inspection. But it is only after palpation, its position should be confirmed and recorded. The apex impulse is shifted to one or the other side in certain respiratory disorders. The causes of this will be discussed later along with those of tracheal

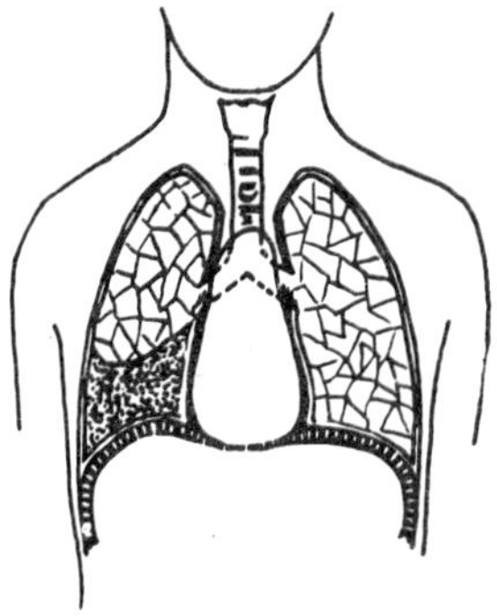

a. Consolidation of lung
Leading to no shift of trachea.

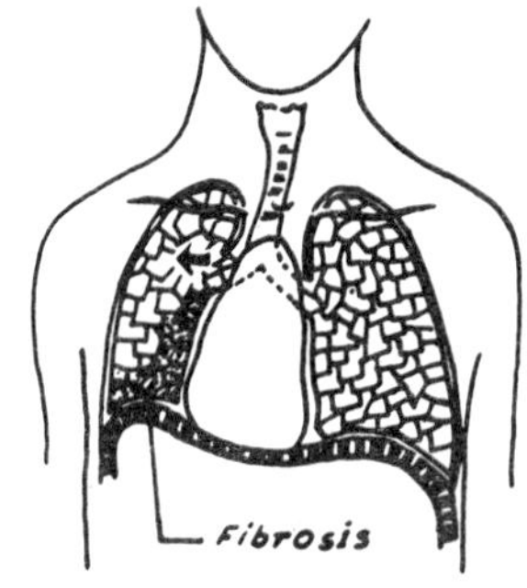

b. Fibrosis of lung
Leading to shift of trachea to same side.

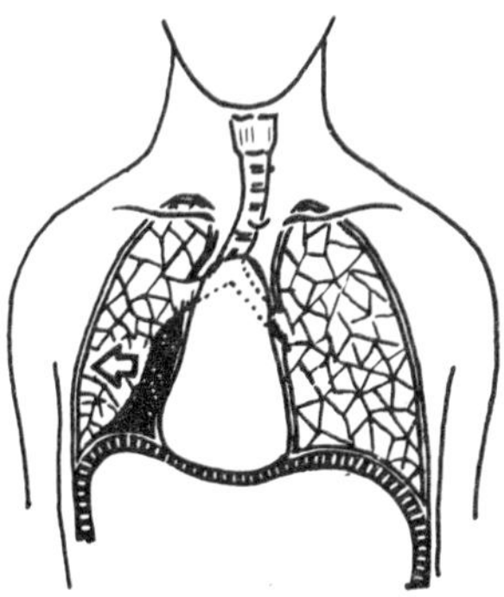

c. Collapse of lung
Leading to shift of trachea to same side.

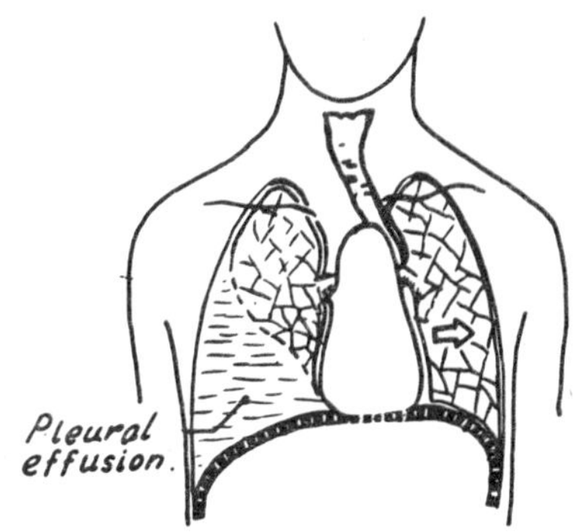

d. Pleural effusion
Leading to shift of trachea to opposite side.

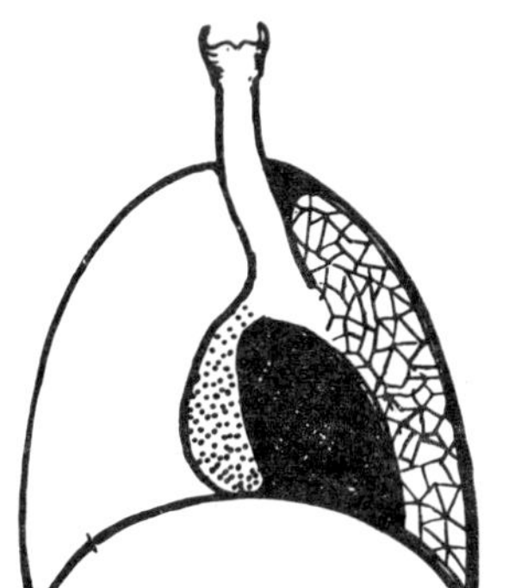

e. Pneumothorax
Leading to shift of trachea to opposite side.

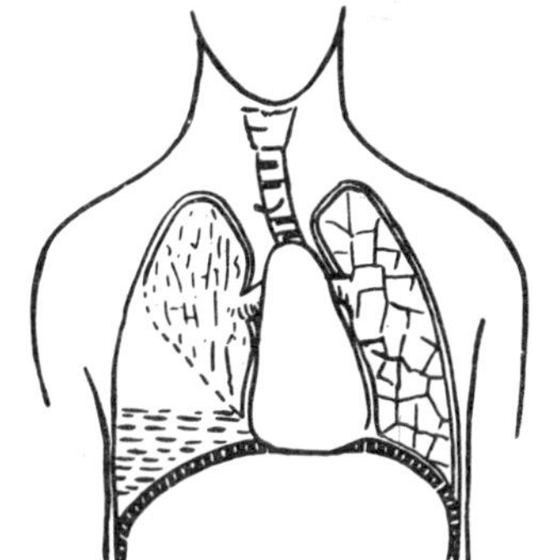

f. Hydropneumothorax
Leading to shift of trachea to opposite side.

Fig. 8.11

Note that whenever collapse of lung is secondary to pleural disease, the shift is to the opposite side. (e.g., d, e, f) and when it is due to primary lesion in lung or bronchial tree, it is on same side (eg. b, c).

shift which is a much more sensitive guide to the shift of the mediastinum.

The position of the trachea can be determined as follows: (Fig. 8.10) The patient is asked to extend his neck. In this position, the pretracheal fascia gets stretched and trachea gets fixed, and it is easy to determine its position. The finger of the examiner is made to follow the trachea and its running is noted. Alternatively, the finger of the examiner is inserted in between the trachea and the sternomastoid muscle on either side and the distance between the two sides is noted.

Normally, the trachea is slightly deviated towards the right side in the upper mediastinum.

The mediastinal shift is due to :-

i. Abnormality of the bony cage of the thorax.

ii. Parenchymal lung disease.

iii. Pleural disease.

iv. Diaphragmatic abnormality.

In abnormalities of the bone cage, the trachea and the apex impulse are shifted to the side of the compressed lung.

In the parenchymal diseases such as collapse or fibrosis of the lung tissue, the trachea is shifted towards the side of the lesion, whereas in pleural diseases such as effusion or pneumothorax the mediastinum is pushed towards the opposite side as shown in Fig. 8.11 a to f.

When the abdominal contents herniate in the thorax the mediastinum is shifted to the opposite side.

3. **Examination of tactile vocal fremitus (T.V.F):**

When certain words are spoken, vibrations are produced by larynx and carried to the periphery of the lungs. These are felt by the palpating hand. These vibrations are called tactile vocal fremitus.

The patient is asked to repeat words like 'one, two, three or ninety-nine' in a clear voice. The examiner's hand or especially the ulnar border which is the most sensitive part of the palm is kept over the chest wall and the vibrations are felt. The two sides are compared over symmetrical areas. The anterior portions, the axillae and posterior regions are symmetrically compared. The vocal fremitus is normally uniform over both the lungs except over the right lung where the larger bronchi are closer to the chest wall.

The T.V.F. is increased whenever the density of the underlying lung is increased and the sounds from the patent bronchi can be transmitted easily to the chest wall. This can happen in consolidation of the lung collapse with a patent bronchus overlying the collapsed portion or when a cavity in the lung is surrouned by an area of consolidation.

The T.V.F. is decreased in -

i. Pleural effusion or

ii. Pneumothorax or

iii. Bronchial obstruction or

iv. Emphysema or

v. Fibrosis of the lung.

In the case of persons having thick chest walls due to either muscle or fat, the T.V.F. is not felt properly. The T.V.F. is decreased when fluid, air, excessive muscle or fat is interposed between the lung and the palpating hand or when the bronchus supplying that area is blocked. T.V.F. is less intense in women and children because their voices are less resonant.

4. **Other findings to be noted on palpation:**

A pleural rub if present can be palpated as a harsh grating feeling below the palpating hand.

Rhonchi and rales if prominent can be easily palpated. They are described as rhonchial fremitus or palpable rales.

Rarely surgical emphysema can be palpated as a characteristic spongy feeling in subcutaneous tissue.

PERCUSSION

Percussion of the respiratory system should be conducted in a systematic fashion. It should begin with the apices and then symmetrical areas on the two sides should be compared. The clavicles should be percussed directly. The anterior areas, the axillae and the posterior surface should be percussed one after another. For percussion of both axilliary and posterior areas, the patient should be made to sit up and he should be asked to fold his hands over the anterior chest wall in such a way that scapulae are pulled forward exposing a maximum area of the lungs posteriorly.

Discussion of some basic principles involved in percussion:

Percussion of the chest produces vibrations of both the chest wall as well as the underlying lung parenchyma. Vibrations so produced penetrate internally and also spread externally over the chest wall. If the stroke is heavier, the penetration is deeper as well as more extensive externally.

The pitch of the sound produced is interpreted to determine the proportion of air containing tissue and solid tissue in the areas which are percussed.

When the air containing tissue is greater than the solid parenchyma (as happens in pneumothorax or emphysema) the note produced is lower in pitch than normal. Hence it sounds hyperresonant.

As opposed to that when the solid tissue is more in proportion to air containing tissue the note on percussion is higher in pitch as the vibrations are rapid and quickly disappear. This results in dull or flat note. The thickness of the chest wall either due to muscular development or obesity does not affect the note produced by percussion except to a slight extent. Light percussion vibrations penetrate to about 6 cms inside the thoracic cavity. If the chest wall is about 4 cms thick any pulmonary lesion below 2.5 cms in the lung tissue will not affect the note on percussion in any way.

Percussion over the normal lungs: The percussion note over the normal lung tissue has a particular character which can be learnt only by experience. It is low pitched note, the sound produced is called the normal lung resonance. It is slightly less resonant over the back as the musculature over the back is heavier as compared to that in the front.

The border of the normal lung resonance is as follows : The anterior border of the right lung can be easily mapped out up to the sternum. However on the left side the cardiac dullness is superimposed over the lung resonance. The area of impaired note over the surface of the heart is referred to as the area of the 'relative cardiac dullness'. If the percussion is continued medially towards the sternum, a flatter or more dull note is produced over the area of the heart which is not covered by lung tissue. This area is known as the area of 'absolute cardiac dullness'. Clinically this area has no special significance.

The lower border of the lung can be percussed up to the sixth interspace in the midclavicular line, the eighth interspace in the mid-axillary line and the 10th interspace in the mid-scapular line. The range of movement of the lungs can be determined by percussing these borders at the end of deep inspiration and full expiration. This percussion is also known as 'tidal percussion'.

The apices of the lungs are frequently affected by tuberculosis. Hence, percussion to map out these areas deserves particular mention. The resonant note over apices extends up to 5 cms above the clavicles and is slightly higher on the right side than the left. This resonance also corresponds to the 'Krönig's isthmus'. (Fig. 8.12) This is an area or a band of resonance connecting the anterior and posterior zones of lung resonance. It is bounded laterally by the dullness of shoulder area and medially by the dull note over the muscles in the neck. It is about 5 cms in width. It is narrowed or absent in apical pulmonary tuberculosis or other lesions involving the apical areas.

Traube's semilunar space is normally in midclavicualr line around the left 7th space. It is bound on the right by left lobe of liver, on the left by spleen and superiorly by heart and inferiorly by left costal margin. The tympanitic note is due to the presence of air in the fundus of the stomach.

Its clinical importance is as follows :

1. If the Traube's space extends laterally to anterior axillary line it indicates massive collapse of left lung or left lower lobe.

2. If the Traube's space is obliterated it indicates pleural effusion on the left side. In case of left-sided pneumonia or encysted effusion,

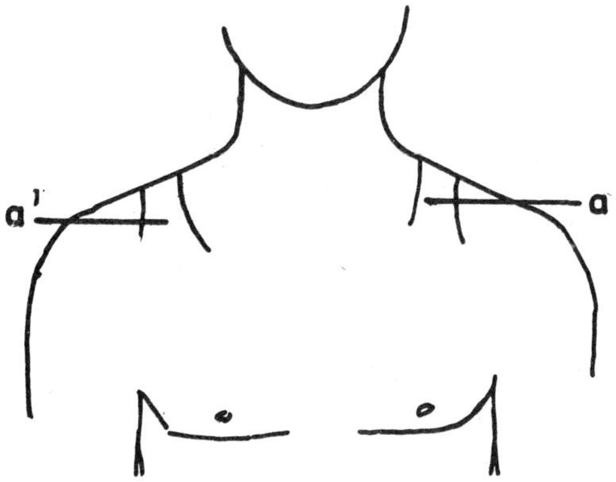

Fig. 8.12
Kronig's isthmus indicated by 'a'.

Traube's space is not obliterated.

Abnormal percussion notes:

As discussed above, the percussion note over the lungs changes according to the proportion of air and the solid tissue. Hence, it can either be hyperresonant or dull.

Varieties of notes with increased resonance:

A. **Hyperresonant note:** It is produced when the lungs are affected by emphysema and pneumothorax.

The emphysema may either be generalised or it could be compensatory in nature near an area of collapse of the lung.

B. **Skodaic resonance:** This is a note encountered above the level of pleural effusion. It is a hyperresonant note with a peculiar quality and is supposed to be due to relaxation of the lung tissue upwards due to the pressure of the effusion.

C. **Tympanitic note:** It is usually present over a tension pneumothorax or over a large cavity or an emphysematous bulla of the lung. It can be compared with the note heard over the normal Traube's space or normal abdomen.

D. **Amphoric resonance:** Sometimes the tympanitic note is encountered in patients with pneumothorax or a large cavity and it has a peculiar hollow quality. The sound produced is low pitched and is characteristic.

E. **Cracked pot resonance:** When a large cavity is communicating with a bronchus, the air is driven out of the cavity into the bronchus during percussion. The note produced at this time can be compared to the note produced while percussing over a broken earthenware vessel.

Varieties of notes with decreased resonance:

A. **Impaired note or dull note:** This is produced over an area of consolidation or collapse due to the fact that the proportion of solid tissue to the air containing tissue is increased. If the consolidation is absolute, the note produced is designated as dull, while if some amount of air is present in the lungs, the note known as impaired note is normally produced over the liver.

B. **Stony dull or flat note:** This is encountered in patients suffering from fluid in the pleural cavity. The note is totally dull. However, the term stony dull is used mainly because the resistance encountered by the finger kept over the chest wall (the plecimeter finger) is increased markedly. Stony dull note can be compared with the note produced by percussing thigh muscles.

Other abnormal changes encountered on percussion:

A. **Abnormal findings on percussion associated with pleural effusion:**

1. The upper level of the fluid in a patient suffering from pleurisy with effusion is not at the same level in the front, in the axilla and in the back. The upper level is higher in the axilla than in the anterior or posterior surface. Hence, the upper border of this dullness represents an 'S' shaped curve which is also known as Ellis 'S' curve.

The reason for the level of the fluid being

highest in the axilla is probably capillary suction. The two layers of pleura are closest in the axillae and as the fluid rises highest in the thinnest capillary, the pleural fluid level tends to rise in lateral portions. The part of the lung below the hilum is attached to the pulmonary ligament and hence cannot retract as easily as that in the lateral region. Hence, the fluid rises more in the axillae as that region is more free to collapse. However, it is now believed that 'S' shaped curve is radiological artefact.

2. A triangle of dullness known as Grocco's triangle can be mapped out in certain patients suffering from pleural effusion. It is on the opposite side of the pleural effusion and is situated posteriorly near the vertebral spine. It is bound medially by the spine and this border extends from the upper level of the effusion to the tenth thoracic spine. The lower border extends along the tenth intercostal space for about 5 to 7 cms. The third side of the triangle is drawn by joining these two boundaries. The dullness is due to the posterior mediastinum. Grocco's triangle is quite a constant sign.

3. A left sided pleural effusion usually obliterates Traube's semi-lunar space. The presence of Traube's space in normal position in patients suffering from left sided pleural effusion may point towards an encysted effusion.

B. Abnormal findings on percussion encountered in pneumothorax and hydropneumothorax : (Fig. 8.13)

i. In patients suffering from hydropneumothorax, the upper level of the fluid is always horizontal. Hence, it will change its position according to the position of the patient. A shifting dullness can be elicited in such patients by the following manoeuvre : The upper limit of dullness is marked when the patient is sitting up. Then he is asked to lie down and the same area is percussed again. It will be found to be resonant, as the fluid slips down to horizontal level in lying down position and the previously dull area will become resonant.

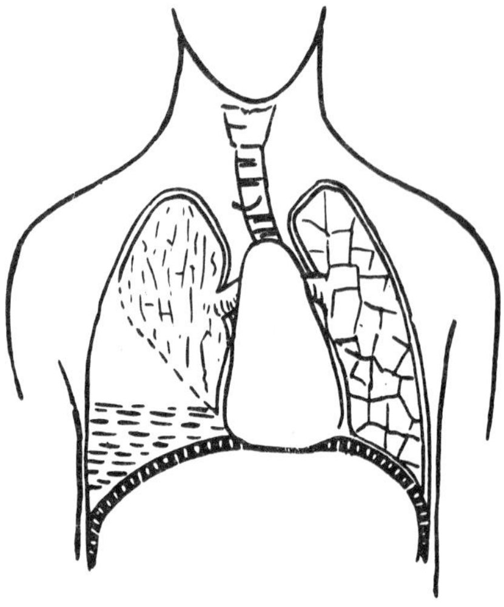

A. In vertical position. The fluid level is horizontal so the dull note corresponds up to the fluid level.

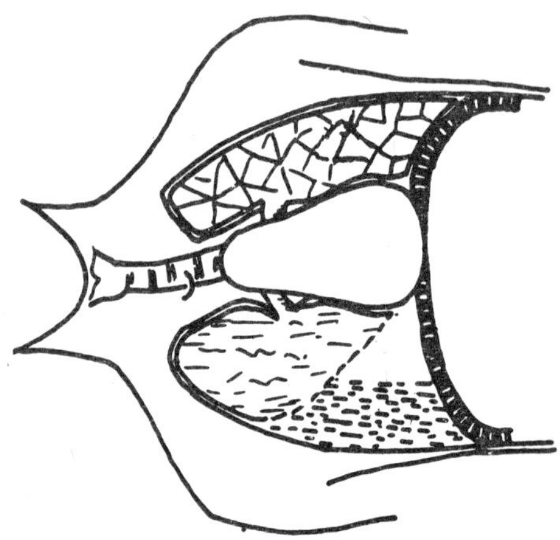

B. If patient lies on the side of lesion, the fluid level is horizontal again and the dull note corresponds up to the fluid level.

Fig. 8.13
Hydropneumothorax - Shifting dullness.

ii **Coin sound :**

In patients suffering from the pneumothorax, the following sign can be elicited. A silver coin (50 paise or a rupee coin) is placed on the anterior chest wall and is then struck by another silver coin. The sound produced is clearly heard over the posterior chest wall with the help of stethoscope. The clear metallic quality is preserved as the sound travels through air and hence the note is unimpaired.

C. **Abnormal percussion findings sometimes associated with a cavity in the lung:**

i. When a lung cavity communicates with the bronchus the percussion note over it changes its character in deep inspiration and expiration. This is due to the fact that during inspiration the cavity becomes more tense due to filling with air.

ii. Wintrich's sign : In a similar situation, when the lung cavity is communicating with the bronchus the note appears more resonant with the mouth open during inspiration than when it is closed.

iii. Gerhardt's sign : When a lung cavity is filled partially with fluid and air, the percussion note over the area above such a cavity changes with posture. This is also known as Gerhardt's sign.

D. **Other rare signs encountered on percussion :**

i. Myotatic irritability : A localised contraction of the muscle bundles is seen sometimes while percussing the chest wall. It was thought to be a sign of tuberculosis in the past. It is now known to be present in any disease causing emaciation or debility.

ii. William's tracheal resonance : A patch of pneumonia in the areas below the first or second intercstal space near the sternum may give rise to a tympanitic note on percussion. This is because of the fact that the consolidation is confluent with the trachea and the vibrations of the percussion note are conducted up to the trachea producing a resonant note.

AUSCULTATION

Auscultation of the sound produced during respiration is the most important part of respiratory system examination.

All the areas of the chest covering the lungs should be auscultated systematically: the front of the chest, the axillae and then the posterior aspect. It is advisable to compare the two corresponding areas on both sides so that any minor variations can be easily detected.

For the auscultation of the front and the axillary regions the lying down position of the patient may be used. However, for auscultation of back ideally the patient should be sitting up with his hands crossed in front of his chest, so that a maximum area of the chest wall posteriorly can be auscultated. Moreover, in lying down position when the patient is turned on his side, the breath sounds are less in intensity on the side on which the patient is turned.

The patient should be instructed to breathe in and out with his mouth open when auscultating the lungs. Ideally, the examiner should demonstrate to the patient what is expected of him.

The following points should be noted carefully when auscultating the lungs:

I. Breath sounds;

II. Adventitious sounds;

III. Vocal resonance. (V.R.)

I. **Breath sounds :** (Fig. 8.14)

Breath sounds are produced by the passage of air in and out of lungs during inspiration and expiration. During inspiration when the air is drawn into the lungs, it passes through the larynx, trachea and bronchi up to the alveoli. The accompanying figure shows the eddies and the turbulance produced when this inspired air strikes the sharp borders of the bronchial bifurcations. During expiration when the air is travelling out of the small bronchi it mixes with air currents coming from other airways, and strikes against the walls of main bronchus and again causes turbulance. The turbulance produced during expiration is less as compared to that produced during inspiration, presumably because outgoing air does not encounter sharp bifurcations of bronchi. This sound produced is because of movement of air and the turbulance caused by the air within tracheobronchial tree. The sounds heard by the stethoscope over chest are the same tracheobronchial sounds but are modified because of alveoli as given below:

When this sound is transmitted to the periphery through the lung parenchyma, it has to pass through the alveoli. The alveolar membranes act as tense vibrating membranes (they are tense due to the negative pressure in the thoracic cavity) and modify the sound travelling in the bronchi. Hence the sounds which are heard over the lungs have a rustling character as compared to the harsh nature of the tracheobronchial sounds.

The breath sounds are represented or drawn by symbols as follows:

The inspiratory sound is denoted by the upstroke and the downstroke denotes the expiratory phase. The thickness of the line denotes the intensity and the length corresponds to the duration of the sound.

The following types of breath sounds are heard over the chest wall in health and disease. (Fig. 8.15)

A. Vesicular breath sounds.
B. Bronchovesicular breath sounds.
C. Bronchial breath sounds.

A. **Vesicular breath sounds :**

These are heard all over the normal lung parenchyma (except in the interscapular region and near the right apex where the sounds are bronchovesicular due to close proximity of the main bronchi).

The inspiratory sound is easily heard and has a rustling quality. It is more prolonged and better heard than the expiratory sound. The expiratory sound is fainter and is about one-third in duration as compared to that of inspiratory sound. There is no gap or pause between the inspiratory and the expiratory sounds.

The vesicular breath sounds are better heard in thin-walled people and in women. They appear diminished in intensity in persons who have thick muscular chest walls or who are very obese.

Pathologically, the vesicular breath sounds are

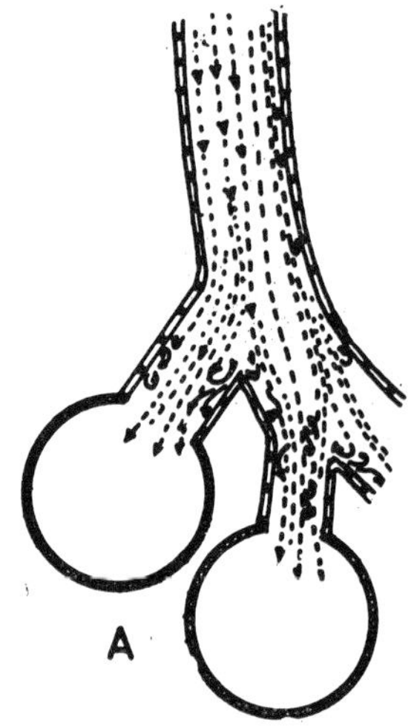

A. Inspiration — Note the turbulance and eddies (air currents in whirling motion) produced when air strikes sharp borders of bronchial bifurcation.

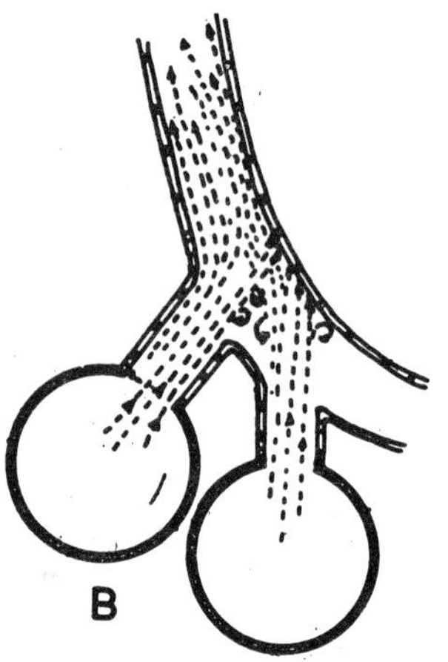

B. Expiration — Air coming out of small airways (bronchioles) mixes with air currents from other bronchioles and strikes against walls of parent bronchus. As the air currents do not encounter sharp bifurcations turbulance is lesser than that in inspiration.

Fig. 8.14
Production of breath sounds.

diminished or absent whenever their conduction to the chest wall is obstructed.

This may be due to -

i. **Complete obstruction of the bronchus:** No air is transmitted to the portion of the lung whose bronchus is totally blocked. Hence, in collapse of the lung where the bronchus is not patent, breath sounds will not be heard.

ii. **Affected elasticity of the alveolar tissues:** If the elasticity of the lung tissue is affected adversely, then the sounds will not be transmitted as usual to the periphery. Hence in emphysema and fibrosis of the lungs, the sounds will not be transmitted to the periphery in the normal intensity and will not be modified.

iii. **Obstruction to the conduction of breath sounds to the chest wall:** This happens when there is a presence of either air or fluid in the pleural cavity which then separates the lung tissue away from the chest wall. Hence, in patients who have either pneumothorax or pleural fluid the breath sounds are diminished in intensity.

Fluid is a good conductor of sound. Still the breath sounds are absent or diminished over pleural effusions. This is due to the fact that the sounds from the lungs have to travel first through air in the alveoli and then through the fluid of the effusion. The sounds are not transmitted well due to this change of media through which they have to travel. In massive pleural effusions, when the air is completely driven out of the lung parenchyma, the bronchi can transmit the sounds directly through fluid and bronchial sounds are heard over the pleural effusion.

B. Bronchovesicular breath sounds:

Before discussing these breath sounds and their characteristics it will be advisable to discuss the physical changes in the lungs which cause the alteration in the normal vesicular breath sounds. The accompanying figure (Fig. 8.15) shows the anatomical changes in the lungs which, change the vesicular breathing to broncho-vesicular type of breathing. It can be said that when the alveoli are filled with fluid (either transudate or exudate) then the character of the vesicular sounds starts changing. When the alveoli contain a mixture of air and fluid, bronchovesicular sounds are heard.

Bronchovesicular breath sounds have an inspiratory phase similar to that of vesicular breathing. The expiratory phase is prolonged and becomes harsher and its duration is equal to that of inspiration. Its harshness depends on the proportion of fluid and air in the alveoli. More the proportion of fluid in the alveoli, harsher is the expiration. However, there is no pause in between inspiration and expiration.

Bronchovesicular breathing is heard whenever there is fluid in the alveoli which does not drive away the air completely from them. Hence in pneumonitis, tuberculosis or congestive cardiac failure when the above mentioned physical state is present bronchovesicular breathing can be heard.

C. Bronchial breath sounds:

Tracheal breath sounds, which are heard while auscultating over the trachea, are similar in

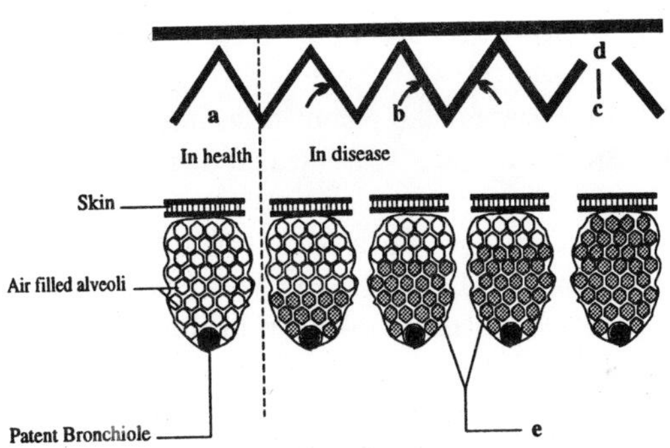

Fig. 8.15
Exudate filled alveoli

To show how the breath sounds change from vesicular to bronchovesicular and thence to bronchial type depending on exudate present in alveoli

a. Vesicular breath sounds, b. Bronchovesicular breath sounds, c. Bronchial breath sounds, d. Pause in between inspiration and expiration, e. Exudate filled alveoli.

character to bronchial breathing except that bronchial breath sounds are less intense. Otherwise whenever bronchial breathing is heard over the chest it is indicative of disease.

True bronchial breathing has the following characteristics: The inspiratory sound is harsh and much louder than the normal inspiratory sound of vesicular breathing. The expiration is harsh and high-pitched and is equal or more prolonged than the inspiratory sound. There is pause between inspiration and expiration. The breath sounds as a whole have a hollow or blowing quality.

As seen from the figure 8.15, bronchial breath sounds are heard whenever a patent bronchus transmits its sounds to the periphery through a solidified lung tissue. Rarely, the transmission may be through a pleural effusion which drives away the air completely from the alveoli.

Hence, bronchial breath sounds (bronchial breathing) are either heard over areas of lobar pneumonia due to consolidation or over collapse of the lung when the overlying bronchus or the main bronchus remains patent as explained later. They are also heard over the area affected by pulmonary infarction of the lung.

Types of bronchial breath sounds:

These depend on two factors :

a. On the size of the patent bronchus through which the sounds are transmitted to the periphery.
b. On the presence of cavities which can act as resonating chambers and hence impart a peculiar character to the bronchial breath sounds.

1. **Tubuar breath sounds:** When the bronchi below the consolidated tissue are smaller in size, the sounds heard are higher pitched and appear shrill. These are called tubular breath sounds and are heard over consolidation due to pneumonia.

2. **Cavernous breath sounds:** These are hollow toned low pitched. They are heard over cavities or when there is a communicating pneumothorax. The sounds are hollow and can be compared to a sound produced by blowing in an empty vessel. (Cavernous breathing can also be compared to sound produced by 'sighing').

3. **Amphoric breath sounds:** This type of breath sounds have a metallic quality. They are heard over cavities which compress the surrounding alveoli and impart this particular type of tone to the breath sounds. They are usually heard over thin-walled tuberculous cavities. They are also heard over a pneumothorax which is communicating with the lung. These sounds can be compared to sounds blown through a blowpipe.

4. **Medium pitched breath sounds:** When sounds are neither tubular nor cavernous or amphoric (i.e., neither high pitched nor low pitched or loud) they are called medium pitched bronchial breath sounds.

II. Adventitious sounds:

Vibrations which are produced by pathological processes in the lungs, tracheobronchial tree or the pleura are known as adventitious sounds. They are always indicative of a pathological process.

They can be divided as follows :

1. Rhonchi or dry sounds;
2. Rales or moist sounds;
3. Other miscellaneous adventitious sounds.

1. **Rhonchi:** (Fig. 8.16 a, b & c) : A rhonchus is a term derived from Greek word which means wheezing. It is a prolonged musical whistling sound produced within the tracheobronchial tree. It is produced whenever a portion of the tracheobronchial tree becomes narrow, either by spasm or sometimes due to presence of an obstructing neoplasm or due to inflammatory swelling as in bronchitis or allergy. Since the bronchi normally shorten and become narrow during expiration, rhonchi are better heard during expiration and during the expulsive phase of coughing.

Rhonchi are divided into two main types;

a. Sonorous
b. Sibiliant

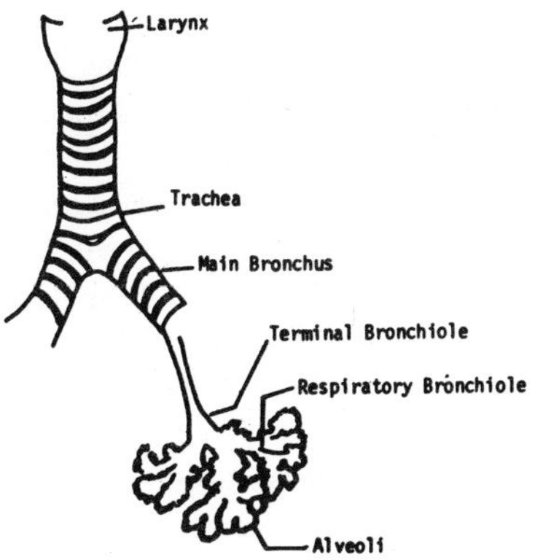

Fig. 8.16 a
Normal laryngo tracheo bronchial tree.

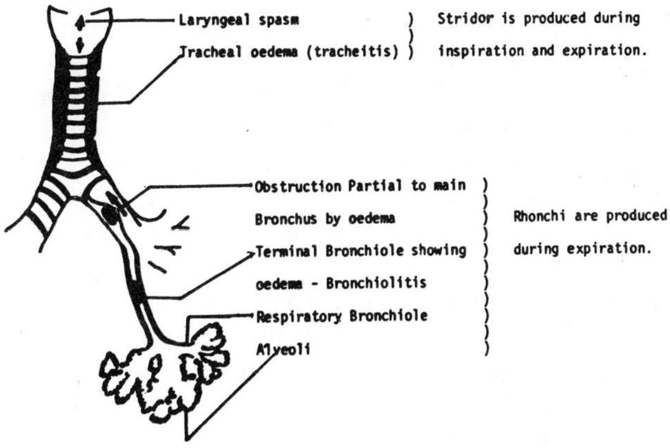

Fig. 8.16 b
Production of stridor and rhonchi.

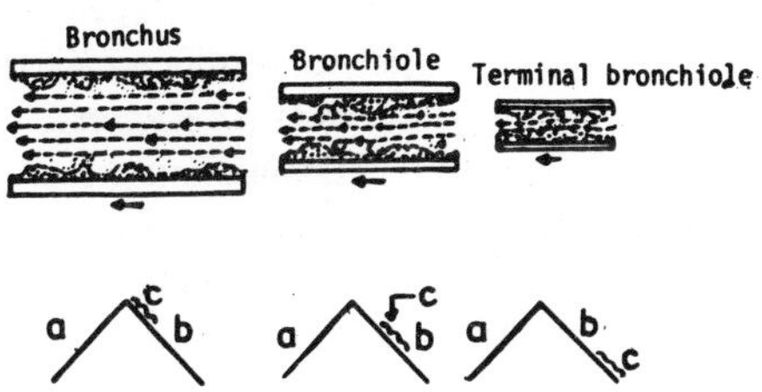

Fig. 8.16 c
Production of rhonchi

a & b Inspiration and expiration, respectively.

c Rhonchi.

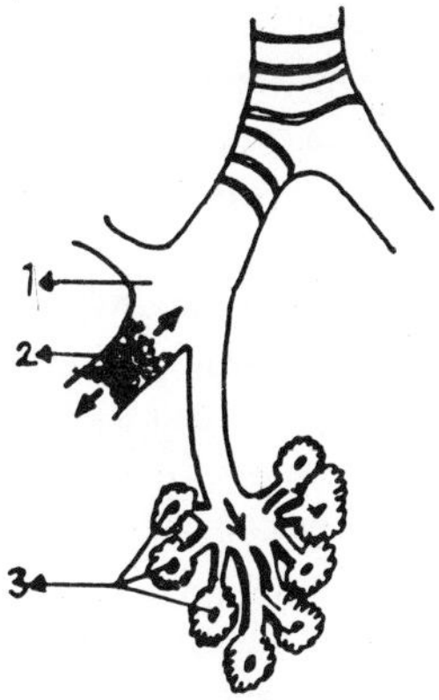

Fig. 8.17 a
Mode of production of rales.

1. Main bronchus,
2. Secretions collected in bronchus make bubbling noise during inspiration and expiration,
3. Exudate or transudate in alveoli, make fine moist sounds during inspiration.

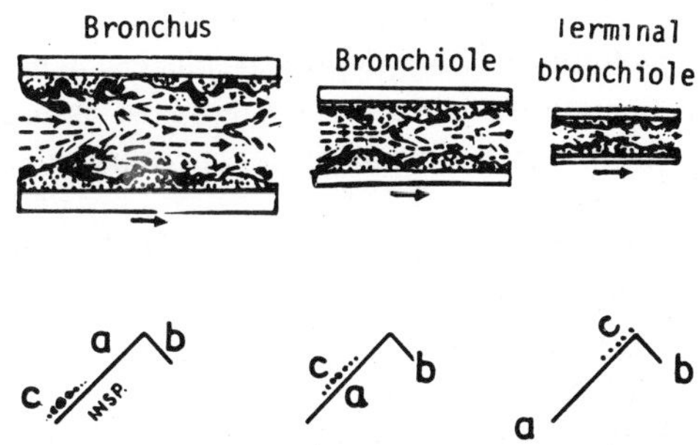

Fig. 8.17 b
Production of "Rales" (moist sounds) during inspiration.

a & b Inspiration and expiration, respectively.
c Rales.

Sonorous rhonchi are produced by sapsm of the larger bronchi and hence have a hollow character and the sound is low pitched in quality. They are heard most easily in the early phase of expiration. Sibiliant rhonchi are produced due to spasm of the smallest bronchi.They are shrill high pitched sounds which are best heard at the end of the expiratory phase.

Narrowing or spasm of the intermediate bronchi produces sounds which are intermediate in pitch, and can be denoted as medium pitched rhonchi.

The relationship of mode of production and character of rhonchi is illustrated in Fig. 8.16 b and c.

Stridor is also a dry sound produced by an obstruction of the large upper air passages like larynx or trachea. It is harsh dry sound heard both in inspiration and expiration more in the former. It is loud enough to be heard without the aid of stethoscope. Indrawing of suprasternal fossa usually accompanies stridor. For mode of production of Stridor refer to Figures 8.16 a, b & c.

2. **Rales:** The term rale is derived from a French word which means bubbling sound. (Fig. 8.17 a & b)

Rales are produced by bursting of the surface films of fluid bubbles inside the bronchi or alveoli. They are more evident during inspiration. The reason for this is two fold. The first is the passage of air during inspiration reaching those areas in which the bubbles are present (as happens in the finest crepitations). The second reason is during inspiratory phase the bubbles are more likely to burst at this time.

The three main types of rales are distinguished:

a. Coarse rales;

b. Medium rales;

c. Fine rales or crepitations.

This classification is dependent on their pitch and so also on the predominant phase of inspiration in which they occur.

The rales produced due to exudate in the large bronchi are coarse or bubbling in nature. They are best heard in inspiration in its initial phase, but also can be heard in expiration and in rare cases can be loud enough to be heard without the aid of a stethoscope.

The medium pitched rales are produced when the smaller bronchi are affected. They are well heard in the mid phase of inspiration and are higher in pitch than the coarse rales. They are heard commonly in patients who are suffering from bronchiectasis.

The fine rales are also known as crepitations. They are high pitched and are heard as crackling sounds. They are due to presence of fluid in the alveoli and hence are heard only at the end of deep inspiration. The sound produced by crepitations can be compared to the sound which can be produced by rubbing a lock of hair in between the fingers.

Crepitations are present in all diseases which give rise to fluid in the alveoli. Hence they are present in patients suffering from tuberculosis, pneumonia, left ventricular failure or pulmonary edema.

Other types of rales:

a. **Post-tussive rales:** These are heard when there is a minimum amount of disease in the alveoli. Hence they are heard during the beginning of inspiration following a cough. They are probably because of separation of sticky alveolar walls by the act of cough which have been stuck together.

b. **Leathery rales:** Rales heard over bronchiectatic areas have a peculiar leathery nature. They change their nature and characteristics after the patient coughs. Though thought to be diagnostic of bronchiectasis, they can be heard over lung cavities.

The relation of the moist sounds and the phase of inspiration which are best heard is shown in Fig. 8.17 (b).

Other miscellaneous adventitious sounds:

a. **Pleural rub:** This is a harsh, grating friction sound produced by two inflamed layers of pleura rubbing against each other. Hence it is most prominent during the latter part of inspiration and early phase of expiration. It is most commonly heard over the lower areas or bases of the lungs as the respiratory excursions are widest over these areas. It is accentuated by increasing the pressure of the chest piece over the wall of the thorax. It is usually associated with local tenderness and sometimes the rub may be palpable as a local friction fremitus. It should be differentiated from rales. (Shown in accompanying table.)

b. **Succussion splash:** This sound was first described by Hippocrates and hence also known as Hippocratic succussion splash. It is produced by shaking a patient when air and fluid are both present in the pleural cavity. The sound produced is splashing sound and can sometimes be heard without the aid of a stethoscope. Rarely this may be the presenting symptom which brings the patient to doctor. This may be accompanied by a tinkling sound when the drops of fluid which are shifted go on falling in the main body of fluid.

c. **Posttussive suction:** This sound is heard after a bout of coughing in a patient who has a thin-walled cavity communicating with a bronchus.

Table 8.1

Rales	Pleural rub
Heard whenever bubbling sounds are produced and not necessarily over base of lungs.	Usually heard at the base of lungs
Interrupted sound	Harsh continuous sound
Heard at the beginning of inspiration and expiration, sometimes throughout both the phases.	Heard at the end of inspiration and beginning of expiration
Change in intensity on coughing	Does not change in intensity on coughing
Not affected by pressure of stethoscope	Louder with pressure of the stethoscope
Spread over a wide area	Localised over a small area
Not associated with local pain	Associated with stitch like pain

During the bout of cough, the air is expelled from the cavity and in the immediate inspiration following the cough, air is sucked inside the cavity producing the sucking sound.

d. **Gurgling sound :** A gurgling sound is heard over the chest wall in a patient who has bronchopleural fistula. It is probably produced by air entering the pleural fluid through the fistula.

III. **Vocal resonance : (V.R.)**

Vocal sounds are produced in the larynx by vibrations of the vocal cord. The sound is carried upwards into the oral cavity and the sinuses and hence its resonance is increased. It is also carried downwards through the tracheobronchial tree up to the chest wall. Major part of the voice is conducted through the lumen of the bronchi while a part of it is conducted in the walls of the bronchi.

The sound when produced in the trachea has vibrations of about 400 cycles per second (c.p.s.). In the terminal bronchiole the vibrations are approximating 1200 c.p.s. Alveoli act as selective transmitters of sound and they damp the higher frequency vibrations. Only sound with vibrations of 100 to 150 c.p.s are allowed to be transmitted to the chest wall. This ability is gradually last when the alveoli becomes affected by the disease. Hence when the alveoli become solidified there is an increase in the transmission of higher frequency vibrations to the chest wall.

These facts govern the production of normal auscultatory vocal resonance (A.V.R.) and its modification in disease.

Normal A.V.R.: (Auscultatory vocal resonance) The patient is instructed to say 'one, two, three' or 'ninetynine' in a clear voice and the examiner auscultates the chest wall with the aid of a stethoscope.

The normal lung parenchyma modifes this sound so that this sound 'one, two, three' is not heard clearly. It is heard as a weak rumbling sound where the syllables of these words merge into each other. The sound also appears distant and appears to be located near the chest piece of the stethoscope.

Normal A.V.R. is loudest at the right apex and interscapular area, as the bronchi are nearest to the thoracic wall in these areas. It is also louder in men than in women due to the natural high resonance of voice in men.

Decreased vocal resonance: In all conditions where the voice sounds produced in the larynx cannot be transmitted to the chest wall, the A.V.R. will be reduced. Hence, excluding diseases of larynx where voice cannot be produced properly, the following disease processes will cause diminished A.V. R.

1. Obstruction of the bronchus-complete or partial.
2. Obstruction of the bronchus with the collapse of the lung:
3. Emphysema or fibrosis of the lung parenchyma;
4. Pleural effusion or pneumothorax;
5. Thickened pleura.

Altered vocal resonance: Vocal resonance is altered whenever the lung parenchyma is affected by disease and becomes more dense. When normal air containing alveoli are reduced in number or are absent, the spoken words and their consonants are heard better.

a. **Bronchophony:** When the A.V.R. is tested over diseased area which is affected as described above, the 'one, two, three' which is spoken by the patient is heard very clearly, and the sound appears to be coming from the ear piece of the stethoscope rather than the chest piece. However syllables of the sound produced are still not clearly heard.

In conditions where the lung parenchyma is completely solidified, the syllables are heard clearly and then the A.V.R. is known as spoken pectoriloquy.

These abnormalities are heard over the area of consolidation, collapse of lung with a patent bronchus, over a large neoplasm or rarely over massive pleural effusions.

b. **Whispering pectoriloquy:** The patient should be explained how he should whisper. When the patient is asked to whisper 'one, two, three' and the examiner auscultates over the normal lung, practically no sound can be distinguished except a rustling sound. This is due to the fact that a whisper is very low in intensity and the syllables have already merged into each other when the sound is produced.

When this whispering sound can be heard clearly it is known as 'whispering pectoriloquy'. It is present in the same conditions which cause spoken pectoriloquy.

It indicates a massive consolidation of the lung or a large cavity which is communicating with a bronchus.

c. **Aegophony :** When the A.V.R. is heard as a nasal sound over the thorax (it can be compared to the bleating of a sheep) it is known as aegophony. It is usually heard over the area above the level of pleural effusion. It is supposed to be due to relaxation of alveolar walls immediately above the level of the effusion and hence a change in their normal selective transmission. It is sometimes heard over consolidation and lung cavities partially filled with exudates.

9. Respiratory System — Common Disorders Encountered

Common disease processes affecting the respiratory system:

PLEURISY

Definition: Inflammation of pleura.

Types of pleurisy: i. Dry pleurisy.
ii. Pleurisy with effusion.

i. **Dry pleurisy:** All the conditions causing pleurisy with effusion can give rise to dry pleurisy either at the onset or during the time of absorption.

ii. **Pleurisy with effusion:** The following discussion includes all the conditions in which fluid is present in pleural cavity. The fluid can either be exudate or transudate. Transudate in the pleural cavity is usually secondary to cardiac failure or it may be associated with generalised anasarca.

A. Causes of transudate: (hydrothorax)

1. Congestive cardiac failure.
2. Hypoproteinemia—
   a. Nutritional,
   b. Renal causes - Nephrotic syndrome,
   c. Cirrhosis of the liver.
3. Polyserositis;
4. Associated with ovarian tumour (Meighs's syndrome);
5. Phantom tumour.

Usually an interlobar effusion associated with C.C.F. disappears and can re-appear depending on the cardiac decompensation.

B. Causes of exudate:

1. **Primary tuberculosis of the pleura:**
   Though labelled as idiopathic in the past, a biopsy of the pleura can be done to demonstrate the typical tubercle lesions.

2. **Secondary:**
   a. **Due to extension of a disease process from the lungs:**
      i. Infective: pneumonia, lung abscess or bronchiectasis.
      ii. Neoplastic : bronchogenic carcinoma, secondary deposits in the lungs.
      iii. Vascular : infection of lungs.

   b. **Extension from the parietes:**
      i. Trauma to the thoracic wall.
      ii. Extension from pericarditis.
      iii. Mediastinal diseases like oesophageal rupture.
      iv. Diseases of the ribs.

      Osteomyelitis either tuberculous or non-tuberculous.

   c. **Sub-diaphragmatic diseases:**
      i. Amoebic or pyogenic liver abscess (sympathetic effusion)
      ii. Acute pancreatitis (peculiarly acute pancreatitis following alcoholic intake leads to left-sided effusion)
      iii. Subphrenic abscess.

   d. **Malignant disease of the pleura:**
      i. Primary mesotheliomas (rare),

ii. Secondary deposits in the pleura.

e. **Obstruction to the thoracic duct:**
   i. Trauma,
   ii. Glands pressing on the thoracic duct,
   iii. Filariasis.

Symptoms:

1. **Onset:** a. Sudden: with high fever, pleural pain and breathing difficulty due to 'catching type of pain'.
   b. Gradual: The first manifestation may be dyspnea due to accumulation of fluid in the pleural cavity causing diminution of the pulmonary vital capacity.

2. **Other symptoms:**
   a. Cough: Usually short bouts of cough.
   Dry unproductive in type.
   May aggravate the pain due to pleural inflammation.
   b. Dyspnea : Gradually progressive.
   Patient may find difficulty in lying down especially on the unaffected side.

3. **Systemic symptoms:** (Due to infection)
   Fever
   Loss of appetite
   Loss of weight
   Asthenia

4. **Past history:** a. May give a history suggestive of pulmonary tuberculosis in the past.
   b. History of the causative lesion in secondary effusion.

5. **Family history:** Tuberculosis in the family members or associates.

6. **Examination:**

A. General:
   i. May show no abnormality.
   ii. Cervical lymphadenopathy may be present.
   iii. Anaemia.
   iv. Clubbing: Mild if associated with pulmonary tuberculosis. Marked if associated with suppurative lung diseases like bronchiectasis, lung abscess, empyema or malignancy.
   v. Edema of feet is present in associated cardiac or other secondary conditions.

B. **Respiratory system:**

Inspection:

1. **Shape and size of the chest:**
   a. Asymmetrical deformity on the side of lesion may be seen as bulging of the intercostal spaces in massive effusion.
   b. Rarely fullness of the hypochondrium.

2. **Respiratory movements:**
   a. Diminished on the affected side.
   b. In small effusions, the only sign may be a slight delay or lag when the respiratory movements are initiated.

3. **Position of the apex beat and trachea:**
   a. Apex beat is pushed to the opposite side of the effusion.
   b. May not be visible if pushed below the rib.
   c. Cardiac pulsation may be seen on the right side as a massive left-sided effusion produces a marked shift.
   d. Trachea is shifted to the opposite side causing a prominence of the sternomastoid muscle on the side to which it is displaced (Trail's sign).

Palpation:

1. Confirmation of the diminished movements and the shift of apex beat.
2. Shift of the trachea should be confirmed by palpation.
3. Palpable pleural rub.
4. T.V.F. is diminished over the effusion.

Percussion:

1. Stony dull note over the effusion.

2. Ellis 'S' shaped curve can be demonstrated.
3. Grocco's triangle—triangle of dullness on the opposite side of the pleural effusion.
4. Garland's triangle—area of resonance above the level of effusion.
5. Obliteration of the normal resonance of Traube's semilunar space in left-sided effusion.

Auscultation:

1. Air entry diminished or absent over the effusion.
2. Character of the breath sounds.
   a. Vesicular (diminished in intensity) when breath sounds are heard,
   b. Rarely bronchial if the effusion is massive,
   c. Pleural rub may be heard,
   d. Diminished A.V.R.
   e. Aegophony immediately above the level of pleural effusion,
   f. Rarely bronchophony and whispering pectoriloquy if the effusion is massive.

Investigations:

1. **Blood count with E.S.R.**
   May show leucocytosis indicating a pyogenic or acute tuberculous infection. E.S.R. raised. It has more of prognostic significance.

2. **X-Ray chest :** PA view : (Pls 9.1 a & b)
   a. Obliteration of the costophrenic angle is the only abnormality in minimal effusions,
   b. Dense homogeneous opacity with a concave margin extending highest in the axilla,
   c. Shift of the mediastinum to the opposite side.

3. **Examination of pleural fluid:**
   Most important investigation as a diagnostic aid.
   Indications for pleural tapping.
   a. **Diagnostic:** Every pleural effusion should be tapped for determining its exact nature.
   b. **Therapeutic:**
      i. When there is associated cardiac / respiratory embarrassment manifested by severe dyspnea, orthopnea or tachycardia.
      ii. Any effusion with the upper level of effusion at the second intercostal space.
      iii. Bilateral pleural effusions.
      iv. Whenever the fluid is infected. (Repeated drainage should be done or a continuous intercostal drain should be used).
      v. Haemorrhagic effusions.
      vi. Effusions which do not get absorbed in a short period of time (to prevent adhesions and permanent collapse).

Treatment:

1. **General:**
   a. Bed rest either in the hospital or in the house.
   b. High protein diet.

2. **Specific:**
   a. Depends on the causative lesion.
   b. Anti-tuberculosis therapy depending on the regime used.

3. **Corticosteroids:**
   Usually added to the anti-tuberculosis treatment to promote rapid absorption of the pleural fluids.

PNEUMOTHORAX

Pneumothorax means presence of air in the pleural cavity.

Etiology:

1. Following rupture of pulmonary tubercle focus.
2. Rupture of an emphysematous bulla.
3. Following trauma to the chest-wall :
   i. Penetrating injury;
   ii. Fracture of the rib and the pulmonary

injury due to the fractured end of the rib;
iii. Crush injury;
iv. Following pleural paracentesis.
4. Rupture of a congenital cyst in the lung.

Types of penumothorax

1. Spontaneous
2. Tension —closed ball valve
   open — brancho pleural fistula
3 Catamenial —a type of spontaneous pneumothorax; occurs at the time of menstruation. Right side more affected than left. Pathogenesis —obscure, may be related to intrathoracic endometriosis.

Symptoms:

Onset:

i. Usually sudden with acute breathlessness and pain in the chest on the affected side (spontaneous or closed).
ii. May be gradual onset of breathlessness if the leak is slow especially when associated with pulmonary tuberculosis (spontaneous or closed).
iii. Rapidly progressive dyspnea may present as peripheral circulatory failure due to marked lowering of cardiac output. It is medical emergency.

The patient will complain of—

i. Progressive dyspnea (especially in case of tension pneumothorax).
ii. Cough - dry non-productive.
iii. Rapid progress to cardiorespiratory embarrassment if the pneumothorax is of the tension variety.

Past history:

i. Suggestive of pulmonary tuberculosis
ii History of chronic bronchitis with emphysema

Signs:

Respiratory system:

Inspection:

i. Shape and size of the chest. Asymmetrical deformity due to bulging of the intercostal spaces if pneumothorax is massive.
ii. Respiratory movements: Diminished on the affected side.
iii. Position of the apex beat and trachea: Shift of the mediastinum on the opposite side. Sternomastoid more prominent on the opposite side.

Palpation:

i. Confirmation of the shift of the apex beat and trachea to the opposite side of the lesion.
ii. Diminished or absent T.V.F.

Percussion:

i. Hyperresonant note on percussion.
ii. May obliterate the cardiac or hepatic dullness depending on the side and extent to which it is affected.

Auscultation:

i. Air entry diminished or absent on the affected side.
ii. A.V.R. diminished or absent.
iii. Coin test can be elicited on the affected side.
iv. Amphoric breath sounds in open pneumothorax.
v. Gurgling sound heard over fistula in open pneumothorax.

Investigations:

X-Ray chest P A view: (Pl. 9.2)

i. Shows a transluscent picture on the affected side.
ii. No vascular markings of the lungs or no lung tissue can be seen in this area.
iii. Sharp clearly defined rib margins as compared to the normal side. Intercostal spaces widened on the affected side.
iv. Lung which is seen as a small rounded opacity near the mediastinum.
v. The other lung may show evidence of pulmonary tuberculosis or emphysema.
vi. Shift of mediastinum to the opposite side.

Treatment:

1. If there is no cardiorespiratory embarrassment
   i. Bed rest;
   ii. Cough suppressants;
   iii. Anti-T.B. therapy should be started if there is evidence of any tuberculous focus.
2. Withdrawal of air from the pleural cavity by means of a needle and syringe or by the way of a needle connected to under water drainage tube if there is any severe or progressive dyspnea and tachycardia (tension pneumothorax).
3. In case of closed (spontaneous) pneumothorax, air should be removed only if collapse of the lung is marked and if air does not get absorbed in seven days.
4. In case of open pneumothorax surgical help is required to drain the air.

HYDROPNEUMOTHORAX

Hydropneumothorax means presence of air and fluid both in the pleural cavity.

Etiology:

1. Any condition which causes pneumothorax may lead to hydropneumothorax. Especially if the opening in the ruptured lung remains patent and the pleural cavity gets secondarily infected.
2. Rupture of a lung abscess or infected lung cyst.
3. Following tapping of pleural effusion or empyema.

Symptoms:

1. Sudden onset of dyspnea.
2. Cough with pleural pain on the affected side.
3. Sudden increase in dyspnea in a patient who is previously suffering from respiratory diseases.
4. Fever if hydropneumothorax is secondarily infected and other constitutional symptoms, so also those pertaining to other systems.
5. May complain of a splashing sound in the chest especially on movement.

Signs:

Inspection and palpation:

Inspection and palpation will reveal the same signs as those elicited in a patient having pneumothorax.

Percussion:

1. There will be an area of dullness with a tympanitic note above the level of dullness. The position of the dull note will vary depending on the position of the patient. If the patient is sitting up, the dullness will be at the base with a horizontal upper level. If the patient is lying down, the dullness will shift as shown in Fig. 8.13 and the tympanitic note will be above the dullness.

The line demarcating these two — that is dull and tympanitic note will be horizontal and not concave (The upper level of dullness in pleural effusion is curved and shows a rise in the axilla).

2. Coin sound can be elicited over the 'pneumo' part of the hydropneumothorax.

Auscultation:

1. Air entry diminished on the affected side.
2. Breath sounds vesicular if heard.
3. Succussion splash followed by tinkling sound which may be heard without the aid of a stethoscope.

Investigations:

X-ray chest PA (Pl. 9.3)

1. Shows a translucent area as seen in pneumothorax above and a uniform homogeneous opacity below.
2. The level of the uniform opacity indicating fluid is horizontal.
3. Shift of the mediastinum to the opposite side.

Treatment:

1. Rest.
2. Paracentesis : a. if the patient is dyspneic.
   b. for diagnostic purposes.

3. Anit-tuberculous line of treatment if the exudate is predominantly lymphocytic.
4. If pyogenic, culture and antibiotic sensitivity of the fluid should be done to find out the most effective antibiotic.
5. Continuous intercostal drainage to prevent permanent collapse of the lung especially in pyopneumothorax.
6. Decortication of the lung (surgical intervention) if the lung does not expand even after drainage for sufficient period of time.

PNEUMONIA

Pneumonia or lobar pneumonia can be defined as inflammation of the lung parenchyma usually affecting one lobe.

Bronchopneumonia is more lobular in distribution, may spread to the parenchyma from the bronchi and is very often bilateral.

Etiology:

1. Age and sex:

Occurs at both extremes of age, i.e., in infants and in old age when the resistance to the infection is poor. Paradoxically healthy adult males are affected especially following exposure to cold breeze or trauma.

The incidence is higher in:

i. Extremely cold climate.
ii. In persons suffering from chronic nephritis, diabetes, cirrhosis and chronic alcoholism.
iii. In persons having chronic upper respiratory tract infections.
iv. Following operations on the upper respiratory tract.
v. In persons suffering from left ventricular failure.

II. Organisms which can cause penumonia:

Streptococcus pneumoniae (pneumococcus)
Staphylococcus aureus
Streptococcus pyogenes
Klebsiella pneumoniae (Friedlander bacilli)
Francisella tularensis (Tularemia)
Escherichia coli
Proteus species
Pseudomonas aeruginosa
Haemophilus influenza
Pasteurella multocida
Mycoplasma pneumoniae
Pneumovirus (Respiratory syncytial virus)
Chlamydia pisttaci
Mycobacterium tuberculosis
Fungal infections : Histoplasma capsulatum
Blastomyces dermatitidis
Coccidiodes immitis.

III. Associated with collagen disorders:

1. With systemic lupus arrhtematosis.
2. Rheumatic fever and rheumatoid arthritis
3. With polyarteritis nodosa.

IV. After exposure to toxic gases.

V. After ingestion of kerosene and paraffin or peleum (aspiration pneumonia).

VI. Radiation pneumonia.

Symptoms

1. May be preceded by a mild upper respiratory infection or coryza.
2. Onset abrupt in 80% of the cases with chills and high fever and tachycardia.
3. Cough with pleuritic pain over the site of affection.
4. Shallow grunting respirations with or without dyspnea.
5. Sputum rusty or frankly blood stained.
6. Cyanosis and sweating.
7. Mental confusion and toxic psychosis.

Signs:

General Examination:

1. Elevated temperature.
2. Rapid respiratory rate with *alae nasi* participating in the respiratory movements.
3. Tachycardia with low B.P.
4. Cyanosis may be present.
5 *Herpes labialis* commonly seen — when

streptococcus pneumoniae are causative organisms.

Respiratory system:

Inspection

1. Size and shape of the chest — normal
2. Respiratory movements — restricted on the affected side.
3. No shift of the apex beat and trachea.

Palpation:

1. Respiratory movements diminished on affected side.
2. Tactile vocal fremitus increased when pneumonic process has progressed to consolidation.
3. Pleural rub may be palpable.

Percussion:

1. A dull or impaired note over the area which is affected.

Auscultation:

1. Bronchial breath sounds of tubular type when consolidation is established, otherwise bronchovesicular or harsh breath sounds are heard over developing consolidation or resolving pneumonia.
2. Crepitation and rales always heard.
3. A.V.R. shows bronchophony and whispering pectoriloquy.

Investigations:

1. **X-ray chest PA :** (Pl. 9.4)
   a. Shows a homogeneous opacity in the affected area.
   b. Usually affecting one lobe and appears triangular in shape.
   c. No shift of the mediastinum.

2. **Blood count:**
   a. Polymorphonuclear leucocytosis if bacterial and nontuberculous
   b. Raised E. S. R.

3. **Sputum:**
   a. Shows polymorphonuclear leucocytes.
   b. R.B.C. in sputum.
   c. Sputum should be cultured for isolating organisms and their sensitivity to antibiotics should be determined.

Complications:

a. **Pulmonary:** 1. Atelactasis of whole or part of the lobe. 2. delayed resolution causing fibrosis. 3. lung abscess.

b. **Spread to the adjacent structures:** 1. Pleural effusion. 2. empyema, 3. pericarditis.

c. **Metastatic spread:** 1. Arthritis. 2. endocarditis. 3. meningitis.

d. **Alimentary:**
   1. Paralytic ileus (toxic). 2. acute dilatation of the stomach. 3. jaundice due to hepatitis.

e. **Toxic:**
   1. Peripheral circulatory failure.
   2. convulsions (especially in infants).
   3. psychosis.

Treatment:

General:

1. Bed rest.
2. Liquid or light diet.
3. Cough suppressants if severe cough giving rise to pleuritic pain or severe discomfort.
4. Oxygen therapy if cyanosis.
5. Tranquilisers
6. Prevention and treatment of peripheral circulatory failure.

Specific:

1. Antibiotics depending on the type of pneumonia.

BRONCHIECTASIS

Bronchiectasis can be defined as a permanent pathological dilatation and distortion of the bronchi in which infection is a very common supervening complicating factor.

Two varietics of bronchiectasis can be seen on pathological examination. (Fig. 9.1)

1. Saccular (cystic) which usually affects the large proximal bronchi.
2. Fusiform (cylindrical) which affects relatively, the smaller bronchi.

Development of bronchiectasis follows an infection or obstruction of bronchi leading to collapse of the affected part of the lung. Most often both these factors play a combined role together in its development. A collapse of a segment or a lobe results in an increased negative pressure pulling on the walls of the bronchi present in that segment. If the walls are weakened by inflammatory process, they are easily dilated and give rise to bronchiectatic changes.

Etiology :

1. **Congenital :**
   a. Associated with cystic fibrosis.
   b. Kartagener's syndrome: a triad comprising bronchiectasis, dextrocardia and sinusitis.

2. **Acquired :**
   a. Childhood: respiratory infections, influenza, measles, whooping cough, pneumonia, acute bronchitis.
   b. Adults: Usually following bronchial obstruction.
      i. Endobronchial obstruction by foreign bodies, or endobronchial tuberculosis or bronchial adenoma adenocarcinoma.
      ii. Compression by hilar lymph nodes or tumours.
   c. Associated with chronic infections in the lungs : Pulmonary tuberculosis or chronic pyogenic infections.

Symptoms:

Depend upon the presence of infection and anatomical locations of the defect in the lungs.

1. No symptoms: Especially if situated in the upper lobes and when there is no secondary infection.
2. Recurrent haemoptysis without any other manifestation like chronic cough and expectoration bronchiectasis sicca, i.e., dry bronchiectasis.
3. Recurrent bouts of cough and expectoration simulating recurrent attacks of bronchitis or penumonia.
4. Classic picture of cough with large amount of expectoration which is maximum early in the morning on waking up. Recurrent haemoptysis with general symptoms of a chronic infection like fever, loss of weight.

(The reason for the expectoration being maximum in amount in the morning is that, during sleep the infected material tends to collet in the bronchiectatic portion. As these areas are lined with squamous epithelium instead of the usual ciliary epithelium, cough reflex is not elicited. On waking up, due to the change of posture, the infected material drains into the normal bronchi eliciting the cough response which results in

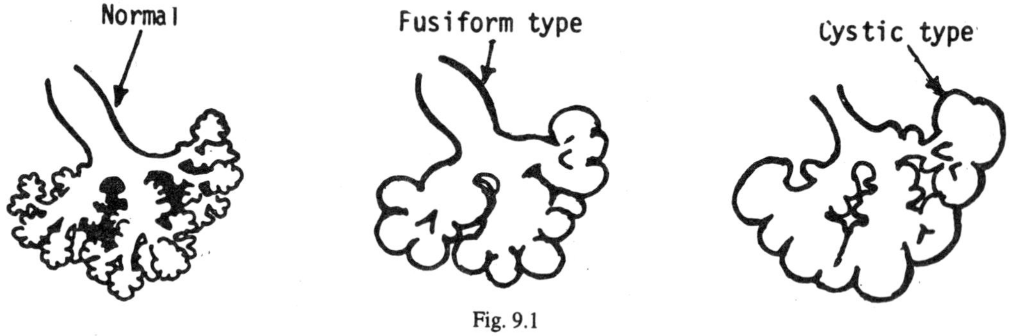

Fig. 9.1
Types of Bronchiectasis.

violent cough and expectoration).

5. Asthenia due to chronic ill health.

Signs:

General Examination:

1. Dyspnea and orthopnea if the disease is extensive.
2. Clubbing of the fingers.
3. Pulmonary osteoarthropathy.
4. Anaemia.
5. Sinusitis.
6. Wasting and aedema of feet due to hypoproteinemia.

Respiratory System:

Inspection, palpation and percussion may not reveal any particular abnormality except that emphysema is very common accompaniment of the long-standing bronchiectasis.

Auscultation:

1. Bronchovesicular (harsh) breathing.
2. Presence of typical coarse rales which are described as leathery in nature.
   These rales change or alter on coughing but do not disappear.
3. Low pitched bronchial breathing — if cystic bronchiectasis (signs of cavity).

Complications:

1. Recurrent attacks of pneumonia.
2. Haemoptysis (Large bouts of recurrent haemorrhage may require surgical intervention).
3. Lung abscess : When infection from the bronchiectatic area spreads to the normal lung, abscess can result.
4. Cor Pulmonale : Extensive bronchiectasis leads to obstruction of the pulmonary circulation resulting in cor pulmonale and later on right ventricular failure (commonest mode of death).
5. Brain Abscess : Most common site for a metastatic brain abscess from bronchiectasis is the right frontal lobe.
6. Empyema and pyopneumothorax : Due to rupture of a bronchiectatic lesion into the pleural cavity.
7. Amyloid disease : Secondary amyloidosis due to the chronic suppurative condition in the lungs.

Investigations:

Blood counts:

i. May show presence of anaemia.
ii. Mild leucocytosis.
iii. E.S.R. may be raised.

Urine:

No abnormality except proteinuria should point towards amyloidosis.

Electrocardiograph: Shows changes P pulmonale and RT ventricular hypertrophy suggestive of cor pulmonale in long standing cases.

X-Ray chest PA (Pl.9.5) It usually is not very helpful in demonstrating bronchiectasis. However, a small triangular opacity indicating secondary pneumonic consolidation may be seen.

Cystic bronchiectasis will produce ring shadows with fluid levels.

Bronchography: It is done to determine the extent of bronchiectasis.

Bronchoscopy: It should be done if bronchial obstruction is thought to be the cause of bronchiectasis.

Sputum : Routine examinations, as well as a culture to isolate the organisms should be done and their sensitivity to the various antibiotics should be ascertained. This is a very helpful measure for chemotherapy.

Pulmonary function tests: These should be carried out particularly in those patients who are to be considered for surgical resection of the brochiectatic area.

Treatment :

1. Diet: Should be high in proteins and calories. (The chronic expectoration results in a loss of proteins and they should be adequately replaced).
2. Postural drainage: Every patient should be taught to cough out the sputum daily in the morning by adopting a posture which will drain the affected portion of the lung. This should be assisted by deep breathing exercises.
3. Expectorants and agents which liquify sputum (mucolytic agents) : These should be used either in conjunction with or without antibiotics to facilitate the drainage of the mucoid materials.
4. Steam inhalation with tincture benzoin may help to liquify the sputum.
5. Antibiotics: Ideally the antibiotic to which the organisms in the sputum are sensitive should be used. The course of any given antibiotic should be given in a full dosage and for a sufficiently adequate length of time so that resistance to that particular antibiotic does not develop. It is also advisable to use a different antibiotic when a second or repeat course of antibiotic is required for recurrence of the infections.
6. Surgical treatment: In general surgery should be advised when the bronchiectatic area is localised to one lobe and there are recurrent bouts of infection or haemoptysis. However, the lung function should be adequate before such procedure is undertaken. More than a lobe can also be removed if these functions are adequate.

COLLAPSE OF LUNG

The term collapse of the lung is used clinically to the two types of conditions:

1. Active collapse.
2. Passive collapse.

The term passive collapse is used to describe the collapse of the lung which is secondary to either pleural effusion or pneumothorax. Here the lung is compressed from outside and hence the collapse is secondary to these lesions.

Active collapse is also known as atelectasis. The term atelectasis derived from Greek, means imperfect expansion. The massive collapse is the term used when the whole lung is affected by obstruction to its main bronchus causing active collapse.

Bronchial obstruction is the cause of this condition. The obstruction could be: (Fig. 9.2)

1. Inside the lumen:
   a. Mucus plug;
   b. Foreign bodies.
2. In the wall of the bronchus:
   a. Bronchogenic carcinoma;
   b. Endobronchial tuberculosis;
   c. Bronchial adenoma.
3. Outside the lumen:
   Compression by enlarged hilar glands,
   Aortic aneurysm,
   Mediastinal neoplasms (mass).

The collapse caused by a mucus plug should be understood in detail as it can cause variable physical signs. (Fig. 9.3)

Initiallly, when the mucus plug blocks a bronchus, the segment or lobe peripheral to it collapses and air does not enter the collapsed segment. Due to the inherent elasticity of the alveolar and bronchial tissues, the lung starts collapsing and the air in the affected segment is absorbed. This results in a progressively greater negative pressure being exerted on the collapsed segment and the plug of mucus in some cases is aspirated peripherally. It breaks down into small mucus particles which block the peripheral terminal bronchi. This results in an anatomical condition where the part of the lung remains collapsed but the main bronchus in the affected segment becomes patent. These two variations, i.e., the main bronchus remaining closed or becoming patent gives rise to varying clinical signs.

Symptoms:

These depend upon the amount of lung tissue involved and whether there is any superadded infection. Usually, a massive collapse has a sudden and dramatic onset with severe dyspnea. Patient also complains of chest pain on the affected side with palpitations. Fever and other general symptoms of infection may be complained of, if there is secondary infection.

(As post-operative collapse is a common condition, a sudden onset of dyspnea in an operated patient who was otherwise progressing well, should make the examiner suspicious of this condition.)

Signs:

General Examination:

1. Patient is usually dyspneic or orthopneic.
2. Tachycardia.
3. Cyanosis depending on extent of collapse and acute mode of onset.

Examination of the respiratory system:

1. Shape and size of the chest : There is an asymmetrical deformity produced by either flattening or retraction of chest wall on the affected side.
2. Respiratory movements: Absent or markedly diminished on the affected side.
3. Position of the apex beat and trachea: Both are pulled towards the side of the lesion.

Palpation:

1. Crowding of ribs on the affected side; the intercostal spaces are narrowed as compared to the corresponding other side.
2. Confirmation of the diminished movements as well as the mediastinal shift.
3. Tactile vocal fremitus absent or may be increased (if the bronchus has become patent as described above).

Percussion:

Dull note over the affected segment or side of the chest. If on the left side, elevation of the gastric tympanitic note may be found. Traube's space is shifted laterally.

Auscultation:

If the main bronchus is obstructed:
1. Absent breath sounds
2. A.V.R. not heard.

If the main bronchus becomes patent:
1. Bronchial or tubular breath sounds.
2. Crepitations may be present.
3. Bronchophony and whispering pectoriloquy present.

Investigations:

X-Ray chest PA:

1. Homogeneous opacity involving the whole lung or segment.
2. Narrowing of intercostal spaces and crowding of ribs on the affected side.
3. Shift of the mediastinum to the affected

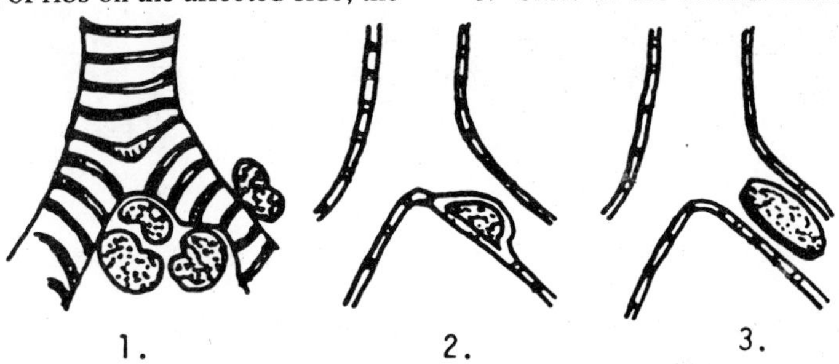

Fig. 9.2
Bronchial Obstruction

1. From outside (extramural) e.g., glands.
2. Within the wall (intramural) e.g., bronchogenic carcinoma, bronchial adenoma, endobronchial tuberculosis.
3. In the lumen (intralumina) e.g., foreign body, mucus plug or thick tenacious secretion.

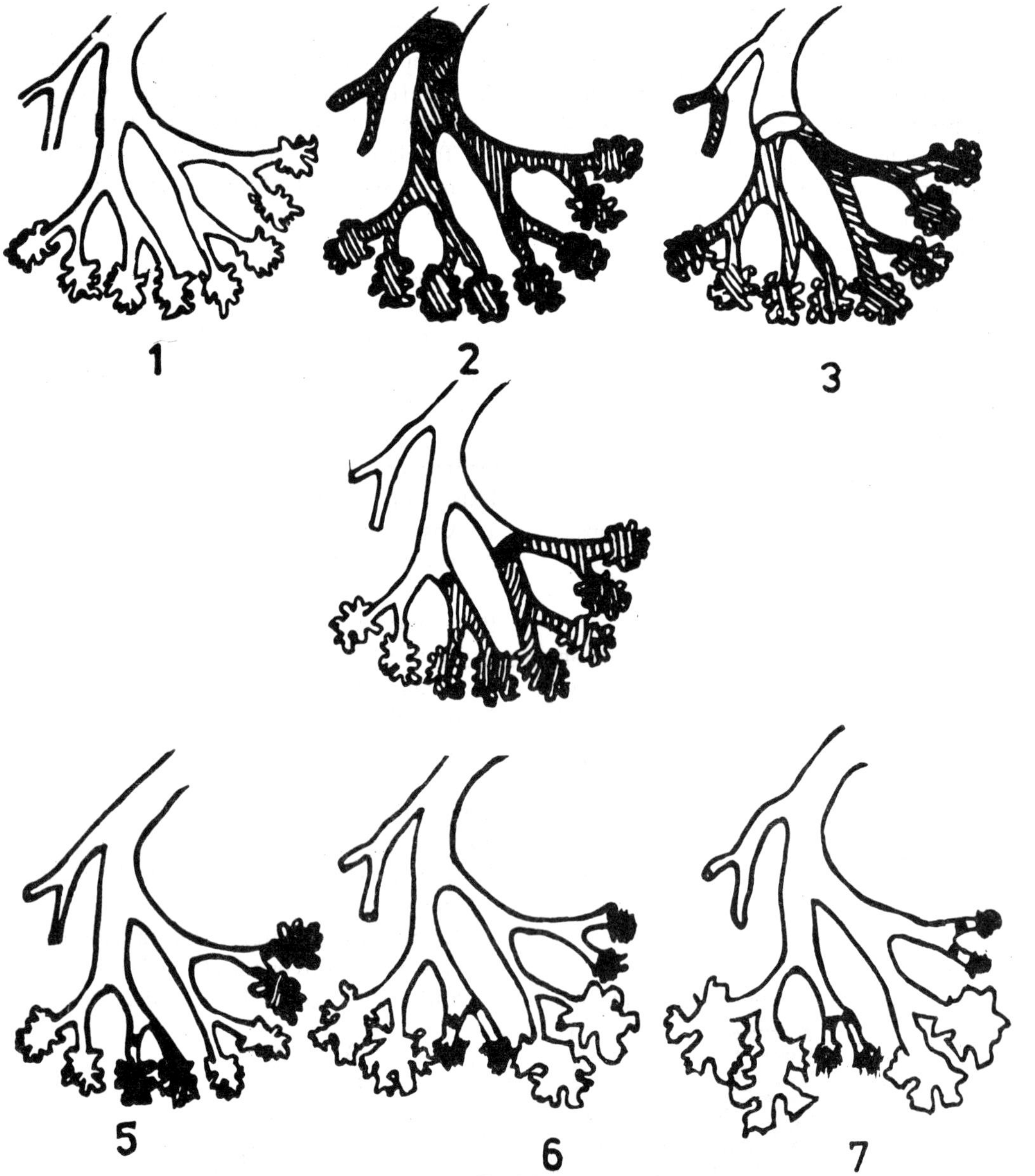

Fig. 9.3

Mucus Plug — causing collapse of lung leading to various sequelae and signs.

1. Normal bronchial tree.
2. Mucus plug completely obstructing the main bronchus, clinically absent breath sounds.
3. Mucus plug moving down the bronchial tree, there is no alteration in size of bronchi.
4. Mucus plug has divided in two parts and obstructed two small bronchii, one segment has escaped obstruction.
5. Few terminal bronchi involved.
6. Mucus plug has not moved further but alveoli are shrinking and unobstructed bronchi have increased in size.
7. Complete collapse of obstructed alveoli and bronchioles with dilatation of bronchi and unobstructed alveoli. Tubular breathing of varying degrees with absence of foreign sounds is seen in stages 3 to 7.

side.

4. In long-standing massive collapse, scoliosis of the spine with concavity towards the affected side.

Bronchoscopy:

1. To determine the cause.
2. If possible to aspirate the mucus plug or removal of the foreigm body which is obstructing the bronchus.

Treatment:

1. Relief of pain and infection if present.
2. Correction of the underlying disease either by medical or surgical means.

LUNG ABSCESS

A lung abscess is described as a lesion in the lung parenchyma containing purulent material.

It is usually a result of a virulent infection. When the

(1) infection is carried in the lungs by way of aspiration of infected material from the upper respiratory tract; or (2) when the inflation of the lung is hampered by mechanical cause; or (3) due to inadequate drainage because of obstruction to the bronchus; (4) due to liver abscess bursting into lung.

Hence, its causes can be classified as :

1. **Necrotising infections caused by specific organisms:**
   Pyogenic:
   Staphylococcus aureus.
   Freidlander's haemolyticus.
   Streptococcus haemolyticus.
   Mycobacteria :
   Mycobacterim tuberculosis.
   Parasitic :
   Entamoeba histolytica.

2. **Due to bronchial obstruction:**
   a. Bronchogenic carcinoma.
   b. Foreign bodies (aspirated from upper respiratory tract).
   c. Mucus plug (either aspirated or from the bronchi).
   d. Bronchostenosis.

3. **Due to vascular embolism:**
   a. Emboli from thrombosed leg veins (prolonged recumbency).
   b. Pulmonary infarction.
   c. Pyaemic lung abscesses.

4. **Traumatic:**
   a. Infected haematoma of the lung.
   b. Penetrating chest injury.

5. **Spread from adjoining structures:**
   a. Spread from amoebic abscess of the liver.
   b. Rarely from paravertebral abscess.

6. Infection in an existing congenital cyst of the lung.

Symptoms:

They depend upon the severity of the condition.

1. Mild rise of temperature with cough, expectoration and mild chest pain or discomfort in chest
2. High hectic fever, severe chest pain, cough, expectoration of foul, large amount of sputum which can be blood stained and symptoms of general toxemia.
   (Lung abscess is three times more common in men than in women).

Signs:

General Examination

1. Fever;
2. Wasting;
3. Anaemia;
4. Foul breath;
5. Marked clubbing of fingers.

Respiratory System:

1. If the abscess cavity is full of infected material, the signs elicited will be similar to those of consolidation.
2. If there is a partial drainage, the following signs will be present:

i. **Percussion:**

A tympanitic note may be elicited if the cavity contains a fair degree of air and if it is superficial. Amphoric resonance may be produced if the cavity is of a large size. If the lung abscess cavity is large and has thin walls and if it is communicating with a bronchus a cracked pot sound may be produced over it on percussion.

ii. **Auscultation:**

Breath sounds will be bronchial in nature and may appear to be having a typical cavernous nature (low pitched). Rales medium and fine are usually heard and rhonchi may also be heard if there is any bronchostenosis.

Investigations:

1. Blood count will show anaemia and a high polymorphonuclear leucocytosis.

2. Sputum: Routine examination will show polymorphonuclear leucocytosis and presence of gram positive cocci or gram negative bacilli.
   Culture and sensitivity to antibiotics must be determined to aid in the management.

3. **X-Ray chest:** (Pl. 9.6) a. Will reveal a homogeneous opacity of consolidation with a radioluscent area in its centre in the initial stages.
   b. After drainage into the bronchus the classical picture of a rounded cavity with horizontal fluid level will be seen.

4. Bronchoscopy should be carried out to determine whether there is any obstruction and if so, to determine its nature. The aspirated material when cultured gives a more correct idea about the nature of the infected organisms.

Treatment:

1. Rest in bed.
2. High protein and high caloric diet.
3. Antibiotic therapy:
   The principles are:
   i. Determining the appropriate antibiotic.
   ii. Should be given in full therapeutic doses.
   iii. Should be continued for an adequate length of time.
4. Physiotherapy:
   i. Postural drainage.
   ii. Deep breathing exercises.
5. Surgical resection:
   Rarely required if early and correct antibiotic therapy is given.
   However, resection should be done in those patients whose cavities do not resolve within a period of 4 weeks.

CHRONIC BRONCHITIS WITH EMPHYSEMA

The word emphysema means an unnatural inflation of a part of lung with air. It means a distension of air spaces distal to the terminal bronchiole with destruction of their septa. It is usually associated with chronic bronchitis.

Pathological classifications:

Two main types of emphysema are described. (Fig. 9.4)

1. **Panlobular:** The alveolar destruction and distension is peripheral and involves the whole of the primary lung lobule. The changes affect the whole of the lung but mainly the bases.

2. **Centrilobular:** Here the distension is restricted to the respiratory bronchiole. Alveolar ducts and the periphery are not involved. These abnormalities are more severe at the lung apices.

Pathogenesis:

There are three important factors in the development of the disease:

1. Lung inflation caused by obstruction to expiration.

2. Loss of elasticity due to stress and strain of coughing or asthma.
3. Lowered resistance of the lung to wear and tear which increases with advancing age.

Hence a combination of chronic bronchitis, bronchial asthma and emphysema is extremely common. Both these processes gradually lead to progressive constriction of bronchi — diminution of vital capacity and secondary cardiac symptoms — Chronic obstructive pulmonary disease. (COPD)

Symptoms:

Progressively increasing breathlessness is the only symptom of emphysema with chronic bronchitis.

Signs:

Patient is orthopneic; Cyanosis may be present; Clubbing of nails.

Signs of CCF
- — Edema of face;
- — Suffused face;
- — Apprehensive look;
- — Edema of feet;
- — Enlarged tender liver.

RS
- — Barrel shaped chest;
- — Widened subcostal angle;
- — Hardly any expansion of chest during inspiration;
- — Rhonchi and fine crepitations may be present;
- — Bronchovesicular breathing.

CVS
- — Heart sounds appear distant and muffled
- — P_2 may be loud

CNS
- — confused mental state

X-Ray

Lungs overinflated
Ribs appear horizontal
Excessive transluscency of lung fields;
Emphysematous bullae present;
Enlarged heart;
Pulmonary conus prominent.

ECG
- — P Pulmonale;
  Rt axis deviation;
  Rt ventricular enlargement.

Blood
- — Routine blood count and blood gas analysis.

Treatment:

No specific treatment;

Symptomatic treatment with diuretics, bronchodilators, tranquillisers and steam inhalation and mycolytic; agents to liquify sticky sputum and antibiotic as and when required.

CAVITATION IN LUNG

A pulmonary abscess is a collection of pus in lung parenchyma resulting from suppurative

1. Alveoli, 2. Respiratory Bronchiole, 3. Terminal Bronchiole

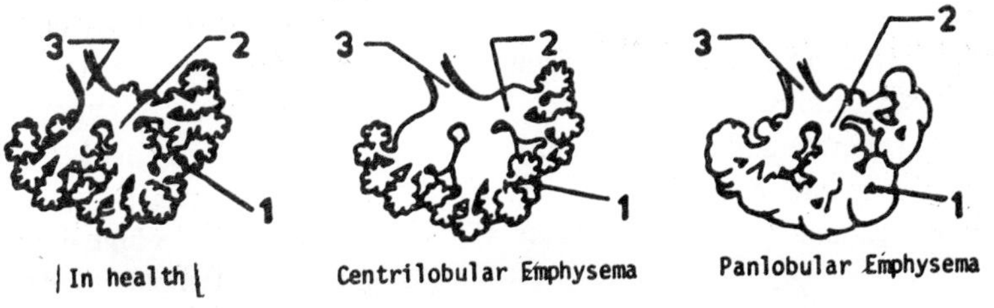

Fig. 9.4
Lung Parenchyma in health, and in emphysema.

necrosis due to bacteria, fungi or parasites. The necrosis which is suppurative may be a result of primary infection or infection secondary to obstruction of the bronchi, or secondry infection of infarcted lung tissue. Cavity is sequelae after the contents are coughed out.

Etiology:

1. Bacteria:
   - *Mycobacterium tuberculosis*
   - Staphylococcus aureus
   - Klebsiella pneumoniae
   - Friedlander's bacilli
   - *Streptococcus* } common at extremes
   - *Pneumoniae* } of age — infancy and old people

2. Fungi:
   Actonomyces israelii
   Histoplasma capsulatum

3. Parasite:
   Entamoeba histolytica
   Echinococcus granulosa. (hydatid cyst infected)

As tuberculous cavity is most commonly seen — more details are given regarding the same.

Prediposing factors:

- Malnutrition
- Increased stress on body as occurs
  During — pregnancy
  — childbirth
  — puberty
- Diabetes mellitus
- Overcrowding and poor sanitary conditions
- Inadequately treated or untreated primary tuberculosis in children
- H/o. recent operation like tonsillectomy.
  H/o. having undergone general anaesthesia (aspiration pneumonia leading to abscess).

Age:

Young people, especially girls around puberty, old persons and diabetics are especially susceptible to tuberculosis.

Symptoms:

In tuberculous cavity:
- Low fever of moderately long duration;
- Night sweats — excessively disproportionate to the rise of temperature;
- Loss of weight;
- Poor appetite;
- General malaise;
- H/o. contact or H/o. tuberculosis in past;
- Recent childbirth.

In other cases
- High hectic fever;
- Cough with blood tinged sputum.

Cough:

Mild to moderate productive in nature — not related to time.

Cough and expectoration become more severe as the disease advances.

Hemoptysis may be just streaks of blood or may be copious in amount and it may be the first symptom which brings the patient to the doctor.

If persistant fever is present in mother after childbirth it should arouse suspicion of tuberculosis. At times fever may be continuous and high (Typhoid onset of tuberculosis).

Common sites of cavitation —
- apex of the lobe (because oxygen supply and drainage of apex of lung is normally less as compared to other parts)
- right upper lobe

General Examination:

- Thin build;
- Skin wrinkled because of recent loss of weight;
- Pallor;
- Clubbing of nails (in tuberculosis and pyogenic abscess);
- Slight fever or high fever;
- Cervical lymphadenopathy;
- Tachycardia;
- Toxic look (acute cases).

RS

— Diminished movements on affected side.

Inspection

— Retraction of intercostal spaces at the affected side.

Palpation

— Diminished movements on affected side;
— Crowding of ribs and narrowing of intercostal spaces may be present on affected side;
— TVF increased.

Percussion

— Hyperresonant note at the site of lesion;
— Note may be impaired if cavity is filled with fluid;
— Kronig's isthmus shows dull note if lesion is at right apex;
— Vocal resonance increased;
— Whispering pectoriloquy may be present.

Investigations:

Blood:

CBC — normal or mild leucocytosis
ESR — raised.

Sputum:

For presence of AFB;
AFB culture and sensitivity especially where the patient has taken irregular treatment in the past or where the patient is in contact with resistant case. Sputum culture and antibiotic sensitivity when superadded infection exists or when other infection is suspected.

X-ray:

Cavity with surrounding infiltration (Pl. 9.8)
Fluid level may be seen.

Activity of the cavity is judged by —

— General symptoms
  — fever
  — malaise;
— Raised ESR;
— Presence of AFB in sputum.

Complications:

— Pneumothorax;
— Empyema;
— Hydropyopneumothorax;
— Cachexia.

Management:

General like
— Reduction of activity;
— Complete bed rest if lesion is extensive;
— High protein diet;

Anti-tuberculous line of treatment.
Improvement is assessed by —

1. Weight gain;
2. General feeling of well being;
3. Lowering of ESR;
4. Regression of lesion on x-ray;
5. Sputum repeated on three successive days showing absence of AFB.

Drugs:

— Antibiotic depending on culture, antibiotic sensitivity.
— Expectorants to liquify sputum and to facilitate cough.
— Anti-tuberculosis drugs.

CHEMOTHERAPY OF TUBERCULOSIS

Principles of therapy:

The anti-T.B. agents owe their effectiveness to specific interference with various vital functions of the tubercle bacilli without harming the host; for example, isoniazid inhibits D.N.A. synthesis and intermediary metabolism of Mycobacterium tuberculosis ad ethambutol and rifampicin interfere with R.N.A. synthesis.

1. The first principle of treatment is to choose drugs to which the organisms are susceptible. The reason for this lies in the natural history of tuberculosis in man. Most cases develop from infections that were implanted years before and most primary infections are acquired from such re-activated cases before any therapy has been administered. In a new case, therapy with two or three drugs may be initiated without awaiting the

results of susceptible studies, though such studies should be performed as a guide to rational choice of drugs as resistance can be found to one or more drugs used.

2. The second principle is always to inflict multiple biochemical lesions on the bacilli simultaneously at the outset. Active tuberculous lesions frequently contain a large number of organisms and thus enough resistant mutants to permit the emergence of clinical resistance to any single drug, is easily possible. This can be avoided only by using several drugs in conjunction at the outset.

3. The third principle is that if the clinician feels that a particular regimen is failing, he should never add only a single drug to the existing drug therapy.

4. The fourth principle is that the therapy must be continued long enough to permit slow healing processes of the body to proceed to completion. This requires 6-18 months depending on the short or long course regime used. If therapy is discontinued as soon as the patient feels well, bacteriologic tests are negative and x-ray shows improvement, likelihood of reactivation is great because anatomic healing lags far behind these favourable signs. For treatment of tuberculosis with different regimes appropriate books may be referred to.

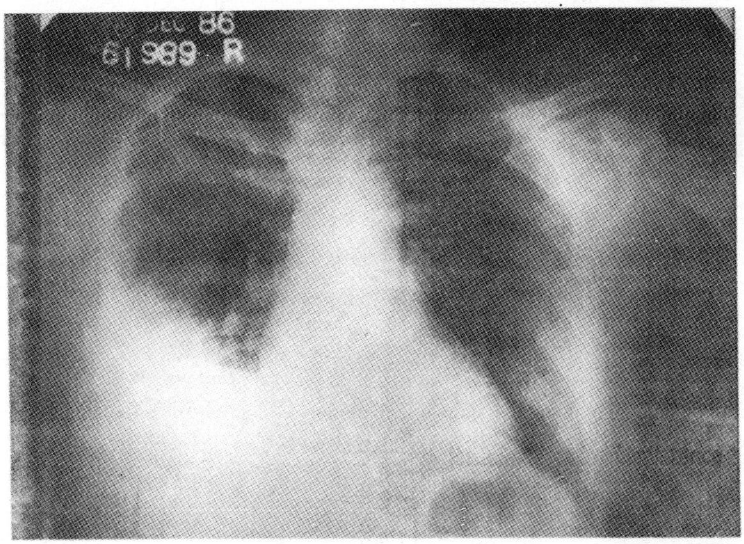

P1. 9. 1a Right sided pleural effusion causing minimal shift of mediastinum to opposite side

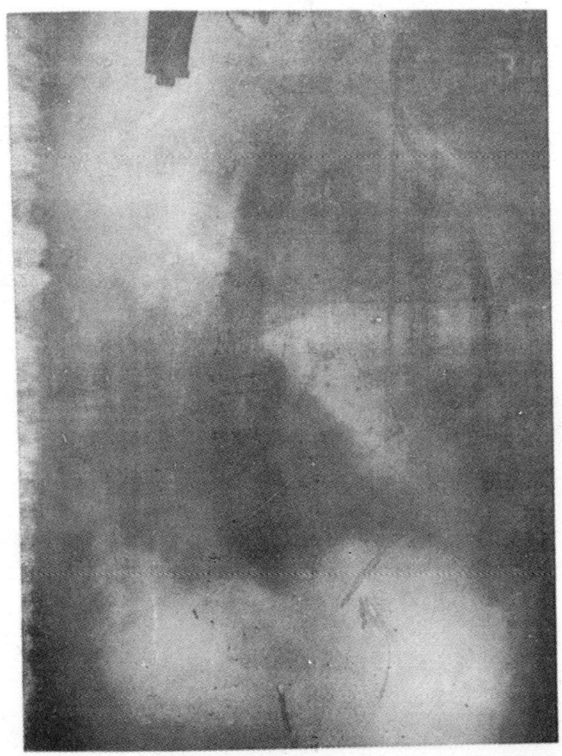

P1. 9.1b Interlobar effusion on right side as viewed from lateral side.

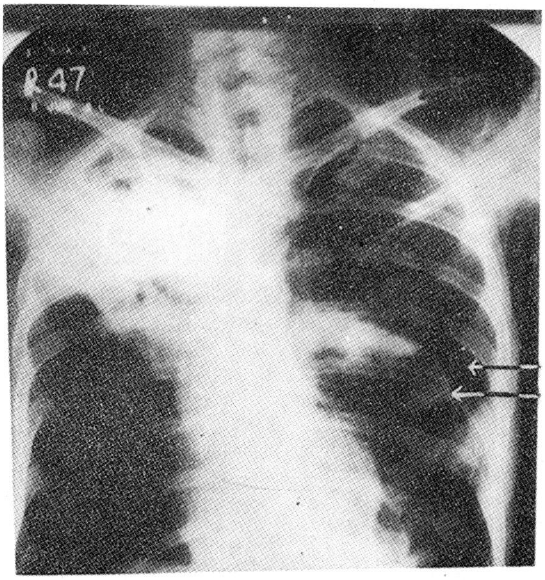

Pl.9.2 Pneumothorax

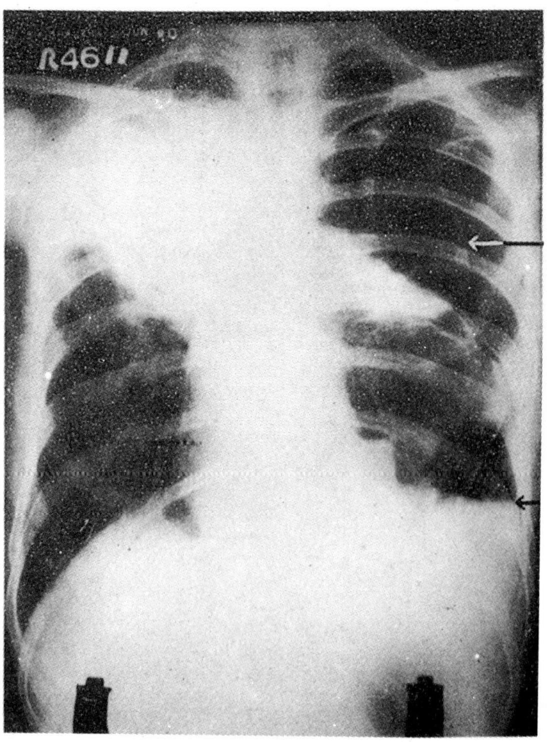

Pl. 9.3 Left sided Hydropneumothorax

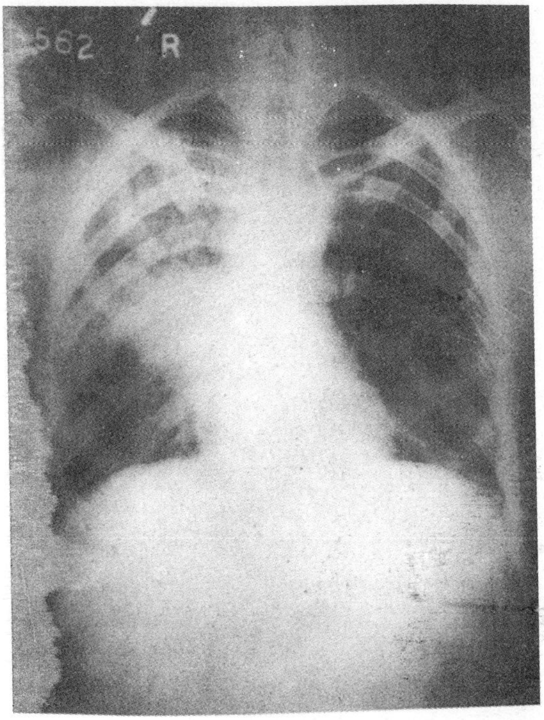

Pl. 9.4 Pneumonia

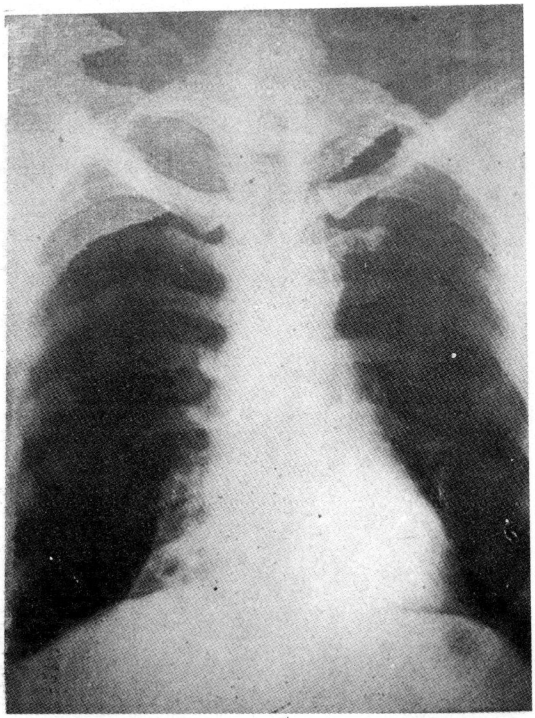

Pl.9.5 Bronchiectasis right base with collapse of related segment.

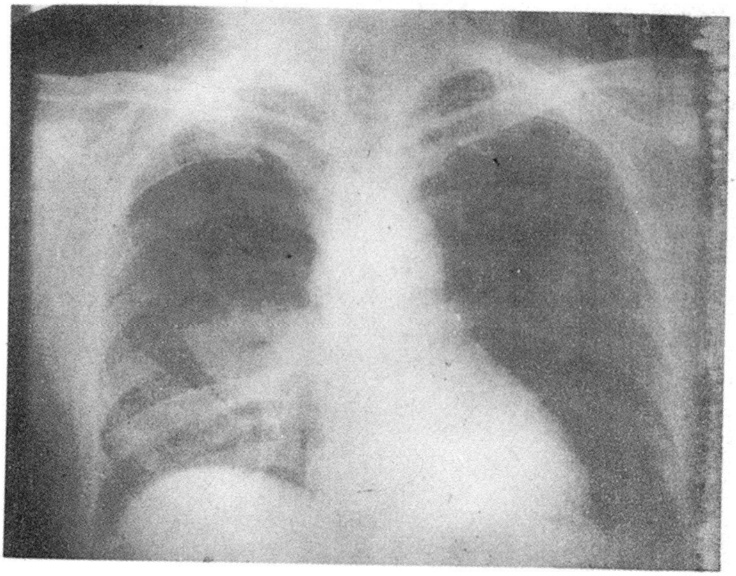

Pl. 9.6 Lung abscess. Note the thick walls of the cavity.

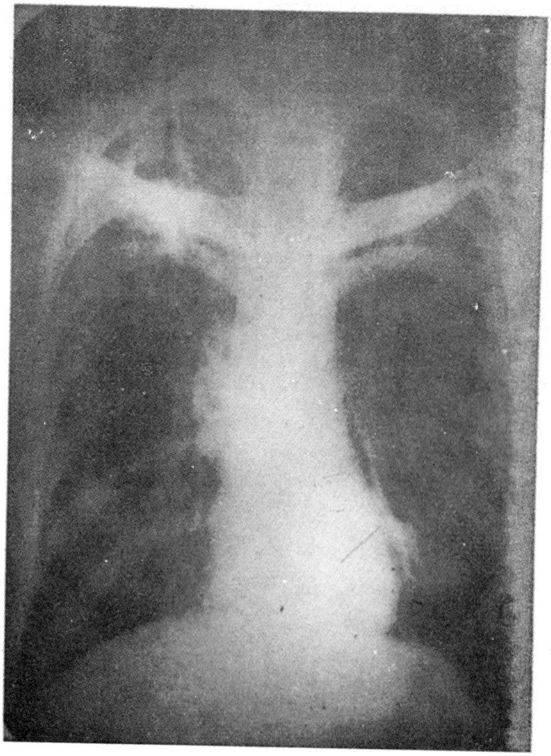

Pl. 9.7 Tuberculosis - Cavity at apex - right lung upper lobe
Note the thin walls of the cavity as opposed to thick walls of lung (abscess), in Pl. 9.6

10. Respiratory System — Common Diagnostic and/or Therapeutic Procedure

Pleural Tapping

I. Indications:

A. Diagnostic

— To confirm the presence and nature of fluid.

To culture the fluid for identifying organisms.

B. Therapeutic

1. Massive effusion when progressively breathless.
2. Tension pneumothorax.
3. Cardiac temponade — manifesting as tachycardia and orthopnea.
4. Bilateral effusions.
5. Any effusion with upper level reaching 2nd intercostal space.
6. Haemorrhagic effusion.
7. If fluid does not get absorbed in short period.
8. To prevent adhesions.
9. Liver abscess bursting into pleural cavity.

II. Method:

i. Patient's consent or consent of the parents in case of minor should always be taken.

ii. Premedication with

1. tranquillizer like diazepam 5-10 mg two hours prior to tapping.
2. Inj.atropine 1/2 - 1 ml IM depending on age to prevent cardiac arrest.

III. **Position:** Patient should be seated with backrest and both his hands should be placed behind his head.

The side to be tapped should be examined to confirm the signs. The lowest area of maximum dullness should be chosen.

The side should be painted with spirit, cetavlon and spirit again. A sterile towel should be placed on all sides of the site chosen for tapping. 2% lignocaine should be infiltrated in skin, tissue and muscle in the intercostal space chosen. A 18 No. needle 150 ml syringe attached (No. 16 in case of empyema) is gently pushed for about 1-1½" depending on thickness of the thoracic wall. Fluid starts entering the syringe. Gradually, fluid should be aspirated. Disposable sterile bivalve connection should be used. Fluid should never be withdrawn rapidly as sudden decompression of lung may cause shock. In case of massive pleural effusion, fluid should be removed till patient is comfortable and till fluid stops coming in case of empyema. Local instillation of 25-50 mg hydrocortisone may be done.

When the fluid is on the right side, care should be taken not to injure liver.

Complications:

Sudden shock :

Lung puncture;

Pneumothorax;

Surgical emphysema;

Introduction of infection.

Section IV: Cardiovascular System (CVS)

11. Cardiovascular System — Symptomatology and History Taking

History Taking

Symptoms related to cardiovascular system are, in most cases, a clear pointer towards the involvement of this system.

However, many presenting symptoms (like edema, pain in the right hypochondrium) may be correlated to CVS only after further questioning. As against this, symptoms relating to CVS (like palpitations, chest pain and even dyspnea) may be due to anxiety, muscular pains or due to respiratory disease. Only careful analysis of the symptoms and examination will reveal the true origin of the disease.

Bearing these points in mind, a gross generalisation can be made as follows :

A patient suffering from cardiovascular disease usually complains of one or more of these symptom complexes.

- I. Chest pain.
- II. Symptoms related to left-sided failure: (a) Dyspnea (b) Cough with expectoration and (c) Hemoptysis.
- III. Symptoms related to right-sided failure: (a) Edema of feet, and (b) Systemic complaints due to venous congestion related to Central Nervous System (CNS), Alimentary System (AS), Respiratory System (RS).
- IV. Palpitations.
- V. Syncope.
- VI. Cyanosis.
- VII. Symptoms of diseases which can lead to CVS disease.
- VIII. Symptoms of complications caused by CVS disease.

Depending on the presenting symptoms or symptoms of the patient a careful analysis of the related points should be made.

Detailed Analysis of the Symptoms

I. Pain in the chest

Pain in the chest is one of the most common complaints. This is because of its ominous significance. However, there is usually no correlation between the severity and duration of pain and seriousness of the condition.

To determine whether the pain is of cardiac or non-cardiac origin, a complete knowlege about the type of pain is essential. The nature and variants of cardiac pain should therefore be analysed and assessed in detail.

Chest pain should be analysed as any other pain elsewhere in the body. Points to be asked are:

1. Site;
2. Character of the pain;
3. Duration;
4. Radiation;
5. Aggravating factors;
6. Relieving factors.

Pain due to CVS diseases can be as a result of:

1. Myocardial diseases;
2. Pericardial involvement

Myocardial diseases:

Classically a myocardial affection is divided into:

1. Anginal pains) Both are due to
2. Pain due to myocardial ischaemia) coronary) insufficiency

3. Pain due to myocardial infarction.

The essential presenting nature of the pain remains the same in these three conditions except for the duration, severity and associated symptoms.

Angina pectoris:

1. Site:

(i) Usually substernal
(ii) Rarely precordial (most precordial pains are due to anxiety or other causes rather than due to angina).
(iii) Rarely the anginal pains may be absent in the chest and may be felt at the site of radiation.

2. Character of the pain:

(i) Usually described as a sensation of squeezing in the chest or as a sensation of heaviness in the chest.
(ii) Could be described as stabbing, sharp, excruciating and likewise.
(iii) The point to be remembered is that whatever may be the description applied to it, the pains are severe and cannot be ignored during the attack.
(iv) Retrosternal burning.

3. Radiation:

(i) Left shoulder;
(ii) Medial border of the left arm;
(iii) To the left side at the angle of the jaw;
(iv) Right shoulder and arm;
(v) Both the arms simultaneously;
(vi) Epigastrium;
(vii) To the back, in the interscapular region.

The diagnostic difficulty arises when the pains are present only at the sites of radiation without being at the original site (substernal).

4. Duration of pain:

(i) Most important point in the diagnosis of angina pectoris is that it does not last for more than two or three minutes.
(ii) Any pain lasting for more than this duration is either non-cardiac or due to ischaemia or infarction.

5. Aggravating factors:

(i) Classically precipitated due to exertion. The patient will complain that when he walks a particular distance (which he is usually able to judge for himself) he gets the typical pain which forces him to stop. Surprisingly, after he gets the attack he can walk for a longer distance, at the same walking speed and on level ground before he gets the second attack.
(ii) Walking uphill or upstairs (against gravity) may be the only exertion which precipitates the attack.
(iii) Emotional upsets : (a) anxiety, (b) anger, and (c) excitement.
(iv) After a heavy meal (as major share of the cardiac output gets diverted to the splanchnic blood supply at this time).
(v) Cold weather which may cause peripheral vasoconstriction (hence increasing the work load of the heart).
(vi) After tobacco consumption.
(vii) Not aggravated by coughing, sneezing or deep breathing.
(viii) Pain at rest is due to spasm of coronary artery. The condition being increasingly recognised as Prinz Metal Syndrome.

6. Relieving factors:

(i) Rest: Anginal pains always disappear when patient rests or stops working.
(ii) Nitrites: Inhalation or sublingual usage of nitrites.

7. Associated factors:

(i) Usually pallor.
(ii) Palpitations and choking sensation.
(iii) Sinking sensation in the epigastrium.

A classic attack of angina:

Usually an elderly male individual complains of constricting pain in the subnsternal region while walking. The patient has to stop walking and usually does so with a hand over his chest in a slightly stooping position.

The pain may radiate to the sites described above and may last for 2 to 3 minutes. It is always relieved by rest. It may be associated with a feeling of sinking and pallor of the face.

Pains of myocardial ischaemia and infarction:

The site, radiation, etc., remains the same but the pain may come at rest. The pain lasts much longer and in patients with infarction, the duration may be for a few hours.

In severe cases the pain is accompanied by all the symptoms and signs of shock. The pains are not relieved by rest. (The full description of ischaemic heart disease is given at the end of this system.)

Pericardial pains:

Visceral layer of the pericardium has no pain endings. But the parietal layer has a few sensory pain endings at the lower portion which are carried through the phrenic nerves. Hence, it is believed that the pain of pericarditis is in most cases due to involvement of parietal pleura next to it. The central part of the diaphragm is supplied by the phrenic nerves. Hence, the pericardial inflammation which irritates this portion is felt along the shoulder and the neck. The lateral parts of the diaphragm are supplied by thoracic 6 to 9 segments. Hence, the irritation is transmitted to this portion of the pleura from the pericardium and is referred to the chest and the upper part of the abdomen.

Pericardial pain has three types of presenta-tion:

1. Pleural type of pain: Sharp cutting pain felt either in the neck or shoulder or on the lateral side of the chest wall. Pain is aggravated by coughing, deep breathing. Sometimes it is aggravated by swallowing as the oesophagus is an immediate posterior relation of the heart.

2. Pain mimicking that of myocardial infarction : Steady, continuous, boring type of pain which is severe in intensity. The exact mechanism of this type of pain is not known. It could be due to inflammatory irritation of efferent cardiac nerve fibres, in the adventitial layers of the coronary arteries.

3. Rarely pain at the left shoulder or the left lateral side of the precordium is felt with every heart beat.

II. Symptoms of left sided failure:

A. **Dyspnea:** As this is one of the most common complaints of patients suffering from cardiovascular disease, a very thorough and systematic questioning should be carried out :

- (i) How long has the patient been suffering?
- (ii) Is the dyspnea present during exertion?
  - (a) If so, is it only while climbing upstairs?
  - (b) Or is it on walking on level ground and how long can the patient walk before experiencing it?
  - (c) Is the dyspnea gradually worsening? (i.e., is the patient unable to walk the distance which he could cover comfortably in the past.)
- (iii) Or is the dyspnea experienced even when the patient is at rest?
- (iv) If the patient is dyspneic at rest —
  - (a) Whether he can lie down flat on the bed,
  - (b) Or does he have to take 2 or 3 pillows when he rests,
  - (c) Is he comfortable only when he is in upright position and has to bend forward or does he feel discomfort on lying down? (orthopnea).

Dyspnea is graded as follows :-

Grade I — Dyspnea on severe (unaccustomed) exertion.
Grade II — Dyspnea on accustomed exertion.
Grade III — Dyspnea on mild exertion.
Grade IV — Dyspnea at rest.

Newer classification or gradation of dyspnea is called NYHA (New York Heart Association). In this classification every symptom of cardiac origin is included. It is as follows :

Class I — Asymptomatic
Class II — Symptoms on unaccustomed exertion
Class III — Symptoms on accustomed exertion
Class IV — Symptoms at rest

As this new classification includes every cardiac symptom, it indicates the degree of cardiac involvement.

(d) Even if he does not give a history of orthopnea at present, whether he had any such episodes in the past.

(v) Does the patient get attacks of acute breathlessness at night which subside on their own or require treatment? If so the patient should be asked to describe the attack.

(vi) Did the patient have any attack in the past of intense breathlessness which did not subside on its own and whether he was bringing out frothy pink sputum, for which he had to be treated at home or hospitalized? (acute pulmonary edema).

This will denote an attack of acute pulmonary edema. As opposed to paroxysmal nocturnal dyspnea, this will not subside without medical treatment.

Pathophysiology and its relation to symptoms of left-sided failure:

Dyspnea, paroxysmal nocturnal dyspnea, orthopnea and acute pulmonary edema are progressive grades of symptoms of left-sided failure.

Dyspnea:

Definition: It can be defined as a subjective feeling of distress associated with breathing difficulty.

Pathophysiology: In the initial stages of left sided failure, the left ventricular output is sufficient to supply the oxygen requirements of the body at rest. Only on exertion when the body requirements are greater, the left ventricular output is insufficient to meet the demands of the body. Hence, the patient feels dyspneic. The same reasoning will explain why the dyspnea in the very initial phases is only on climbing upstairs or on unaccustomed exertion. To supply the increased demands for oxygenation the accessory muscles of respiration have to act. There is also an increased rate of respiration. Both these factors are important in the subjective feeling of discomfort in breathing.

Paroxysmal nocturnal dyspnea:

A typical attack of paroxysmal nocturnal dyspnea is described as follows :

A patient after going to bed normally wakes up in the early hours of the morning. He may attribute his waking up to a bout of cough or a bad dream. However, on waking up he is intensely restless and breathless and usually has to sit up fighting for gulps of air. He may even throw open a window if possible and try and inhale air as rapidly as possible. Usually, this breathlessness is associated with anxiety and cough which is non-productive or is with pink frothy sputum. Depending on the severity, the attack subsides on its own within a few minutes to half an hour.

Pathophysiology: (i) During sleep, respiratory rate is slow and left ventricular output is also reduced. So lessor amount of blood is carried to respiratory centre in medulla. Slow respiration causes CO_2 retention; this along with diminished blood flow to respiratory centre increases the respiratory rate. The accumulation of CO_2 takes a few hours to develop during sleep. So paroxysmal nocturnal dyspnea occurs during early hours of the morning.

(ii) Due to diminished left ventricular output there is diminished renal blood flow resulting in reduced glomerular filtration and increased tubular re-absorption of sodium. This along with mobilisation of edema fluid from dependent parts (i.e., feet) to lungs causes congestion in pulmonary circulation.

(iii) Pulmonary circulation is overloaded because of back pressure. Left side of the heart cannot pump blood (due to failure) in spite of adequate pulmonay venous return.

Due to back pressure in pulmonary circulation there is pulmonary congestion, which leads to diminished gaseous exchange. This contributes to difficulty in breathing.

Orthopnea:

Definition : Orthopnea is a state of dyspnea where the patient is unable to lie down comfortably and is comfortable when he sits up in bed. (Pl. 11.1)

This is because:

(i) In the upright sitting position there is shift of blood volume to the dependent areas due to gravity. Hence, more blood is present in the splanchnic circulation and the blood vessels of lower extremities. Hence, the venous return to the right ventricle falls, and consequently the right ventricular output is reduced which relieves the pulmonary congestion to some extent.

(ii) The diaphragm is at lower level in the sitting position. This increases the vital capacity which allows better oxygenation.

(iii) The accessory muscles of respiration (especially those at the back) can act much more efficiently in the sitting position than when the patient lies down.

(iv) The decreased vital capacity in the lying down position also contributes to the dyspnea by permitting less amount of gaseous exchange in the pulmonary fields.

Acute Pulmonary Edema:

Definition: Acute pulmonary edema is a symptom complex in which patient feels acutely and intensely breathless, brings out pink frothy sputum, the underlyilng cause being left-sided failure (left atrium and/or left ventricle).

As the left atrium is congested, back pressure is built up in the pulmonary veins which is reflected in the lung fields. Due to this congestion an excessive amount of fluid is poured into the alveoli as transudate. This normally is re-absorbed by the pulmonary lymphatics. However, the excessive fluid acts as an irritant in the alveoli which the body attempts to cough out as pink frothy sputum.

Due to congestion in the alveoli the gaseous exchange suffers. There is also a marked increase in the rigidity of pulmonary tissues. These two factors contribute towards the intense dyspnea of acute pulmonary edema.

(B & C) Cough with expectoration and haemoptysis

Questions to be asked as follows :

i. Does the patient have cough?

ii. If so, is it dry or associated with expectoration? Cough due to left ventricular failure is usually dry or accompanied with minimal expectoration.

iii. Does he give a history of hemoptysis?

iv. Has he noticed any bluish discolouration of his nails or lips? If so when? (Whether during an attack of breathlessness or recently.)

Pathophysiology of cough, expectoration and haemoptysis is as follows: Due to congestion of the pulmonary capillaries, there is some degree of exudation of fluid in the alveoli. This reflexly stimulates cough as a protective mechanism and the body ineffectively tries to throw it out.

So also the congestion promotes attacks of infection as it provides a better medium for the organisms to grow. This results in recurrent attacks of bronchitis (more common in winter and hence termed 'winter bronchitis') which is another reason for the cough.

There is haemoptysis due to the increased exudation from the alveolar capillaries and sometimes rupture of these capillaries.

III. Symptoms of right sided failure:

A. Edema

i. Does the patient complain of swelling of the dependent parts? Mostly swelling will be seen in the feet around the ankles and the patient may complain of increase in swelling after exertion. However, the edema will first be noticed on the face and then on the feet, in patients suffering from pericardial effusion (ascites is also usually present).

ii. Has the edema gradually progressed or is

there any history of massive generalised edema which has now responded to treatment?

iii. Is there any complaint of abdominal distension which has followed the edema of feet?

B. Symptoms due to venous congestion and oligemia in the various systems:

i. **C.N.S. :** Is there history of insomnia, decreased mental activity or headaches?

ii. **A.S. :** Does the patient complain of acute pain over the right hypochondrium? or is there any complaint of anorexia and nausea with a sensation of fullness in the abdomen?

iii. **R. S. :** There is no congestion in the lungs in right ventricular failure. However, there is oligemia due to right ventricular failure which results in poor oxygenation. Does the patient complain of tiredness on walking? Does he feel a shortness of breath or tightening in the chest after exertion which makes him stop the exertion?

Pathophysiology of right sided failure and its correlation to the symptomatology:

Due to the diminished output of the right ventricle there is a congestion in the right atrium which is then transmitted to the vena cavae. This increase in the venous pressure raises the hydrostatic pressure in the capillary tree on the venous side resulting in a transudation of fluids in the tissues in the extracellular space of the extravascular compartments. The decreased output of the right ventricle results in diminished pulmonary venous return hence decreased left ventricular output, resulting in renal oligemia. This causes extravasation of the fluid in the extra vascular space and sets into motion two reflex mechanisms to keep the blood volume constant.

a. increased re-absorption of sodium (Na) and water from the renal tubules, and
b. aldosterone secretion which also promotes re-absorption of Na and hence water.

Due to these reasons more water is re-absorbed which increases the blood volume and hence aggravates venous congestion. This propagates the vicious cycle which increases the edema.

The other symptoms related to various systems as described above are all on the basis of venous congestion due to poor drainage.

The complaints like insomnia and others related to CNS are due to cerebral venous congestion. They have to be specially inquired into since they may be considered by the patient as insignificant (as these symptoms are present commonly in association with any disease process).

The complaint of acute pain over the right hypochondrium is due to hepatic venous congestion. Liver parenchyma has no nerve endings and the pain nerve endings are all situated in the hepatic capsule. The pain felt is due to acute stretching of this capsule. After chronic congestion, which results in a fairly long period of stretching of the capsule, the pain may completely disappear.

Anorexia, nausea and vomiting are present due to congestion of the gastric mucosa and due to portal venous congestion.

IV. Palpitations:

Definition : Subjective feeling of awareness of one's own heart beat is *palpitation*.

The following points should be looked into :

i. Does the patient have palpitations?
ii. If so do they increase during exertion?
iii. Can the patient make out whether they are regular or irregular?
iv. Do they start suddenly, continue for some time and then disappear equally suddenly; either spontaneously or after some particular physical exertion or when external stimulus ceases.

Palpitations can be produced by tachycardia and cardiac arrhythmias.

Extrasystoles may be felt as sudden thumps in the precordium, and if innocent, they may disappear on exertion and increase if they are pathological.

Atrial fibrillation may be experienced by a

patient as irregular palpitations in the chest.

Paroxysmal supraventricular tachycardia is a condition where the patient who is alright will complain of very sudden onset of palpitations which stop spontaneously or after vagal stimulation. However palpitations are so commonly produced by non-cardiac causes like anxiety, excitement that their presence in most of the cases may have no diagnostic significance.

V. Syncope:

Definition : Attacks of sudden transient blackouts are called syncope. Inquiry should be carried out whether the patient complains of transient loss of consciousnes? If so, is the complaint long-standing or of a short duration? Syncope in cardiac causes is due to cerebrovascular ischaemia. It can happen in valvular diseases with diminished output, myocardial failure (especially causing acute left ventricular failure) or in arrhythmias including heart block.

VI. Cyanosis:

Following questions should be asked about the patient.

i. Does he complain of cyanosis? If so, how long is it present?
ii. Whether from birth or of a recent origin. If from birth, is it accompanied by attacks of squatting on exertion?
iii. If it is of recent origin then for how long and what is the progress?

Cyanosis from birth or for a very long time will indicate a congenital defect in the heart. Attacks of squatting on exertion are typical of Fallot's tetralogy — one of the most common congenital cardiac defects causing cyanosis.

The above one is an analysis of the various symptoms which the patient can complain of. A patient may present with dyspnea coming on only during exertion. It is the examiner's duty to analyse it further by asking him the relevant questions whether he has any other symptoms of left ventricular failure. The patient in such a case may not volunteer the information of attacks of paroxysmal nocturnal dyspnea unless he is directly questioned. Important negative points should be noted.

He should also be asked regarding all the other points described above. An inquiry about right ventricular failure, chest pain, palpitations, syncope and cyanosis should be conducted when the patient comes with exertional dyspnea. After the presenting complaint is analysed thoroughly, the examiner will have to inquire about two points : a. History of diseases which can lead to cardiovascular disease. b. History of complications produced by the cardiovascular disease.

VII. History of diseases which can lead to cardiovascular disease:

This of course will entail a knowledge of the various disease processes encountered. This will only come with experience. Certain questions (which are described below) will be irrelevant, in one condition, while they may be extremely important in the other, for example if a young male 15 years old comes with a history of chest pain and breathlessness pointing towards a valvular disease a history of syphilis and diabetes will be irrelevant. However, if he is 50 years old then both these questions will have very important bearing. History of rheumatic fever in the past is very important in valvular diseases of the heart.

1. Classical History of Rheumatic Fever: Patient will complain of pain in the joints which fleets from one major joint to the other. Usually a history of sore throat or upper respiratory tract infection before the onset of joint pains is available. The joint pains are accompanied by fever and other symptoms of systemic infection. However, rheumatic fever can be present without joint pains.

The so-called 'growing pains' are of ominous significance. They are usually due to rheumatic fever and passed off by ignorant parents as of no significance. Such history in childhood may lead to rheumatic valvular diseases in adulthood.

2. History of syphilis: Male patients should be asked whether there was an exposure to this infection, followed by a local sore. In females, the

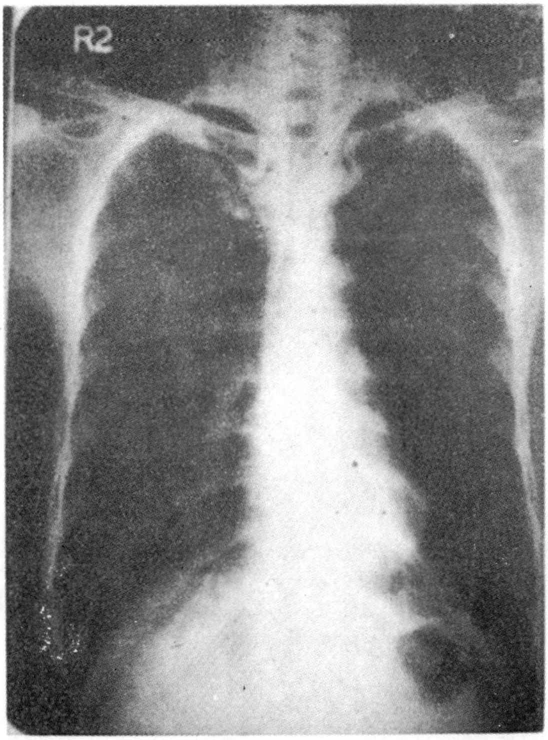

Pl. 9.8 Emphysema

Note widened intercostal spaces. Narrow elongated heart and increased transluscency of lungs

history may be indirectly available by asking about history of repeated abortions. Syphilitic aortitis, aortic regurgitation are common sequales of syphilis.

3. **History of hypertension and diabetes:** The patient should be asked whether his blood pressure was ever recorded in the past and if so whether he was told that he has high blood pressure.

This is the only way by which a history of hypertension can be asked as the so-called symptoms caused by hypertension (like headache, dizzy spells) are present in various other diseases. History of diabetes can be confirmed by asking about polyuria, and nocturia, polydipsia and polyphagia. Hypertension and diabetes are very often the causes of ischaemic cardiovascular disease.

4. **History of tobacco consumption:** History of smoking or any other method of tobacco consumption should be inquired into. The importance of course is in atherosclerotic cardiac disease.

VIII. **History of complications produced by the cardiovascular diseases:**

a. Does the patient give history of embolisation? i.e.,
   i. Sudden monoplegia or hemiplegia due to cerebral emboli.
   ii. Hematuria with renal colic.
   iii. Sudden shooting pain in a limb with local swelling, pain and cyanosis.
   iv. Left hypochondrial tenderness, splenic infarction.
   v. Sudden blindness due to occlusion of ophthalmic artery.

b. History of pressure symptoms due to enlargement of chambers of the heart.
   i. Left atrial hypertrophy can produce hoarseness of voice and dysphagia due to pressure of enlarged left atrium on right recurrent laryngeal nerve and oesophagus.
   ii. Aneurysm of arch of aorta will produce the same symptoms in addition to pressure on the sternum.
   iii. Erosion of the spine with local pain and even paraplegia in patients with aneurysm of descending aorta.

12. Cardiovascular System — Clinical Examination

A systematic examination of the patient must be carried out before examining the CVS proper — peripheral vascular system and heart.

The method to be followed has been explained in the chapter on general examina tion.

The points of particular interest in the general examination (Peripheral Vascular System) which are related to the CVS are :

I. Examination of the pulse.
II. Blood pressure.
III. Jugular venous pressure and pulsations.
IV. Edema of dependent parts.

I. Examination of the pulse:

Definition : It is a wave of expansion felt due to systolic ejection of left ventricle in already filled arteries.

The radial artery is usually examined at first for pulse. This is because of the ease of palpation of this artery and convenience both to the examiner and the patient.

Pulse should be examined for the following:

a. Presence or absence of peripheral pulses;
b. Equality on both sides;
c. Rate;
d. Rhythm;
e. Force;
f. Tension;
g. Volume;
h. Condition of the arterial wall.

a. **Presence or absence of peripheral pulses:** Routinely all the peripheral pulses should be examined. It should be an ingrained habit of examiner to palpate radial, dorsalis pedis, popliteal, femoral and carotids. Method and sites of palpating peripheral arteries is shown in the photographs. (Pl. 12.1)

Conditions like

1. Pulseless disease (Takayashu's syndrome)
2. Peripheral vascular diseases
3. Diabetic arteriopathy
4. Subacute aortitis
5. Peripheral embolisation can be diagnosed by the absence of peripheral pulses.

b. **Equality on both sides :** If volume and force of the pulse (explained below) are unequal on both sides they are indicative of :

1. Coarctation of aorta, or
2. Aneurysms of the aorta, or
3. Cerebrovascular disease (carotids are felt unequal on both sides).

c. **Rate:** Pulse rate should be counted foı at least one minute so that extrasystoles are not missed. The habit of holding the pulse for 15 seconds and then calculating the rare should be deplored, as occasional extrasystoles or other irregularities are likely to be missed. It should be simultaneously correlated to heart beat, so that any beat that is too weak to be transmitted to radial pulse can be judged. Normal rate in adult is abut 60-90 beats/minute.

d. **Rhythm:** Normally sinus rhythm is present and beats are regular.

e. **Force :** Force of the pulse denotes systolic pressure. It is judged by amount of pressure required to obliterate the pulse.

Clinically it is judged as follows. The radial pulse is palpated by 3 fingers of the examiner. The most distal finger (towards the periphery) is kept tightly pressed to prevent any back flow of the blood. The most proximal finger then slowly compresses the pulse until the pulse is no longer felt by the middle finger. The force exerted in this way is the force of the pulse.

f. **Tension:** Tension of the pulse denotes diastolic pressure. Clinically it is judged as follows : The artery is compressed by the examining finger till the pulse is best felt. A very heavy pressure is required to feel the high tension pulse indicating high diastolilc pressure. Moderate pressure is required for medium or normal diastolic pressure and light pressure for low diastolic pressure.

g. **Volume:** Volume denotes stroke output of heart, i.e., left ventriculalr output per beat. It is also described as amplitude of the pulse.

It is judged by the uplift of the palpating finger when pulse wave passes through the artery.

h. **Condition of arterial wall:** This can be judged by rolling the artery especially brachial artery in between two fingers. In old age or when artery is markedly atherosclerotic it can be rolled as a cord in between fingers.

Abnormalities of pulse:

Normally the pulse rate corresponds accurately to the heart rate. However, in certain conditions like atrial fibrillation or multiple extrasystoles cardiac beats fail to produce a pulse wave as the contractions are not strong enough to open the aortic valves. In such cases there will be an apex pulse deficit.

Abnormalities of pulse rate —

— fast rate - tachycardia, i.e., above 100 per minute.

— slow rate — bradycardia, i.e., below 60 per minute.

The pulse rate can either be fast (tachycardia) or slow (bradycardia) with a normal sinus rhythm.

Causes of tachycardia: 1. Physiological: (a) In children, (b) in emotional upsets, (c) after a hot bath, (d) after exertion.

2. Pathological: i. Non-cardiac : (a) fevers, (b) anaemia, (c) thyrotoxicosis, (d) beriberi.

ii. Cardiac : (a) paroxysmal tachycardia, (b) atrial fixed block (2.1 or 3.1), (c) Cardiac failure, (d) myocarditis, (e) pericarditis with effusion, (f) infective endocarditis.

Causes of sinus bradycardia: Physiological: a. In athletes, b. A familial trait.

Pathological : a. vagal stimulation, b. viral infection and enteric fever, c. raised intracranial tension. d. hypothermia, myxoedema, e. early myocardial infarction.

Abnormalities of rhythm of the pulse: (Fig. 12.1)

The pulse is usually regular but may show the following abnormalities : Sinus arrhythmia is a physiological variation in the pulse rate with the phases of respiration. During inspiration the pulse

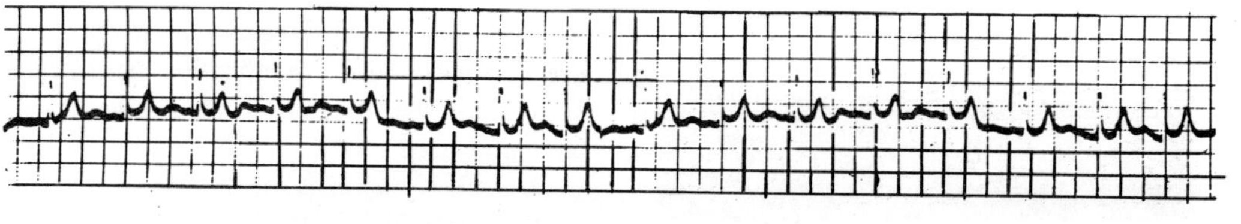

Fig. 12.1
Sinus arrhythmia.

rate gradually increases and during expiration the rate slows down.

Normally it is seen in infants and children but may persist in adults. It is of vagal origin. The irregularities of the rhythm which otherwise are seen, can either be regular or irregular.

Irregularly irregular: (Fig. 12.2 a, b, & c)

1. Occasional dropped beats : (a) due to occasional extrasystole (premature beats), (b) early heart block (Wenchebach's phenomenon), (c) sino atrial block (very rarely).

2. Multiple irregularity: (a) multiple extrasystoles, (b) atrial fibrillation.

3. Atrial flutter with changing block.

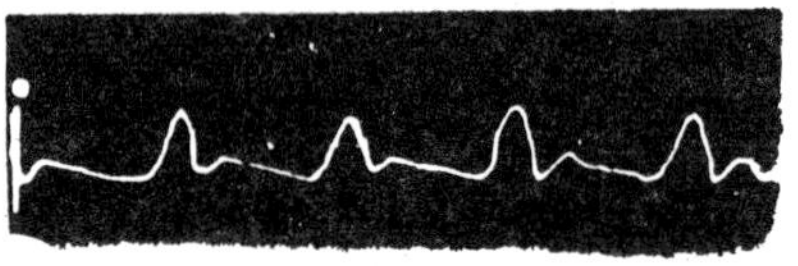

Fig. 12.2a
Regular pulse

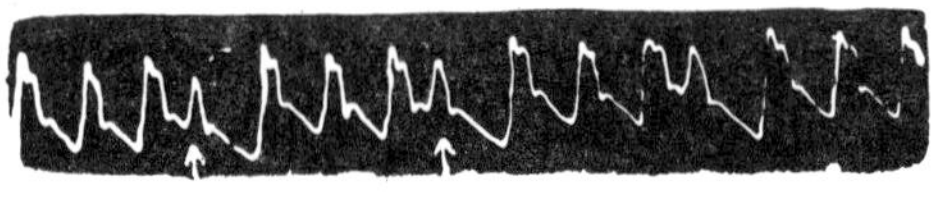

Fig. 12.2b
Premature contractions

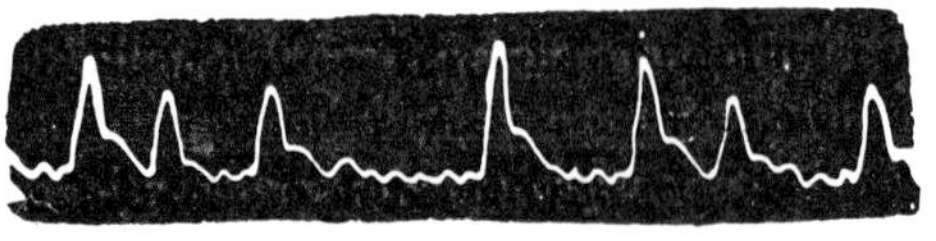

Fig. 12.2c
Irregulary irregular pulse of atrial fibrillation

Regularly irregular:

1. Extra systoles appearing regularly after fixed normal beats: bigeminus (couplings of beats), trigeminus, quadrageminus, etc.

Pulsus bigeminus: (Fig. 12.3 a & b)

This pulse is also described as coupling of beats. This type of pulse is a result of regularly repeating extrasystoles. After every normal beat there is an extrasystole. Hence on palpation two beats are felt in succession followed by a pause. This sequence is repeated again and again.

Digoxin toxicity is one of the most common causes resulting in this abnormality.

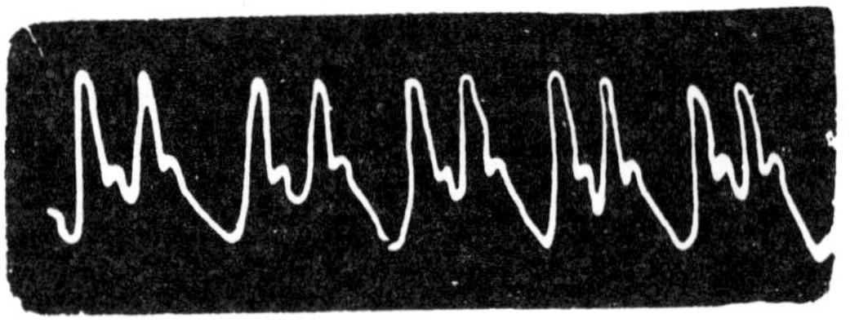

Fig. 12.3a
Pulsus bigeminus

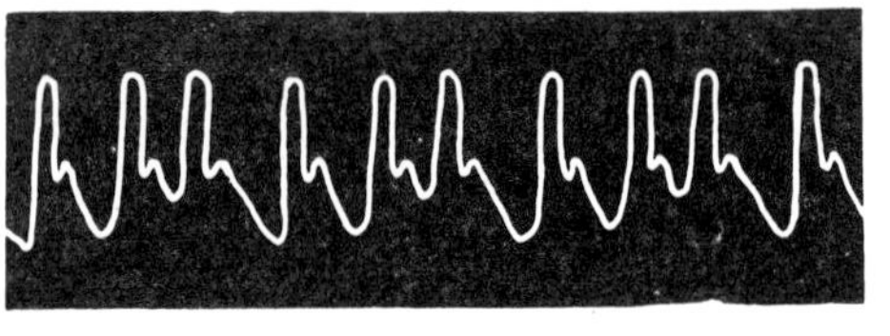

Fig. 12.3b
Pulsus trigeminus

Abnormality of force:

Abnormalities of force can cause apparently irregular pulse but on examination the rhythm is normal and the variation in force gives a false feeling of irregularity.

a. Pulsus alternans
b. Pulsus bisferiens
c. Dicrotic pulse
d. Anacrotic pulse

a. **Pulsus alterans :** (Fig. 12.3c.) Here the rhythm is normal (i.e., every beat comes after the same interval) but every alternate beat is weaker than the previous beat. This should not be confused with pulsus begeminus, where there is a distinct pause after two beats.

Pulsus alternans can be checked very easily by taking the blood pressure (B.P.) of the patient. When the systolic pressure is checked at the highest level where the sounds are audible by the auditory method, only alternate sounds are heard. When the pressure is brought down then all the sounds become audible. This is because the alternate weaker beat produces a pulse wave which is not sufficient to register the highest systolic pressure.

This type of pulse is felt in severe left ventricular failure. If usually indicates a grave prognosis.

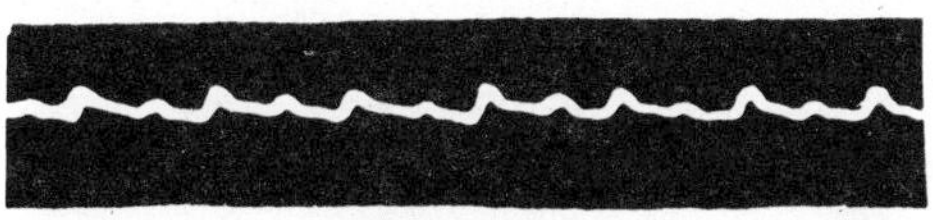

Fig. 12.3c
Pulsus alternans

b. **Pulsus bisferiens :** (Fig. 12.3 d) In this type of pulse, every pulse beat is distinctly felt to have a double impulse. This happens when both aortic stenosis and incompetence coexist. The water hammer pulse of aortic incompetence (described later) and slow rising and slow falling pulse of aortic stenosis can be said to be superimposed on each other giving rise to this picture.

c. **Dicrotic pulse :** (Fig. 12.3e) A double wave may be palpated when there is very low output and high peripheral resistance, e.g., severe congestive cardiac failure (CCF), cardiac temponade.

d. **Anacrotic pulse :** (Fig. 12.3f) Rarely seen in patients having obstructive lesions of the aortic valve or in hypertensives. The initial tidal wave may be more prominent than the main wave. Though described as clinically present, it is more easily recognised by pulse tracing recordings, as it is difficult for inexperienced hand to judge it clinically.

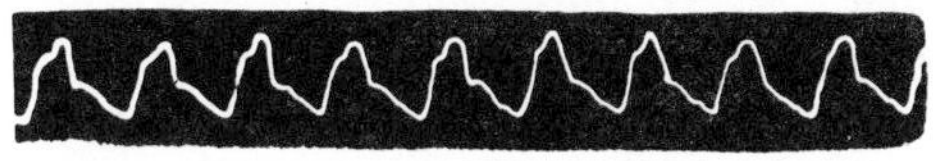

Fig. 12.3d
Pulsus bisferiens

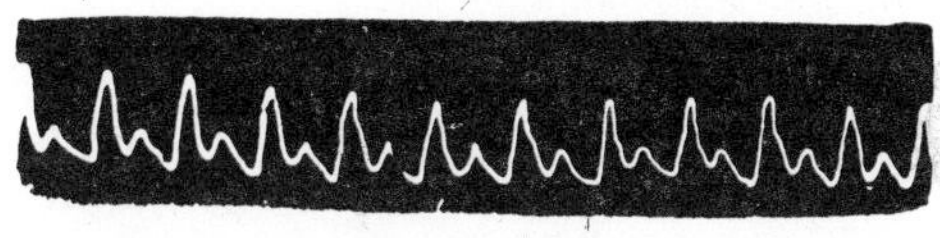

Fig. 12.3e
Dicrotic pulse

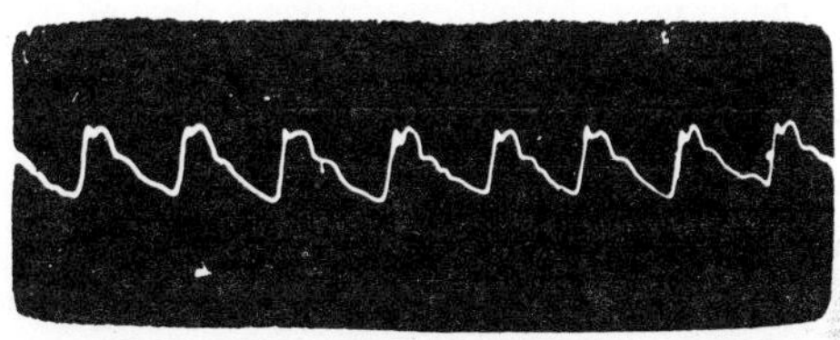

Fig. 12.3f
Anacrotic pulse

Abnormalities of volume of pulse:

In this condition, the volume of the pulse is markedly reduced during inspiration and is increased during expiration. In severe cases the pulse may be practically absent in deep inspiration.

Usually seen in patients suffering from cardiac temponade due to conditions as pericardial effusion or constrictive pericarditis.

Pulsus paradoxus is really a misnomer as it is an exaggeration of the normal phenomenon of an imperceptible reduction in the pulse volume during inspiration.

Cardiac tamponade means cardiac embarrassment. Both filling and contraction are affected, in conditions like pericarditis with effusion, constrictive or adhesive pericarditis, massive pleural effusion and mediastinal tumour, tension pneumothorax, and massive emphysema.

Abnormalities of pulse due to variations in force, tension and volume:

These will be considered together as they are closely interrelated.

a. **The water hammer or Corrigan pulse or collapsing pulse :** (Fig. 12.3g) The pulse shows a combination of increased force, low tension and also increased volume.

In its milder form it is also called as bounding pulse. In Corrigan pulse, the pulse is felt to rise suddenly and fall equally rapidly. If the forearm is held in its middle portion by the examiner a distinct palpable shock is felt. This can be made more prominent by raising the arm which brings the radial artery in line with the aorta.

The name water hammer pulse is derived from a toy used in the past. The toy consisted of a glass tube sealed at both ends and had water in a vacuum. When the toy was held in the hand and inverted, a sudden thump was felt.

Bounding pulse has the same characteristics of a force, tension and volume. But as these changes are not very advanced, it does not give the thump as described above.

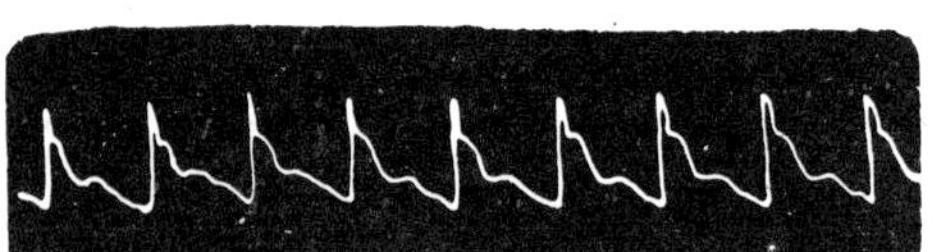

Fig.. 12.3g
Water hammer pulse

Cause of collapsing pulse :

1. Aortic incompetence.
2. Temporary after hot bath or in pregnancy.
3. In anaemia, thyrotoxicosis, beriberi, cirrhosis of the liver and corpulmonale.
4. Arterio-venous shunts and AV aneurysms.
5. Complete heart block.
6. Persistent ductus arteriosus.
7. Aorto-pulmonary window.

b. **Thready Pulse:** Rapid pulse with low volume and low force is seen during any condition producing shock.

c. **Slow rising and slow falling pulse** (Pulsus *parvus et tardus*): Seen classically in aortic stenosis. The pulse characteristically has a slow rise and fall.

d. **Pulsus parvus:** (Fig. 12.3h) A pulse with the above characteristics but without the slow rise and fall. This is seen commonly in tight mitral stenosis.

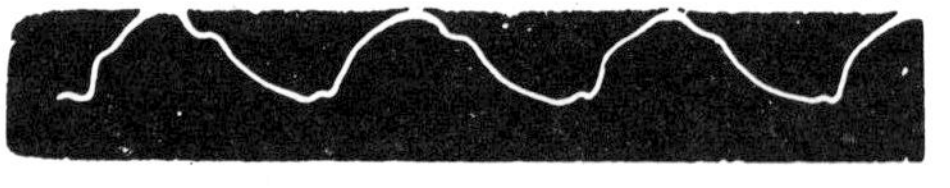

Fig. 12.3h
Pulsus parvus

II. **Measurement of the blood pressure:**

It is the lateral pressure exerted by column of blood onto the arterial wall. Blood pressure (BP) is measured by the technique of sphygmomanometry and the instrument is known as sphygmomanometer.

Various types of instruments are used but the best one is mercury type. The aneroid and the electronic instruments are easy to use and more easily portable but they require frequent checks and calibrations.

The most important point in the technique of measuring the B.P. is the size of the B.P. cuff and the method of tying it onto the arm of the patient (especially in hypertension). The standard cuff is about 12 cms wide. If a smaller size of the cuff is used, the readings recorded will be higher. The cuff should be so tied that the rubber bag is on the inner aspect of the arm so that it can compress the brachial artery properly. The cuff (lower border) should be about 2 cms above the elbow. The cuff should be tied firmly. It should neither be too tight nor too loose.

After tying the cuff as described above the blood pressure is checked as follows :

Palpatory method:

The examiner's fingers are kept on the radial pulse and the pressure in the cuff is raised until the pulse is no longer felt. Then the cuff is gradually deflated by releasing the pressure.

The systolic pressure is the pressure when the pulse is felt at first. Palpatory method should always precede the auscultatory methods as certain patients with high blood pressure show what is termed as auscultatory gap.

Auscultatory method:

The chest piece of the stethoscope is placed over the front of the elbow just below cubital fossa over the brachial artery. The pressure in the cuff is then raised above the level of systolic pressure as determined by the palpatory method.

The pressure is then gradually released. The following sounds are then heard in succession.

They are also known as Kortkov's sounds.

1. Sudden appearance of a clear sound (which can be faint but is distinct). This marks the systolic pressure.
2. These sounds persist for the next 10 mm fall in pressure.
3. The sounds become murmuring in nature for the next 15 mm fall.
4. They are followed by short, loud and distinct tapping sounds for next 10 to 15 mm fall.
5. The sounds suddenly become muffled. This is the level of diastolic pressure.
6. The sounds disappear.

Auscultatory gap: In some patients with hypertension the first sound denoting the systolic pressure appears as described. Then it disappears after reducing the pressure and reappears after a further fall. This gap between the appearance of the first sound and re-appearance is called auscultatory or silent gap. The cause of silent gap is not known. If the palpatory method is not used for checking the level of the systolic pressure, the mistake of inflating the cuff pressure only above the second level (when the sounds reappear) can be made by the examiner. This will give a misleading low systolic blood pressure reading.

Normal range of B.P. recordings:

Normal systolic B.P. recorded is between 95 and 150 mm Hg and the normal diastolic pressure is between 60 and 90 mm Hg in adults.

Systolic B.P. in infants and children can be calculated roughly by the following formula: $90 + \frac{\text{age in years} \times 5}{3}$. Diastolic pressure tends to be 60 ± 10 at all ages in infants and children.

The first reading taken during the examination may be unduly high as the patient may be worried and tense. Hence, in such cases the B.P., cuff should be left in position and the readings checked again after some time. Reassurance of the patient which puts him at ease helps in bringing down such types of increased readings.

Hypertension and hypotension:

There is no sharp dividing line between normal and high blood pressure; but an arbitrary definition is given as when a resting supine adult has arterial pressure of 160/95 mm or higher hypertension is said to be present. This definition is based on deleterious effect of the pressure on different tissues and organs of the body.

Diastolic pressure is more important and sustained diastolic high pressure needs careful evaluation and treatment. Systolic pressure changes with age, excitement, emotions, etc., and therefore is very labile.

Hypotension: When pressure recordings are systolic less than 100mm Hg diastolic less than 60 mm Hg hypotension is said to exist. It may be acute as in the case of diuretics, myocardial infarction, pulmonary embolism septicaemia, cardiac tamponade, etc.

Chronic hypotension may exist following deficiency of adrenocortical hormones. Orthostatic hypotension may be due to drugs or idiopathic, diabetes mellitus, peripheral neuropathy, multiple sclerosis, motor neuron disease, syringomyelia., tabes dorsalis. In short it is due to any cause leading to interference in neural pathways between vasomotor centre and efferent sympathetic nerve endings. Idiopathic or neurogenic hypotension needs no treatment. Only high salt diet may be of use.

The B.P. recordings from two arms may vary by as much as 5 mm of Hg and the difference is considered significant or abnormal when it is more than 10 mm (B.P. in both the arms should be recorded at the same occasion). B.P. in the legs is recorded to be higher than in the arms and the difference may be as high as 20 to 40 mm Hg. This is partly due to : 1. Size of the cuff, the muscle mass of the thighs is larger and as the same cuff is used, the size of the cuff used is relatively smaller, and presses a shorter column of blood in femoral artery. 2. As one takes B.P. recordings in arteries away from the heart, recordings are higher than those recorded in arteries nearer the heart.

In a standing position, the systolic B.P. in the upper extremities may be lowered by 10 to 15 mm Hg. as compared to that in the lying down position. The diastolic B.P. may be raised or lowered or there may be no change in it, when it is recorded in the upright position.

The systolic B.P rises and the diastolic B.P. falls during exercise. The systolilc rise is due to the increased cardiac output while the diastolic fall is due to the fall in peripheral resistance.

III. Examination of jugular veins:

These should be checked both for their pressure and pulsations. (The term J.V.P. may mean either jugular venous pressure or jugular venous pulsations and should not be used as a general descriptive term.)

Jugular venous pressure : The internal jugular veins are usually used to estimate this pressure. The external jugular veins may be used but they may give a false reading due to presence of valves (which are absent in internal jugular veins) or they may be kinked at the base of the neck due to their superficial position.

In examining these veins, the position of the patient is very important. The sternomastoid muscles must be relaxed and should not be rotated for more than a few degrees as excessive rotation can tense the sternomastoids and obscure the internal jugular veins. The trunk should usually be inclined at an angle of 30^0 to 40^0. If the pressure is very high it may be necessary to raise the angle up to 90^0 so that the top of the venous pulsations is visible. The patient should be breathing gently. The height of the column of blood should be checked at the end of expiration.

The height is measured from the sternal angle which is a convenient bedside reference point. It does not accurately correspond to the mid-point of the right atrium in all positions and so the best point of reference is one-half of the anteroposterior diameter of the chest in the fourth or fifth interspace as shown in Fig. 12.4 which corresponds to right atrium. The vertical distance between level of right atrium and sternal angle is about 5 cms in all positions (see Fig. 12.4). The vertical distance between the sternal angle and the highest point of filling in the jugular veins is recorded along with the degree of elevation as jugular venous pressure. Normally it is about 3 to 4 cm at 30^0 to 45^0 angle of elevation (Fig. 12.4). The internal jugular veins on both sides should be examined. The pressure is rarely elevated only in the left jugular vein due to pressure of an atherosclerotic arch of aorta on the innominate vein.

Venous pressure can also be recorded by observing a prominent vein on the dorsum of the hand. The patient's head should be elevated at 30^0 to 45^0 angle. The hand should be first lowered so that the vein becomes distended. Then it is gradually raised passively without excessive flexion at the elbow or shoulder to avoid kinking of the veins. The veins normally will collapse at the level of the sternal angle. If the pressure is raised, the vertical distance above the sternal angle should be recorded along with the angle of elevation of the arm. It gives a rough idea about the venous pressure. The results may not be accurate as there may be peripheral venous vasoconstriction associated with congestive cardiac failure (CCF) or the pressure may be elevated due to local obstruction to venous return in the arm.

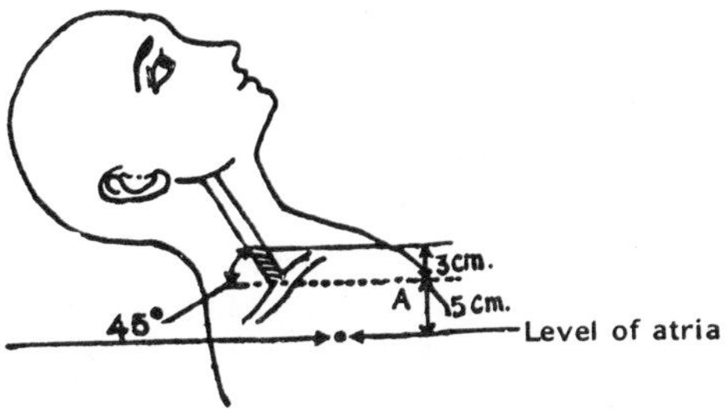

Fig. 12.4
Judging venous pressure

A
Reference point (sternal angle) from where vertical height of engorged veins is measured.
Note that the head is raised to 45^0.
The column of vein engorged is shaded.

Hepato jugular reflex (or reflux):

This procedure is used to confirm the presence of rise of venous pressure.

The patients's head is elevated at an angle of 30^0 to 45^0 so that the top of the venous pulsations is clearly seen. The patient is asked to breathe in and out quietly throughout the procedure as sudden intake and holding of breath which occurs reflexly when pressure is applied over the abdomen is avoided (this Valsalva's manoeuvre is the most common cause of false positive results). A gentle but steady pressure is applied for 30 to 60 seconds and the jugular venous pressure is observed. If there is a rise of more than one cm it is of positive significance indicating right ventricular failure.

Another method of eliciting hepato-jugular reflux is as follows:

Ask the patient to lie flat and not to raise the head. He should breathe in and out slowly. Press gently over right hypochondrium. The jugular veins naturally get distended even in normal persons. Now, if the pressure over the liver is maintained for more than a minute the distension of veins disappears in normal persons; but in presence of early or residual right ventricular failure, the distension of neck veins persists as long as the pressure is maintained.

This can be explained as follows: According to Sterling's law, the more cardiac muscle fibre is stretched, the more powerful is the contraction up to a certain limit. When the right atrium is normal and venous ring (i.e., opening of superior and inferior vena cavae) is normal, any pressure over the hepatic area temporarily increases the venous return and stretches the venous ring and right atrial wall. As a result of stretching the musculature contracts and the jugular veins do not remain distended even though the pressure over liver is maintained. But in the case of right ventricular failure (RVF) the musculature of right atrium and venous ring are already stretched beyond the limit and any extra strain or load with respect to the venous return does not have any effect on contraction. Hence the jugular veins remain distended as long as pressure over hepatic area is maintained. Hepato jugular reflex is of no significance when jugular venous pressure is raised 3 cm or above. It is significant in cases of early and/or residual (recovering) right-sided failure.

Causes of increased J.V. pressure:

1. After exertion-transient.
2. Excitement : May be due to increased tone of the vessel walls (transient).
3. Hyperdynamic conditions : Fever, beriberi, corpulmonale, anaemia, thyrotoxicosis, cirrhosis of liver and pregnancy.
4. Congestive cardiac failure or right ventricular failure.
5. Increased intrathoracic pressure : Physiological: cough, Valsalva manoeuvre; Pathological: Pleural effusion.
6. Increased intra-pericardial pressure : Peri-

cardial effusion, constrictive pericarditis.
7. Increased intra-abdominal pressure: Pregnancy, ascites.
8. Superior vena cava obstructions: J. V. pressure is increased without pulsations in complete obstruction of superior vena cava due to mediastinal mass.
9. Bradycardia (more commonly in heart block).
10. Tricuspid stenosis.

Jugular venous pulsations:

The right internal jugular vein is usually observed for venous pulsations. The position of the patient is extremely important and should be carefully adjusted as described before. In most normal subjects the optimum angle of elevation of the trunk is less than 30^0 but when the J. V. pressure is raised it may be necessary to prop up the patient at 90^0. The sternomastoids should be relaxed. A tangential beam of light from a torch may make the pulsations more prominent and palpation of the carotid artery on the left side helps in assessing the timings of the venous pulsations.

The venous pulsations in the neck must be distinguished from the arterial pulsations in the neck.

The following points help to distinguish one from the other as seen in Table 12.1.

Table 12.1

Venous pulsations	Carotid arterial pulsations
1. Better seen than felt	1. Better felt than seen.
2. Slow and undulating	2. Brisk and forceful.
3. Obliterated by gentle pressure at the base of the neck (as this blocks retrograde transmission of waves).	3. Unaffected by applying pressure at the base of the neck.
4. Change with posture.	4. Do not change with posture.
5. Change with respiration	5. Do not change with respiration.
6. Abdominal pressure or pressure over liver increases venous pulse.	6. Unaffected by abdominal pressure.
7. More than one wave in one cardiac cycle.	7. Only one wave in one cardiac cycle.

Changes in venous pulse with respiration:

Normally deep inspiration increases the venous return to the heart because of increase in the intra-thoracic negative pressure. Hence the veins collapse (empty) during inspiration and the level of pulsations decreases. But the amplitude of the pulsations is increased by full inspiration. In patients with increased venous pressure due to cardiac failure, there is a paradoxic increase in the J. V. pressure during inspiration (Kussmaul's sign). The Valsalva's manoeuvre increases the intra-thoracic pressure and the J.V. pressure rises.

The jugular venous pulsations reflect the pressure changes in the right atrium (Fig. 12.5). The normal jugular venous pulsations consist of three positive (A, C and V) and two negative pulse waves (X and Y). The wave is produced due to distension of a pressure pulse during atrial contraction. It is the largest wave in normal persons. When compared with the timings of the heart sounds, it begins just before the first sound (because first sound = closing of A.V. valve).

The venous pulse pressure starts descending from the top of the wave due to atrial relaxation = X descent. The descent is interrupted by a 'C' wave. This wave is produced by the carotid artery pulsation impacting on the jugular vein and due to the retrograde transmission of a positive wave in the right atrium due to ventricular systole.

In timings it corresponds to the end of the first heart sound and reaches its peak after the first heart sound. After the 'C' wave which interrupts the descent is produced by the ventricular systole causing a fall in right atrial pressure and due to continued right atrial relaxation.

This is followed by the V wave which is positive deflection produced due to continued filling of the vena cava and right atrium during ventricular systole.

After the peak of V wave, there is another decline in the right atrial pressure due to decreased bulging of the tricuspid valve as a result of right ventricular isovolumic relaxation and later on by opening of the tricuspid valve. Hence, its timing corresponds to the interval between the first and second sound.

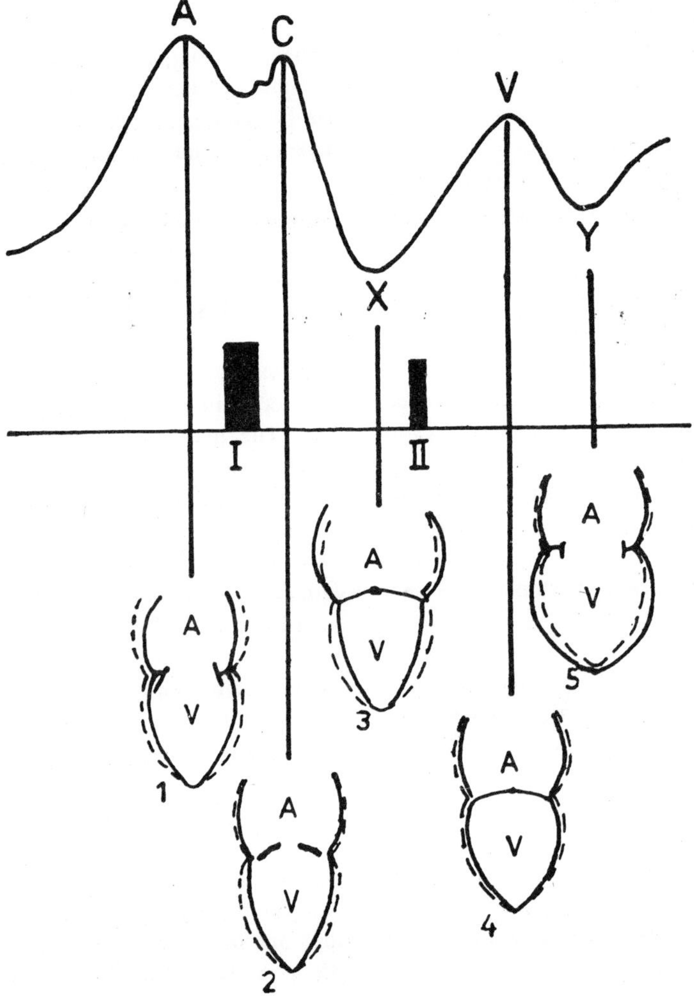

Fig. 12.5

Hemodynamics of venous - pulse changes in R atrium - AV valves and R ventricle. Dotted line indicates normal shape and size of atrium and ventricle when the chambers are neither contracting nor fully relaxed.

A-Atrium V-Ventricle

1. A - wave Produced by contraction of atrium. It precedes 1st heart sound. A-V valves are open and it is the last filling phase of ventricle.
2. C-wave Produced by increase in pressure in atrium caused by bulging of A-V valves in atrium due to ventricular systole.
3. X-wave Produced by isometric relaxation of atrium causing fall in intra-atrial pressure. Ventricle - having phase of isometric contraction. A-V valves are closed and do not bulge in atrium. It precedes 2nd heart sound.
4. V-wave Produced by active filling of atrium from vena cavae leading to increase in intra-atrial pressure.
5. Y-wave When ventricular systole is over and intraventricular pressure falls - A V valves open and blood flows from atrium to ventricle causing fall in intra-atrial pressure.

Common abnormalities of jugular venous pulsations:

a. **A Wave**

1. Absent in atrial fibrillation.
2. Large A waves are present whenever the right atrium is contracting against increased resistance.
   i. Tricuspid stenosis;
   ii. Right atrial myxoma;
   iii. Pulmonary stenosis;
   iv. Pulmonary hypertension.
3. Cannon A waves or grand A waves occur whenever the right atrium contracts against a closed tricuspid valve.
   i. Irregularly in complete heart block, ectopic beats and ventricular tachycardia.
   ii. Regularly in nodal rhythm.

b. **Prolonged A.C. interval**

Due to first degree heart block the time interval between the atrial contraction and the ventricular systole is prolonged resulting in this abnormality.

c. **X descent**

i. Obliteration of the normal X descent is seen in tricuspid regurgitation.
ii. Large X descent is seen in patients with constrictive pericarditis.

d. **Y descent**

i. Slow in tricuspid stenosis.
ii. A sharp deep Y descent is seen in tricuspid regurgitation.
iii. Large Y trough which a sharp Y descent is seen in constrictive pericarditis.

IV. Edema of feet: (dependent parts)

Edema of feet occurs in patients who are ambulatory. It can be judged by pitting (pressing) over skin of tibiae or dorsum of feet.

Edema over sacrum occurs in patiens who are lying down, as sacrum is the most dependent area. On pressing over sacrum, 'pit' can be seen over the pressed area.

(Pitting edema should be distinguished from non-pitting edema. Causes of non-pitting edema are lymphatic obstruction, e.g., filariasis and myxoedema and sometimes angioneuritic edema).

Examination of the heart:

A knowledge of important landmarks, position of valves and corresponding auscultatory areas of heart is essential.

Land marks:

Precordium is the area which overlies the heart. The ribs and the intercostal spaces are used as reference points.

The sternal angle (the angle of Louis) is the junction of the manubrium with the body of the sternum. The second costal cartilage articulates with the sternum at this level and hence the second rib can easily be located. The space below it is obviously second interspace and then the succeeding intercostal spaces may be easily counted.

The midsternal line is the central line of the sternum and the lateral sternal line is the lateral border of the sternum. The midclavicular line is a line drawn vertically from the mid-point of the clavicle. The parasternal line is a line midway between the midclavicular and the lateral sternal line. The anterior axillary and the mid axillary lines are lines corresponding to the anterior axillary fold and middle of the axillary fossa. (Fig. 12.6)

Auscultatory areas: (Fig. 12.7)

The heart is auscultated over four areas, which are designated as mitral, aortic, pulmonary and tricuspid areas.

The mitral area corresponds to the apex and hence is in the fifth intercostal space about 3½ inches (9 cms) from the midline.

The aortic area is at the right of the sternum over the right second costal cartilage.

The pulmonary area is at the left of the sternum in the second intercostal space. The tricuspid area is at the lower end of the sternum.

It should be remembered that these are not the anatomical locations of the corresponding valves.

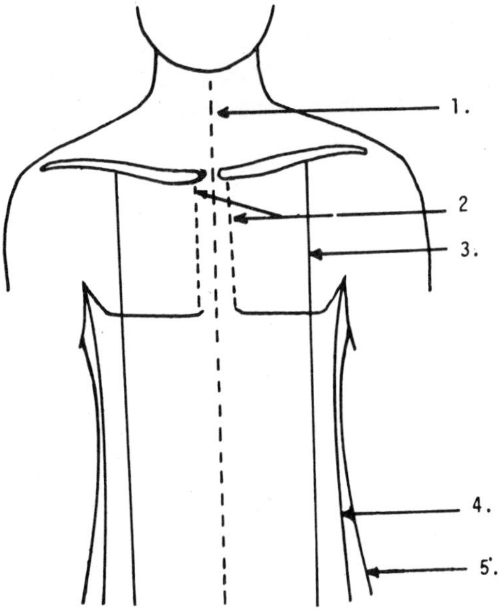

Fig. 12.6

Reference lines in examination of heart

1. Midline
2. Lateral sternal border
3. Mid clavicular line
4. Anterior axillary line
5. Mid axillary line
6. Parasternal line

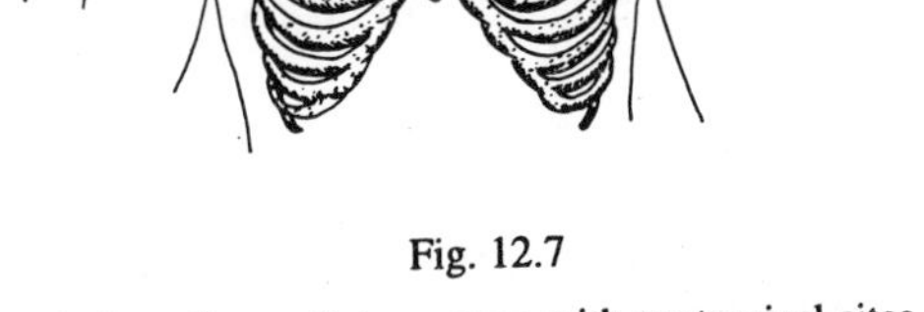

Fig. 12.7

Relation of auscultatory areas with anatomical sites of valves:

A = Aortic area,	P = Pulmonary area,
a = aortic valve.	p = pulmonary valve.
T = Tricuspid area,	M = Mitral area,
t = tricuspid valve.	m = mitral valve.

The relation of these areas and the corresponding valves are seen in the accompanying figure. (Fig. 12.7)

Inspection

The points to be carefully looked for in inspection of the cardiovascular system are:

1. Shape and size of the precordium and tho racic cage.
2. Position of the apex beat
3. Any other pulsations or retraction over the precordium.
4. Pulsations to be seen outside precordium (suprasternal notch and epigastrium)
5. Any distended veins over the precordium and chest.

1. Shape and size of the precordium and thoracic cage:

a. A bulging precordium where both the bony cage and intercostal spaces are prominent indicates a cardiac hypertrophy. It is usually due to rheumatic or congenital heart disease. (Pl. 12.2)

b. A bulging of only the intercostal spaces will be seen in pericardial effusion.

c. Pectus excavatum or depressed sternum is a congenital deformity where there is a funnel shaped deformity of the anterior aspect of thorax. In addition to the inward drawing of the precordium in its medial part, it also pushes the apex impulse laterally. (Note :- Pectus excavatum does not alter function of heart or lungs, it also needs no treatment).

d. A localised bulging to the right side of the sternum or near the manubrium sterni could be due to an aortic aneurysm eroding these structures.

2. **Position of the apex beat:** Apex beat (or apex impulse): Though the term impulse should be reserved for the apex, apex impulse is the lowermost and outermost point where the cardiac pulsations are seen.

Normally in adults it is seen in the fifth intercostal space about 3 ½ inches (9 cms) from the midsternal line. It is also described in relation to the midclavicular line and the normal apex beat is about ½ inch (1 cm) medial to this line. It should not be described in relation to the nipple as the position of the nipple is widely variable.

Abnormalities of the cardiac impulse as seen on inspection:

I. **It may not be visible:** (a) when it lies behind a rib, (b) in an obese individual, (c) in myocardial failure, (d) in pericardial effusion, (e) if covered by a pendulous breast, (f) in extreme shift to the right side when the apex beat lies behind the sternum, (g) diffuse apex beat and (h) emphysematous chest.

II. **The apex beat may be visible but displaced or shifted from its normal position :** (a) due to deformities of the thoracic cage, (b) due to extracardiac causes and (c) due to cardiac causes.

(a) **Due to deformities of the thoracic cage:** (i) Scoliosis or kyphoscoliosis of the spine shifts the apex impulse to one side depending on the curvature of the spine, (ii) pectus excavatum shifts the apex laterally by compressing and flattening the heart.

(b) **Due to extracardiac causes:** Due to respiratory diseases the heart can either be pulled or pushed to one side. Pleural effusion and pneumothorax are the diseases which push the apex beat to the opposite side while pulmonary fibrosis and collapse of the lung pull it towards the side of the disease. Rarely a massive tumour of the intra-thoracic structure may be the cause of the shift. A massive ascites can also shift the impulse upwards.

(c) **Due to cardiac causes:** (i) Dextrocardia where the apex impulse will be on right side in the fifth intercostal space, (ii) left ventricular hypertrophy may cause the apex to shift downwards and outwards and (iii) right ventricular hypertrophy causes the apex beat to be shifted outwards. Though time honoured hypothesis states this, in practice, right ventricular hypertrophy can shift the apex downwards and outwards.

3. **Any other pulsations or retrations over the precordium:**

Left parasternal pulsations indicate a right ventricular hypertrophy. Pulsations in the pulmonary area are seen rarely in pulmonary hypertension. Retraction of the apex along with parasternal pulsation is present in massive right ventricular hypertrophy (right ventricular rock).

Prominent apex beat and retraction of the parastemal area (left side) will indicate massive left ventricular hypertrophy (left ventricular rock). Prominent apical and left parasternal impulses with retraction in between means bi-ventricular hypertrophy (bi-ventricular rock).

An aortic aneurysm may be seen as a pulsating mass either at the base of the heart on the right side in second intercostal space or rarely when it erodes through the sternum. Pulsations in second right space can also be due to aortic regurgitation.

4. **Pulsations to be seen outside precordium:**

(a) Pulsations in the suprasternal notch should be looked for. The common causes of such pulsations are:

(1) Hyperdynamic circulation as seen in anaemia.

(2) Aortic dilatation due to syphilitic aortitis or aneurysm or a high aortic arch,

(3) Abnormal course of the innominate artery or anomalous subclavian artery.

(b) Pulsations in the epigastrium should lbe checked and the common causes of these are:

i. Asthenic individual in whom you can normally see the pulsations of the abdominal aorta,

ii. Aneurysm of the abdominal aorta,

iii. Transmitted aortic pulsations through a tumour situated anterior to it.
iv. Right ventricular hypertrophy causing epigastric pulsation, and
v. Hepatic pulsations in tricuspid valve diseases (either incompetence or stenosis).

5. **Dilated blood vessels over the precordium or the chest wall:**

In the superior vena cava obstruction dilated veins may be prominent over the chest wall. In coarctation of aorta there are dilated arteries over the chest wall. However, they are more commonly seen on the back than in the precordial region. They become more prominent when the patient bends forward.

Palpation:

Palpation should be carried out in a systematic manner. A routine should be followed which will cover all the parts to be examined during palpation of the cardio-vascular system.

The following procedure step by step should cover all the important points:

At first the palm of the hand should be placed so as to cover the left ventricle and the apex area. This will localise the apex which should then be palpated by a finger to note its character, position, etc. The palpating hand will also note any thrills felt over the mitral area. Then the hand should be kept over the parasternal area in the precordium with the base of the palm in the epigastrium and the central portion and the fingers in the left parasternal area (Dressler's method). (Pl. 12.3)

This will palpate the right ventricular pulsations as a heave. Any thrills in the tricuspid area or those due to ventricular septal defect may be felt at the same time. Then the pulmonary area should be palpated for presence of any palpable sounds indicating pulmonary hypertension or any thrill in this area.

Lastly, the aortic area should be palpated for the presence of any thrills. As these manoeuvres cover all the precordial area, any other adventitious palpable sounds like pericardial rub can be felt if they are palpable, and tender areas due to inflammatory pericardial diseases can be automatically noted.

Points to be noted on palpation are:

1. Confirmation of the position of the apex beat and determining character of the same.
2. Presence or absence of right ventricular heave.
3. Palpable sounds.
4. Thrills over the various cardiac areas.
5. Pericardial rub.
6. Tracheal tag.

1. **Confirmation of the position of the apex beat and noting its character:**

Apex beat is the area where maximal thrust is felt by the palpating finger held perpendicular to chest wall. The lowermost and the outermost point which was taken as the position of the apex impulse should not be taken as a landmark, as transmitted pulsations from the apex may erroneously locate the impulse more laterally than its actual position.

After locating the apex beat the force and the character of the apex should be noted. Apex beat is felt properly in thin individuals, children and young adults. The normal force and character of an apex beat is understood only by experience. The changes in its nature described below are in comparison to the normal character.

I. Forceful apex beat: (a) **Heaving apex beat:** An increased thrust of the apex which is forceful and sustained indicates an impulse which is increased both in force and amplitude. Most commonly seen both in aortic stenosis and incompetence. Heaving apex impulse is suggestive of a left ventricular enlargement.

b. **Hyperdynamic apex beat:** In this type of impulse, the force or the amplitude of the apex impulse is increased but the duration is not prolonged. The impression to the palpating hand is that of a quick forceful thrust.

Classically present in aortic incompetence it is

also produced by mitral incompetence or any condition in which the heart is hyperdynamic (thyrotoxicosis, beriberi, severe anaemia, Paget's disease of the bone, pregnancy).

II. **Feeble apex beat:** In any condition where the myocardial contraction is feeble, the apex impulse will also be feeble. Hence in myocarditis or myocardial infarction, the feeble apex is easily explained. Shock due to any cause will have the same effect. In myxoedema as the cardiac muscular contractions are feeble due to infiltration of the cardiac muscle with myxoedematous tissue the same result is produced.

In pericardial effusion or constrictive pericarditis, due to the interference with transmission of the cardiac impulse the apex is felt poorly or not at all.

III. **Tapping apex beat:** In mitral stenosis, a distinct and clear tap can be felt in the position of the apex. This is really a palpable accentuated first heart sound. The left ventricle fills slowly and not to its full capacity during diastole and hence its contraction is poor.

Thrills which can be felt at the apical region will be discussed later.

2. **Palpation of right ventricle heave:**

After palpating the left ventricle and the apex as described above, the right ventricular area (left parasternal area) should be palpated by the method described previously.

This manoeuvre (Dressler's manoeuvre) will also palpate the pulsation of the hypertrophied right ventricle in the epigastrium.

Right ventricular impulse is normally not felt (except in persons with thin chest wall where it can be felt as a part of the generalised palpable cardiac impulse).

Forcible right ventricular pulsations can be felt as either a heave or a hyperdynamic impulse with the same criteria for diagnosis as those for left ventricular heave and hyperdynamism.

Classically right ventricular heave is felt in patients with pulmonary stenosis. However, in severe and long-standing cases of mitral stenosis, the same heaving right ventricular impulse is felt. A hyperdynamic right ventricular impulse is felt commonly in patients with ventricular septal defect.

3. **Palpable sounds:**

Palpation of the loud pulmonary component of the second sound in the pulmonary area should be always undertaken. It is known as the diastolic shock and indicates pulmonary hypertension. Aortic component of the second sound can be palpated in the aortic area in cases of severe hypertension. Same component can also be felt as a palpable shock in syphilitic aortitis or aortic aneurysm provided there is no associated aortic incompetence. Mitral opening snaps and aortic ejection clicks can also be palpated when they are prominent enough.

Triple rhythms including gallop rhythms can be easily diagnosed on palpation (if the triple rhythm is appreciated on palpation). If palpated in the apical area it is left ventricular gallop rhythm and if in the left parasternal area it is the right ventricular gallop rhythm.

4. **Palpation of thrills:**

Thrills can be defined as vibrations felt by the palpating hand when it is placed over the heart or the blood vessels. Detection of a thrill and its accurate description is extremely important. A thrill is never present without a murmur. As murmurs can be defined and interpreted much more easily undue importance should not be given to their presence. In fact an inexperienced examiner is carried away by a palpable thrill ,and tends to forget to analyse the more important findings on palpation.

Thrills are produced due to either obstruction to the blood flow (as by stenosed valves) or by abnormal direction of flow (as in septal defects and regurgitation). They can also be produced by a rapid and increased flow in the normal direction (blood flow in dilated chamber).

Once a thrill is detected, it should be examined for its site, nature and timing. The timing of the thrill can be accurately judged by comparing it with the apex impulse.

Thrills at the base of the heart are more commonly systolic. This is due to the fact that the soft diastolic murmurs which are produced by incompetence of aortic and pulmonary valves are usually not accompanied by thrills. Thrills at the apex and in between apex and base can either be systolic or diastolic depending on the nature of the lesion.

Common thrills encountered on clinical examination:

In the mitral area : Systolic thrill in this area is usually due to mitral incompetence. A diastolic thrill in this area can be a short one or it could be a prolonged one with a typical presystolic accentuation ending in the 'tapping apex' described before. It is pathognomonic of mitral stenosis.

In the parasternal area: A systolic thrill in the third and fourth interspace could be due to ventricular septal defect. A systolic thrill of tricuspid incompetence will also have practically the same site and nature. A diastolic thrill in this area is due to tricuspid stenosis.

In the pulmonary area: A short but prominent systolic thrill is usually due to pulmonary stenosis or atrial septal defect. A continuous thrill may be due to persistent ductus arteriosus but sometimes in early stages, this disease will give rise to only a short systolic thrill. A diastolic thrill may be felt in this area. This could be due to pulmonary incompetence but is more commonly due to aortic incompetence. This thrill is better felt if the patient is asked to bend forward.

In the aortic area: A rough systolic thrill which can also be palpated over the neck vessels is felt in patients with aortic stenosis. However, a flow murmur due to hyperdynamic circulation may produce a thrill in this area.

5. **Pericardial rub:**

This is felt as a harsh grating palpable sound anywhere over the precordium. It may be associated with tenderness. It is diagnostic of a pericardial inflammation.

6. **Tracheal tag:**

The chin of the patient should be raised and firm pressure should be applied in upward direction with fingers of one or both hands on circoid cartilage. A downward pull (tag) is felt by the fingers with each heart beat. It is suggestive of aneurysm of arch of aorta or mediastinal tumour (the downwards pull on left bronchus which is transmitted to trachea and cricoid cartilage). (P1.5)

Percussion of the heart:

Percussion is rough bedside guide of the size and enlargement of chambers of the heart. Though superseded by radiological examination, percussion is valuable where there is lack of these facilities or in a bedridden patient, where radiological examination may not be possible.

The principles in cardiac percussion (in fact in any percussion) which should be followed are : (a) Always percuss from a resonant area towards a dull area. (b) Do not use an unnecessarily heavy stroke on percussion. The stroke used should be sufficient to produce a clear sound. Unnecessary heavy percussion may dampen the minor differences in the sound produced. (c) Percussed finger should be parallel to the border of heart.

Percussion is used to delineate the margins of the heart. At first, the left border of the heart should be percussed. In those patients where apex beat is palpable, the sixth interspace should be used. If it is not palpable, the sixth interspace may be conveniently used as a starting point. The percussion should be started in either the anterior axillary line or sometimes the midaxillary line and then gradually be approached medially towards the cardiac border. The change from the resonant to the dull note over the cardiac musculature should be noted.

Then the left border is mapped out by repeating this procedure in the fourth and third interspaces. The second intercostal space should be percussed on both sides, right and left for any abnormal dullness.

The right border of the heart is mapped out as follows: The percussions should start in the second or third intercostal space in the mid-clavicular line and then should be continued in the same line downwards until the liver dullness is encountered. Then the examiner should choose the space above this (i.e., liver dullness) and then proceed medially until either the right border of the heart or the right border of the sternum is reached.

The normal cardiac borders are as follows: (a) No dullness in the second interspace on either side. (b) Left border : In the third interspace 3 cms from the midline. In the fourth interspace 4 to 5 cms from the midline. In the fifth interspace 8 to 9 cms from the midline. (c) Right border does not cross the right sternal border.

Common abnormalities which can be diagnosed by percussion:

(a) A gross enlargement of the heart is found in patients with cardiomegaly due to cardiomyopathy or any other valvular disease.

(b) A Pericardial effusion will be easily diagnosed by an enlarged area of cardiac dullness with the typical stony dull note. (Stony dull indicates that the resistance to the finger which is kept on the chest wall is markedly increased in addition to the dull note.) If the patient is asked to sit up, it will be seen that the dullness at the base of the heart will be reduced in size as compared to what it is when the patient is lying down. (Suggestive of pericarditis with effusion.)

(c) Dullness in the second right interspace and around may point towards an aortic aneurysm.

(d) Dullness in the third and second left interspace may point towards an enlarged pulmonary segment or pulmonary artery aneurysm.

(e) An enlarged right atrium may give rise to dull note in the third and fourth interspace on the right side.

Relative and absolute cardiac dullness:

A stress was laid previously that the area of the lung covering the heart should be mapped out by percussion. The area which was not covered by the lung was the area of absolute cardiac dullness and the area covered by the lung was known as the area of relative dullness. The only important point to be remembered is, in emphysema, cardiac dullness is reduced or absent as the hyperaerated lung tissue covers the major surface of the heart. Area of absolute cardiac dullness is reduced.

Auscultation of the heart:

This is one of the most fascinating and at the same time confusing parts of the cardiological examination for a beginner as well as an experienced examiner. A rigid method of examination, thinking and interpretation should be ingrained from the very beginning of one's medical career.

Places of cardiac auscultation:

The four cardiac areas which should be examined in a serial manner are :

a. **Mitral area :** At the apex beat or in the fifth left intercostal area inside the mid-clavicular line.
b. **Aortic area:** Second right costal cartilage.
c. **Pulmonary area:** Second left intercostal space near the sternal edge.
d. **Tricuspid area:** Fourth left intercostal space near the sternal edge.

However, various other areas may have to be auscultated as typical signs of certain diseases do not correspond to these areas, so also a friction rub may be present anywhere over the precordium. Hence all the precordial areas should be quickly auscultated after listening to the above mentioned four areas.

Heart sounds:

These must be heard and analysed at the above spaces. A common mistake of a novice is, to give more importance to murmur than to the heart sounds. Whenever heart sounds are to be described the correct method is as follows :

a. Area where the sounds are auscultated.
b. Presence or absence and the nature of the heart sounds.
c. Description of abnormal sounds if any.

Normally if the heart sounds are recorded phonocardiographically four sounds are heard regularly. However, clinically two or rarely three of these sounds are heard.

The most common sounds are the first and the second heart sounds. (Fig. 12.8)

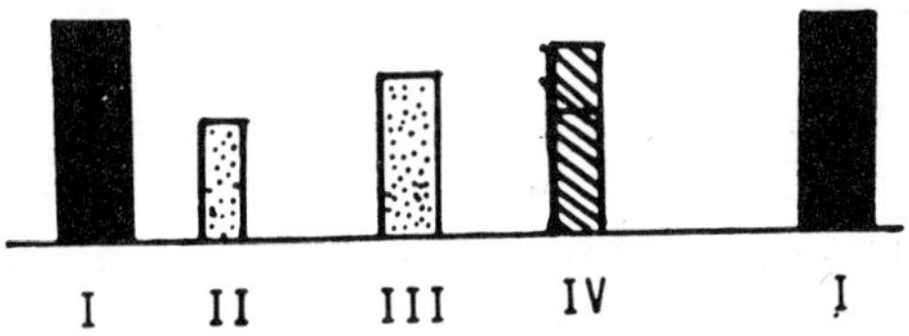

Fig. 12.8
Heart sounds. Note IVth heart sound is normally clinically not heard but can be recorded phonocardiographically.

The first sound is produced at the onset of the cardiac systole. It is produced due to the closure of the mitral and tricuspid valves at the beginning of the systole. The contraction of the ventricles also contribute to this sound production. Phonetically, it is pronounced as 'lub' and is normally a single sound. The second heart sound is produced by closure of the aortic and pulmonary valves.

Normally a single sound, phonetically is pronounced as 'dup'. It is sharper than the first sound.

The interval between the first and the second heart sound is shorter than that between the second and the following first sound. Hence, they can be reproduced phonetically as lub/dup. (pause)

The third and fourth sounds are not normally heard with the stethoscope. They are significant in pathological conditions.

The third heart sound (physiological) is heard near the apex beat and may be accentuated when the person lies in the left lateral position. The sound is produced due to the rapid filling of the ventricles in mid-diastolic phase and coincides in the cardiac cycle with the descending limb of the 'V' wave of the venous phlebogram. It is soft, low pitched sound.

The fourth heart sound is produced because of atrial contraction.

Heart sounds and their relation to cardiac cycle:

Before describing the abnormalities produced by the variation in the character of these sounds a complete description of the cardiac cycle and the various sounds produced will not be out of place.

The first sound is produced by the closure of mitral and tricuspid valves due to ventricular systole. This is followed by the increase of ventricular tension and pressure within the ventricles for a short duration. During this period of isovolumic contraction no flow in or out of the ventricles can occur as all the valves are closed. When the ventricular pressure exceeds the pressure in the aorta and the pulmonary artery, the semi-lunar valves open and systolic ejection phase begins. At this point an ejection click can be heard immediately after the first sound.

Systolic flow begins with a slow flow shortly after the first heart sound and then rapidly increases to a maximum during the mid-portion of the systolic ejection phase and decreases at the end of systole when the ventricles empty. Due to the anatomical arrangement, the semi-lunar valves are folded in the aorta or the pulmonary artery during ventricular ejection and they do not interfere with the flow of the blood.

At the end of this ejection phase, the pressure in the ventricles falls below that in the aorta and the pulmonary artery, and forces the aortic and pulmonary valves to close with an audible snap, producing second heart sound. Aortic and pulmonary valves close rapidly in succession and the aortic component is the louder and earlier of the two. So normally the second sound can be heard as either a single sound or a closely split sound.

At this time (early diastole) the pressure in the ventricles is still higher than that in the atria and hence the atrio-ventricular valves remain closed. During this phase of isovolumic relaxation, there is no flow of blood in or out of the ventricles.

At the end of this phase, the pressure in the ventricles falls below that of the atria and the mitral and the tricuspid valves open and the atria rapidly empty in the ventricles. This can produce the normal low pitched third heart sound.

The ventricular filling flow gradually decreases as the ventricles fill up and is augmented by the atrial contraction at the end of diastole which produces the fourth heart sound (which is recorded only on the phonocardiograph).

This description will help the student to understand the abnormalities which will be described.

Abnormalities of first sound:

1. Feeble or diminished first sound.
2. Accentuated first sound.
3. Reduplication of first sound.

1. **Feeble or diminished first sound:**

(a) The most common cause of a feeble first heart sound is a defect in its conduction to the periphery. Physiologically emphysema of the lungs or pericardial effusion and rarely a pleural effusion can obstruct the conduction.

(b) A feeble myocardial contraction due to myocarditis or ischemic damage to myocardium causes a feeble first heart sound.

In these conditions the first heart sound loses its particular character (lub) and both the sounds appear to be of the same character. This rhythm (lub-dub) along with the tachycardia is known as tic-tac rhythm or embryocardia (as the heart sounds can be compared to the heart sounds of the foetus).

(c) A prolonged P. R. interval which is a feature of first degree heart block and also a feature (variably) in complete heart block produces a feeble first heart sound.

(d) In any condition where the venous return to the heart is impaired and hence the diastolic filling is poor, the first sound will be feeble. This happens in peripheral circulatory failure or shock due to any cause.

2. **Accentuated first sound:**

(a) Physiologically in any condition where there is tachycardia with hyperdynamic circulation the first sound is accentuated. This is because a high filling pressure keeps the cusps fully open until the last possible moment. The common examples of this condition are exercise and fever. Thyrotoxicosis, beriberi and advanced cirrhosis of the liver are other examples of this type of circulation.

(b) Any condition where the atrioventricular conduction time is shortened, first sound is accentuated. This is because the cusps of mitral and tricuspid valves are widely separated and then suddenly closed by the ventricular contraction. The shorter the A.V. conduction time, louder is the first sound.

The cannon sounds (very loud first heart sound) heard in complete heart block are due to the same reason. When the atrial and ventricular contractions practically coincide, a very loud booming first sound is heard. Another rare condition which will shorten the atrio-ventricular conduction is Wolffe-Parkinson white syndrome. Here the first sound is accentuated at every beat.

(c) The first sound is short, sharp and loud in mitral stenosis. It is produced as a result of high pressure gradient between the atria and the ventricles which keep the mitral valve open to the last possible moment before systole and the changes in the valve (which is fibrosed and calcified) combine together to give the typical first heart sound of mitral stenosis.

3. **Reduplication of the first sound:** (Fig. 12.9)

(a) In health, the two components of the first heart sound (mitral and tricuspid) may be heard as two separate sounds.

(b) Contraction of the two ventricles may not occur at same time (separated by a fraction of a second). It occurs in bundle branch block. Theoretically it is possible that a split first sound is heard in this condition.

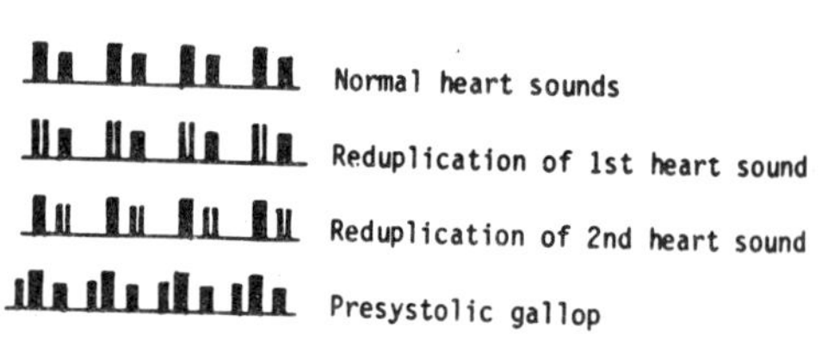

Fig. 12.9
Relation of all these variations with normal heart sounds is well seen.

(c) Ebstein's disease (where there is a deformation of tricuspid valve) is the only condition where a wide pathological splitting of the first heart sound is heard properly.

Abnormalities of the second sound: 1. Feeble or absent second sound. 2. Accentuated second sound. 3. Splitting and its variation. 4. Single second sound.

1. **Feeble or absent sound:** (a) Both the components of the second sound, i.e., the aortic as well as the pulmonary, are feebly heard when the patient has a thick chest wall or has emphysemalous lungs.

(b) The aortic component of the second sound is poorly heard in aortic stenosis where the valve is fibrosed, calcified or deformed. It is also very feeble or may be absent in aortic incompetence where the valves are destroyed by the disease process.

In hypotension of the systemic circulation this component is feebly heard because of the low diastolic pressure.

(c) The pulmonary component is feeble or absent in pulmonary stenosis, Fallot's tetralogy as well as pulmonary incompetence (if not secondary to pulmonary hypertension).

2. **Accentuation of the second sound:** (a) The aortic component is accentuated in hypertension where sometimes it can have a typical musical tambour characteristics in syphilitic aortic incompetence. It is fairly loud in syphilitic aortitis and aortic aneurysm.

(b) The pulmonary component is loud in either secondary or primary pulmonary hypertension (mitral stenosis is one of the most common causes of acquired pulmonary hypertension).

3. **Splitting and its variations:** (Fig. 12.10) The second sound has two components. The aortic component is better heard in aortic, mitral and tricuspid areas, while the pulmonary component is better heard in the pulmonary area.

Both these sounds are heard together in the second and third parasternal area. This is the normal splitting of the second sound. The split narrows during expiration and widens during inspiration. It is best heard in children and young adults. The aortic component is heard before the pulmonary component.

This normal splitting may be absent in elderly people or in patients with emphysematous lungs.

(a) **Wide and fixed splitting:** This is diagnostic of atrial septal defect. There is a wide split in the two components and the gap does not narrow on expiration.

Here the pulmonary component is delayed due to overfilling of the right ventricle (about 3 times) its usual capacity, and consequent delay in its emptying. Because of the magnitude of left to right shunt, the filling of right ventricle remains constant in expiration and inspiration (filling in inspiration occurs due to systemic venous returns). The resultant delay in closure of pulmonary valves is not altered by phases of respiration.

Widening of split may be reduced when pulmonary hypertension supervenes but widening does not alter with phases of respiration.

(b) **Wide splitting** (Variable) : Here the split in the two components is wide but varies with respiration. It is caused by right bundle branch block with a resultant delay in closure of the pulmonary valve. In pulmonary stenosis, due to the delay in the closure of the valve, the pulmonary component is delayed and has an altered quality. Ventricular septal defect also shows a fairly wide splitting which varies with respiration.

(c) **Reversed splitting:** This is due to delayed closure of the aortic valve. Here the aortic component comes after the pulmonary component and hence the interval between them is short during inspiration and wide during expiration. Left bundle branch block is the most common cause of this condition. Aortic stenosis gives rise to the same clinical picture due to delayed closure of the aortic valve.

Persistent ductus arteriosus can give rise to reversed splitting if the shunt is large enough. Rarely severe myocardial ischaemic affection in

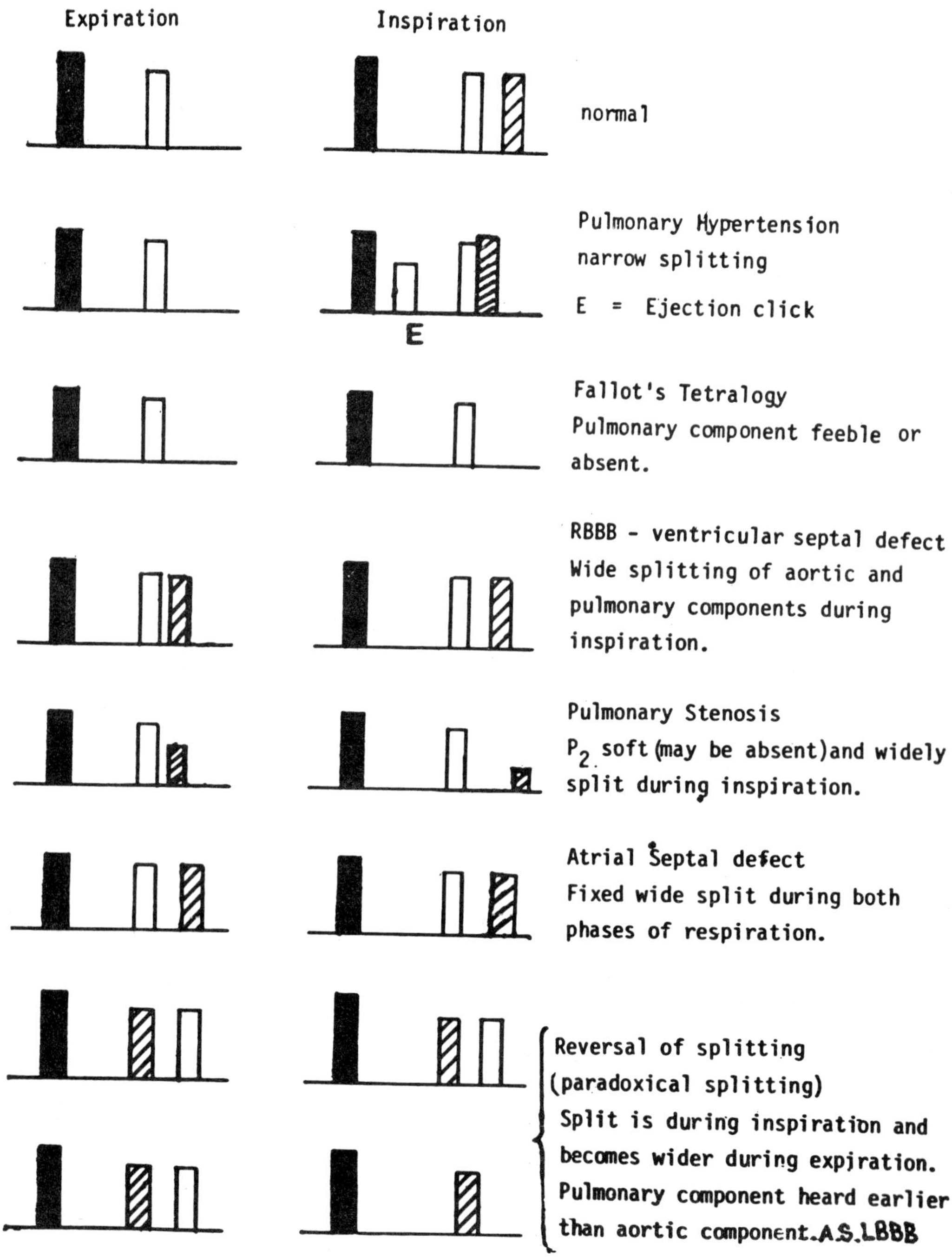

Fig. 12.10
Variations of splitting of pulmonary second sound in various conditions.

absence of left bundle branch block can produce this picture.

(d) **Narrow splitting:** Pulmonary hypertension causes early closure of pulmonary valve.

4. **A single second sound:** Abnormal single second sound can be produced either by fusion of the aortic and pulmonary components or due to one of them being absent.

In aortic stenosis, the aortic component may be delayed and hence both the components may be heard simultaneously. The aortic component may be absent when the valves are calcified and fixed in aortic stenosis. The pulmonary component is absent in Fallot's tetralogy, pulmonary atresia and pulmonary stenosis.

Triple rhythm and abnormally produced sounds in cardiac cycle:

By definition whenever three heart sounds are heard it is called triple rhythm. Hence triple rhythm can be caused by:

1. Duplication of the first heart sound (de scribed above).
2. Duplication of the second heart sound (de scribed above).
3. Opening snap in mitral stenosis.
4. Opening snap in tricuspid stenosis.
5. Systolic ejection clicks.
6. Pericardial clicks.
7. Gallop rhythm a. Presystolic, b. Protodiastolic and c. Summation.

1 & 2. Duplication of the first and second heart sounds has already been described.

3. **Opening snap in mitral stenosis:** (Fig. 12.11) This is a high pitched, sharp sound heard immediately after the second sound in the mitral area. It can usually easily be diagnosed due to its peculiar character which can be best described as a snaper click. It occurs immediately after the isovolumic relaxation phase of the ventricles. The mitral valves which are partly calcified and fibrosed lose their normal elasticity. They also open against a higher pressure gradient between the atria and the ventricles. These two factors combine to produce the classic sound. The opening snap disappears or is absent when the valve is completely ankylosed or calcified; and its presence shows pliable cusps of the valve.

4. **Opening snap in tricuspid stenosis:** Tricuspid stenosis if present is always of rheumatic origin. The snap of the tricuspid stenosis is produced in exactly the same way as the opening snap of mitral valve. However, it increases during deep inspiration. Clinically, it may be impossible to differentiate from mitral opening snap unless the other associated features of the disease like presystolic liver pulsation are taken into consideration.

5. **Systolic ejection clicks:** These are produced by opening of either the aortic or the pulmonary valves at the end of isovolumic (isometric) contraction following the beginning of systole. Hence, they follow very closely the first heart sound.

Aortic ejection clicks are best heard at the apex, the left parasternal border, the aortic area or sometimes over the right carotid artery. They are sharp and high pitched and do not vary with phases of respiration. The aortic ejection clicks are heard when the aorta is dilated. Hence, they are present in patients with aortic aneurysm, syphilitic aortitis or abnormal dilatation of the aorta, coarctation of aorta, hypertension or aortic stenosis with post-stenotic dilatation.

Pulmonary ejection clicks have a peculiar me-

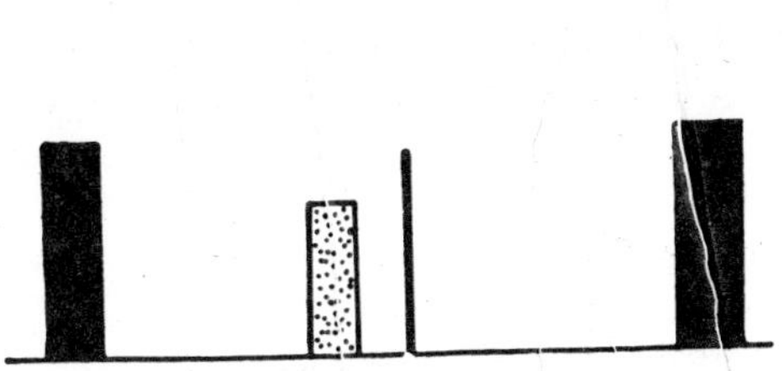

Fig. 12.11
Opening snap - in mitral stenosis after 2nd sound. Smaller the gap between 2nd sound and opening snap, tighter the stenosis.

tallic character and they are best heard in the pulmonary area. They change their character during phases of respiration. They are associated with dilated pulmonary artery, pulmonary stenosis, pulmonary hypertension or idiopathic pulmonary artery dilatation.

Both aortic and pulmonary clicks are usually associated with dilatation of the corresponding vessels. Hence, their mode of production is thought to be due to the vibrations caused by sudden distension of vessel walls (vascular theory).

The other probable cause of their mode of production is the sudden opening of the aortic or that of pulmonary valves (valvular theory).

6. **Pericardial clicks:** These are heard very frequently in cases of chronic constrictive pericarditis. (The term pericardial click should not be confused with pericardial rub.) There is an extra sound during diastole which is again at the end of isovolumic (isometric) relaxation period. This is supposed to be produced by the rapid filling of the ventricles against resistance at this time. The rapid filling is necessary as the constriction offers a resistance to filling of the ventricles. Nowadays so-called pericardial clicks are believed to be due to mitral valve prolapse.

7. **Gallop rhythm:** Potam in 1876 used the term gallop rhythm to describe the triple rhythm which is associated with ventricular failure.

(a) **Presystolic gallop:** This is produced due to fourth sound becoming audible. Phonetically it can be described as 'lub-lub-dup'. When there is a stress on the ventricles due to an increased pressure load, the atrial contractions become stronger to help the efficiency of the ventricles. As a result of more powerful atrial contractions there is an increased filling of the ventricles resulting in more stretching of the muscle fibres at the end of the diastole. The force of the ventricular contraction depends on this and diastolilc length of its muscle fibres (Sterling's law). These strong atrial contraction produce the gallop rhythm by making the physiological fourth sound audible.

If the gallop is left ventricular, these sounds are heard at the apex and if right ventricular they are better heard in the left parasternal area. The gallop is much better heard if the atrioventricular conduction time (P. R. interval in the electro-cardiograph) is prolonged or if there is a left bundle branch block.

Another theory put forward is that the extra sound, which if heard, is due to premature closure of either the mitral or the tricuspid valve depending upon whether the gallop is left or right ventricular. The left ventricular presystolic gallop is usually heard in hypertensive heart disease, aortic stenosis and myocardial infarction.

The right ventricular presystolic gallop is due to pulmonary stenosis. The interval between the gallop sound (extra sound) and the first sound can have a prognostic value. With improvement in the cardiac decompensation interval between the extra sound and the first sound shortens. With deterioration reverse takes place.

(b) **Protodiastolic gallop rhythm:** This term is a misnomer and should be replaced by the term diastolic gallop rhythm. Protodiastolic is the first part of ventricular relaxation while the extra sound in this type of gallop is heard after the phase of isovolumic relaxation.

The extra sound is caused by the sudden distension of ventricles and is produced at the end of the rapid filling phase. It is more common in ventrices with dilated musculature, having no elastic recoil.

The left ventricular diastolic gallop is best heard at the apex in the left lateral position and the right ventricular diastolic gallop is best heard in the fourth left parasternal area.

Common causes of this condition are:

i. Myocardial infarction with dilatation, ii. hypertension. iii. aortic incompetence, iv. mitral regurgitation and v. cardiomyopathies.

The prognosis of these two types of gallop rhythms can be summed up as follows: Gallop rhythm is the cry of the failing heart for help. The presyostolic gallop denotes a heart under stress which is trying to help itself while the protodiastolic gallop denotes a heart which has practically no further reserves left.

(c) **Summation gallop:** When there is marked tachycardia, the presystolic and the third heart sounds can be overlapping each other and the extra sound is heard in mid diastole. If this gallop disappears when the rate slows down, it is of no clinical significance. After slowing of the heart rate, the true nature of the gallop may be evident (i.e., either presystolic or diastolic).

(d) **Quadruple gallop:** If presystolic gallop of one ventricle is combined with the diastolic gallop rhythm of the other ventricle, this rare effect of four sounds being heard in one cardiac cycle can be produced.

Cardiac murmurs:

Murmur is an extra sound produced during the cardiac cycle usually caused by abnormal vibrations of the valves or vessel walls due to either an anatomical defect of these structures or abnormal flow of blood through them.

Mode of production of murmurs: Various theories have been put forward to explain the production of murmurs.

If the flow of blood at a particular part of CVS is turbulent then a murmur will be heard at that area. The turbulent sound is a modification of the smooth laminar flow. A turbulence is caused by two main factors,

1. The velocity of the blood, and
2. The calibre of the blood vessels.

Any abnormal alteration in these two will produce a murmur. Hence, a high velocity of blood flow due to forcible ejection or a dilatation of a particular chamber can produce a murmur. Similarly anaemia can produce a murmur by reducing the viscocity of blood and increasing flow of blood which occurs to meet the demands.

Any abnormal flow due to either high velocity or obstruction may cause bubbling due to liberation of water vapour and blood gases. This produces what is termed as cavitation. This will also produce a murmur. However, this mechanism is not acceptable due to lack of evidence.

The most accepted theory is the formation of eddies (or abnormal currents in a circular direction) due to either obstruction, back flow, flow in a dilated chamber or abnormally rapid flow. This hypothesis serves to explain all the murmurs produced and hence is most acceptable.

Physical abnormalities producing murmurs: Whatever explanation is accepted, murmurs are produced when the following physical abnormalities exist:

1. Hyperdynamic or rapid flow of blood
2. Obstruction to the flow of blood due to stenosis or due to a loose structure (atheromatous plaque or ruptured valve cusp or vegetation as in infective endocarditis).
3. Regurgitation of blood flow in a reverse direction.
4. Flow in an abnormally dilated chamber or vessel.

Description of murmurs: Whenever a murmur is heard the following points must be noted :

1. Timing: (a) Whether systolic or diastolic, (b) Whether it occupies only a particular part of systole or diastole or present throughout or particular phase of cardiac cycle, and (c) Whether continuous, i.e., throughout both systole or diastole.
2. Site: (a) Where it is best heard, (b) Whether localised or diffuse.
3. Intensity and character.
4. Direction of conduction if any.
5. Effect of respiration, posture, exercise and drugs.

1. **Timing:** Systolic murmurs are heard between the first and the second heart sounds and diastolic murmurs between the second and the following first heart sounds.

A systolic murmur may occupy the whole of systole when it is known as pansystolic murmur. It may obscure partly both the first and the second heart sounds and is usually of the same intensity throughout.

An ejection systolic murmur (also known as mid-systolic murmur) starts after the first heart sound. It gradually increases in intensity and then fades out before the beginning of the second sound (diamond shaped murmur). A long systolic murmur starts with the first sound and hence masks it. It may continue even after the first component of the second sound when it is split.

In general it can be said that systolic murmurs may be indicative of heart diseases or they may be innocent. Usually, the pansystolic and long, systolic murmurs indicate a disease process while a short ejection systolic murmur may be indicative of disease process or it may be innocent.

A diastolic murmur usually does not continue throughout diastole. There is no pandiastolic murmur as a rule. But rarely pandiastolic murmur is heard in severe aortic incompetence.

Early diastolic murmur occupies the first part of the diastole and starts immediately after the second sound.

A mid-diastolic murmur may be short — immediately after third heart sound or it may be prolonged when there is an obstruction to the atrioventricular flow (i.e., mid-diastolic murnur may continue as presystolic murmur).

A late diastolic murmur (presystolic) precedes the first sound and may end at the first sound. It usually has a crescendo or rising character when the atria are contracting normally. A diastolic murmur may combine the mid-diastolic timing with the presystolic crescendo character. A systolic and diastolic murmur can be present at the same time when they are called as to-and-fro or see-saw murmurs, e.g., aortic stenosis and incompetence.

A continuous murmur without interruption with an accentuation in the early diastole is heard in patients with patent ductus arteriosus.

2. **Site:** The site of maximum intensity of a murmur should be found out as it will point towards the accompanying cardiac pathology.

Knowledge of cardiac murmurs, and the site where they are best heard is essential to interpret the findings (for example murmur of aortic incompetence is best heard in the left parasternal area).

Whether the audibility of a murmur is restricted to a small area or whether it is heard diffusely over a wide area should be checked.

3. **Intensity and character:** A murmur may be very faint or very loud. Levine has classified and graded them into six categories. Grade I is faintest audible murmur, while grade VI is a murmur which may be heard even when the chest piece of the stethoscope is slightly removed from the chestwall. Grade III murmurs and above are usually accompanied by a thrill.

A crescendo murmur is one which progressively increases in intensity, e.g., presystolic murmur or mitral stenosis and a diminuendo or decrescendo murmur is the one which goes on waning in intensity, e.g., early diastolic murmur of aortic incompetence.

A murmur which increases in intensity and then diminishes is known as crescendo-decrescendo murmur or diamond shaped murmur, e.g., ejection systolic or midsystolic murmurs of aortic and pulmonary stenosis.

Character of murmurs depends on gradations of pitch with varying intensity. Hence a murmur may be described as blowing harsh, rumbling or cooing, in addition to its loudness. These characterisfics should be noted carefully as the very character of the murmur sometimes suggests the nature of the underlying defect.

4. **Direction of conduction:** The murmurs are conducted usually in the direction of the blood flow producing the murmur. Hence, a murmur of mitral incompetence is conducted laterally in the axilla and a murmur of aortic stenosis is heard over the neck vessels.

A very loud murmur may be heard diffusely in all directions because of its loudness itself. It is transmission of murmur and not conduction. This should not be confused with conduction (the two terms are not synonymous). When a murmur is conducted, its intensity is the same at the parent site and at the site where it is conducted, and when it is transmitted, its intensity at the parent site is more than that at the site where it is transmitted.

5. **Effect of respiration, posture, exercise and drugs:** Inspiration increases the blood flow through the tricuspid and pulmonary valves (due to the increased intra- thoracic negative pressure causing increased venous return). Hence, the murmurs produced by defects on right side of the heart are heard louder during inspiration. As opposed to this, the murmurs on the left side of the

heart may become softer during inspiration. Murmurs caused by left to right side shunts may become softer during inspiration.

During inspiration, a larger portion of the heart is covered by the pulmonary tissue and hence during this phase of respiration there may be a mechanical muffling of the murmurs.

Posture may affect the character of the murmurs. Certain murmurs are best heard when the patient is lying down in a particular position (left lateral position makes the murmur of mitral stenosis more prominent), while other murmurs may be best heard when the patient is sitting up and bending forward (murmur of aortic incompetence).

Exercise increases the rate of circulation and hence faint murmurs are better heard after exercise. It may also augment a thrill which was previously doubtfully palpable.

Amylnitrite lowers the peripheral vascular resistance and hence it makes ejection aortic murmurs prominent and the regurgitant left sided murmurs fainter. Phenylephrine and nore-pinephrine increases the peripheral resistance and have an opposite effect.

Pathogenic & Non-pathogenic Murmurs

A. **Non-pathogenic:** Systolic murmurs. (I) Innocent murmurs : Usually mid-systolic (Apparently no cause detected). (II) Flow murmurs : Found in hyperdynamic circulation — Exertion, anaemia, fever, beriberi, thyrotoxicosis, pregnancy and Paget's disease of the bone rarely with arterio-venous fistula.

B. **Pathogenic : I. Systolic :** (I) Due to forward flow: (ejection or mid-systolic). (a) Aortic area : (i) Increased flow — aortic incompetence or rarely in complete heart block. (ii) Obstructive: aortic stenosis (including infundibular). Supra-aortic stenosis, coarctation of aorta. (iii) Dilatation of distal chamber (syphilitic aortitis, aortic aneurysm; atheromatous dilatation). (b) Pulmonary: (i) Increased flow: In left to right shunt, ventricular septal defect and atrial septal defect. (ii) Obstructive : pulmonary stenosis. (iii) dilatation of distal chamber (pulmonary artery). Primary or secondary pulmonary hypertension. (2) Due to regurgitation: (pansystolic or holo systolic). (a) Atrio-ventricular (A-V) valve incompetence : Mitral incompetence (pathological or functional). Tricuspid incompetence (pathological or functional). (b) Left to right shunt : Ventricular septal defect. Early cases of patent ductus arteriosus.

II. **Diastolic murmurs** (all diastolic murmurs):

(1) **Early diastolic:** (a) Aortic : (i) Valvular incompetence, (ii) dissecting aneurysm (causing dilatation of the valve ring) and (iii) bicuspid aortic valve (congenital). (b)Pulmonary : (i) due to pulmonary hypertension either primary or secondary (Graham Steel murmur, (ii) Pulmonary incmpetence, (iii) aneurysm of pulmonary artery (very rare).

(2) **Mid-diastolic:** (a) Atrioventricular (A.V.) valve stenosis : mitral or tricuspid stenosis. (b) A.V. Valve obstruction : ball valve thrombus or atrial myxoma. (c) Increased flow across A.V. valves : (i) Across mitral valve—mitral incompetence , ventricular septal defect (V.S.D.), patent ductus arteriosus (P.D.A.) (flow murmur). (ii) Across tricuspid valve : A.S.D. Anomalous pulmonary venous drainage. (d) A.V. valve inflammation : Carey Coombs murmur occurs in rheumatic carditis to be differentiaed from mitral stenotic murmur by the fact that in rheumatic carditis heart sounds are muffled, the murmur changes its character from time to time. In mitral stenosis 1st sound at mitral area is loud and sharp and the murmur does not have changing character.

(3) **Presystolic or late diastolic:** (a) A. V. valve stenosis; (i) mitral stenosis, (ii) tricuspid stenosis. (b) A. V. valve obstruction : (i) due to ball valve thrombus or atrial myxoma, (ii) due to the regurgitant blood flow from aortic incompetence impinging upon mitral valve cusp (Austin flint murmur).

III. **Continuous murmurs** (all continuous murmurs) : (1) Innocent continuous murmurs: Venous hum. (2) Due to communication between left and right side of the heart of systemic and pulmonary circulation. Patent ductus arteriosus, aorto-pulmonary window, arteriovenus fistula.

(3) Murmurs simulating continuous murmurs : Combination of pansystolic and diastolic murmurs. Aortic stenosis with incompetence. Mitral stenosis with incompetence.

The accompanying table has classified all types of murmurs. Essential features of the important murmurs commonly encountered in clinical practice will now be discussed.

Innocent murmurs: (Fig. 12.12a)

Usually these are detected on routine medical examination when the patient does not have any cardiac symptoms. They do not denote any structural change in the heart or great vessels. They are usually mid-systolic or of ejection types. The common sites at which they are usually heard are: 1. Pulmonary area. 2. Left parasternal area. 3. Rarely at the apex.

Their intensity is mild to moderate except sometimes in young children where they may be quite loud.

They are usually not accompanied by any palpable thrills. They are not conducted but sometimes they are heard all over the front of the chest. They are commonly affected by respiration and change of posture. Valsalva's manoeuvre usually has no effect on them.

They are not associated with any other evidence of cardiac disease like chamber enlargement (though there is generalised cardiac enlargement in anaemia and thyrotoxicosis). To confirm the absence of any abnormality, 2 D-ECHO may be undertaken.

If due to hyperdynamic circulatory states, they disappear when the cause is treated.

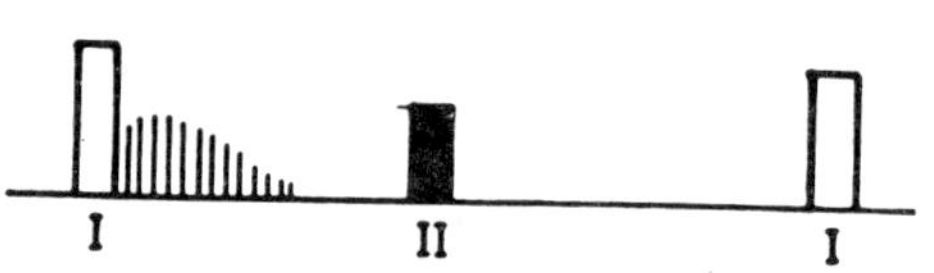

Fig. 12.12a

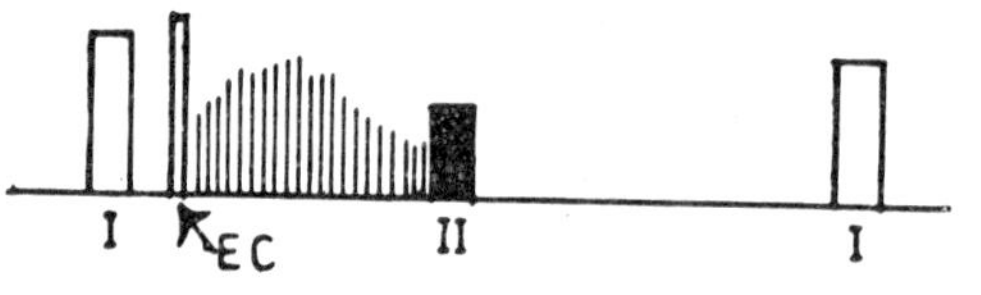

Fig. 12.12b

Pathogenic murmurs (Systolic murmurs) : (Fig. 12.12b)

(1) **Ejection or mid-systolic :** (a) **Due to aortic stenosis (A.S.) :** This is a loud, harsh, ejection systolic murmur best heard in the second right intercostal space in the parasternal area.

It is usually accompanied by a thrill. It is well conducted to the neck and may be widely heard over the precordium. The aortic component of the second sound is usually absent or very faint.

The murmur begins shortly after the first sound and may be preceded by aortic ejection click. More severe the stenosis, harsher is the murmur. Also with severe stenosis, the murmur reaches its maximum intensity later in systole as the left ventricular ejection is prolonged.

Etiology is : (i) Rheumatic, (ii) Congenital, (iii) Idiopathic calcific, or (iv) Atherosclerotic.

(b) **Aortic ejection murmur accompanying aortic incompetence (A.I.) (in-absence of stenosis) :** This is also a harsh systolic murmur in mid-systole at the aortic area. It is usually not heard at the apex but is well transmitted to the neck vessels. It may be difficult at times to distinguish the murmur from that of accompanying aortic stenosis. The points which will differentiate it from that of aortic stenosis are:

i. Flow murmur associated with A. I. is not accompanied by a thrill.
ii. If due to aortic stenosis with aortic incompetence, the pulse will have a classic bisfariens character.
iii. When due to combined valvular AS and AI the murmur may be preceded with an ejection click, while it is absent in AI with a flow murmur.

(c) **Ejection murmurs associated with dialtation of aorta:** A short systolic ejection murmur is heard over the aortic area which is conducted to neck vessels. Maximum intensity occurs in early or mid-systole. To distinguish it from the two murmurs described above (i.e., murmurs of either AS or a flow murmur along with AI) careful attention should be given to the second sound. It is accentuated and may have classic tambour quality (ringing in nature).

Etiology of aortic dilatation: Syphilitic aortitis, aortic aneurysm, atherosclerotic aorta, hypertension, rarely post-traumatic and congenital abnormalities of aorta.

(d) **Murmur associated with coarctation of aorta:** Usually loud systolic murmur best heard at the base of the heart is aortic ejection murmur. There is a long systolic murmur heard over the back in the interscapular area due to narrowing of the aorta.

(e) **Systolic ejection murmur over the pulmonary area:** (Fig. 12.12c) Pulmonary stenosis produces an ejection systolic murmur which may be preceded by an ejection click. The murmur may continue up to the pulmonary valve closure and hence can cross the aortic compoment of the second sound. It is usually accompanied by a thrill. Pulmonary component or second sound at pulmonary area is diminished or absent.

Increased blood flow to the right side of the heart due to septal defects will increase the volume of the blood to be ejected by the right ventricle and ejection systolic murmur over the pulmonary area. Pulmonary hypertension will produce an ejection systolic murmur with a loud pulmonary component of the second sound (helps to differentiate from systolic murmur of pulmonary stenosis).

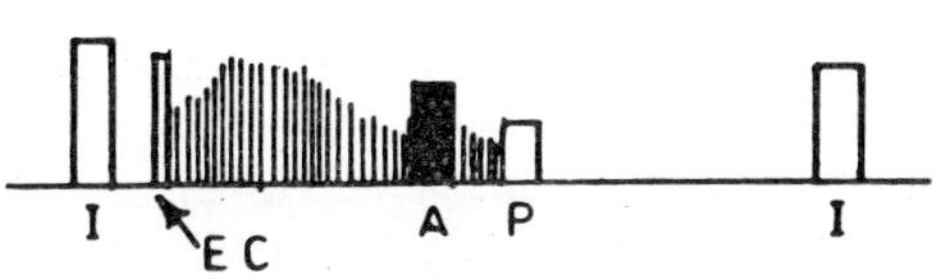

Fig. 12.12 c

2. **Pansystolic murmurs : (Fig. 12.12 d)**

a. **Due to mitral incompetence (MI) :** This pansystolic (also known as holosystolic) murmur is best heard at the apex. It is frequently loud, grade IV-VI. It starts with or immediately after the first sound. It continues throughout the systole and does not wax or wane during any part of systole. It has the same intensity throughout. It may continue partly in early diastole. It is usually accompanied by a thrill and is well conducted to the axilla in a lateral direction.

Quite frequently both the heart sounds are not heard properly in a patient having MI. The absence of second sound is easy to understand as it is due to the murmur masking of the second sound. The first sound may be poorly heard or buried in the murmur due to either rigidity of the cusps of the valve or due to their destruction by the disease process causing the incompetence.

The murmur starts with the first sound. This is due to the immediate regurgitation of blood when the systole begins. Normally there is a period of isovolumic (isometric) contraction when the systolic begins. During this phase both AV valves and aortic and pulmonary valves are closed. Due to the incompetence of valves this phase is not present in the ventricles and the murmur continues up to the second sound.

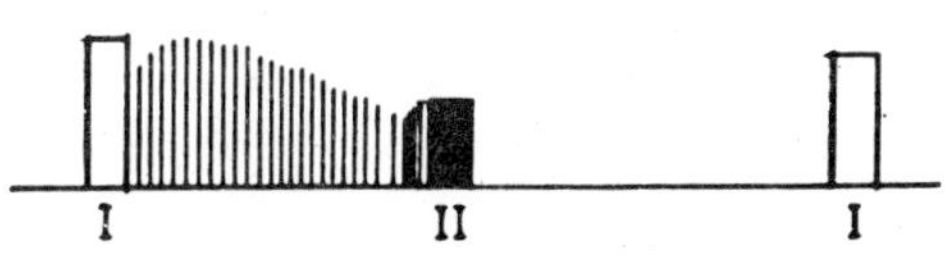

Fig. 12.12d

For the same reason the murmur can spill over in early diastole. When the ventricles relax, the pressure in their cavity falls rapidly and aortic and pulmonary valves close. On the left side, the aortic valves close when the mean pressure in left ventricle falls below 70 mm. Normally there is no back flow. However, in diseased states causing incompetence, the pressure in the ventricle allows the blood to regurgitate in the atrium causing the continuation of murmur in the early diastole.

Etiology Of MI : (i) Mainly rheumatic. (ii) Infective endocarditis. (iii) Traumatic or spontaneous rupture of a valve cusp. (iv) Mitral valve prolapse (MVP).

(b) **Murmur due to tricuspid incompetence :** A murmur similar to that of MI is heard over the parasternal area which becomes louder with inspiration. However, it is very difficult to differentiate it clinically from that of mitral incompetence especially when the heart is rotated in a clockwise fashion.

Etiology : Most commonly encountered along with a tight mitral stenosis causing pulmonary hypertension and dilatation of the right ventricle. The imcompetence can be designated as functional in these cases.

(c) **Murmur due to ventricular septal defect :** (Fig. 12.12e) This murmur is best heard in the third and fourh interspaces on the left side in the parasternal line. It is louder in expiration.

The murmur is quite often associated with a thrill. The louder the murmur, smaller is the defect. The loudest murmur is heard with a very small defect and this does not alter the hemodynamics of the heart in any way. This condition is known as Maladie de Roger or Roger's disease.

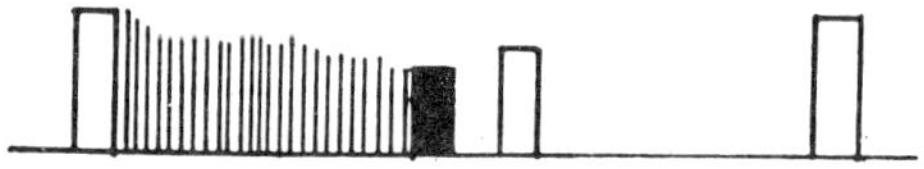

Fig. 12.12e

Diastolic murmurs:

(1) **Early diastolic : (a) Aortic incompetence (AI):** (Fig. 12.13a) The early diastolic murmur of AI starts immediately after the aortic component of the second sound. The aortic component itself is diminished in intensity. The murmur is high ptiched and is loudest initially and then fades away (diminuendo). It can be heard in the aortic area but is usually best heard at the left border of the sternum and sometimes at the apex. The duration of the murmur is short when the leak is slight and longer and louder when the leak is massive.

It is best heard by the chest piece of the stethoscope. It is more easily heard when the patient sits up and bends forward and especially holds the breath in expiration.

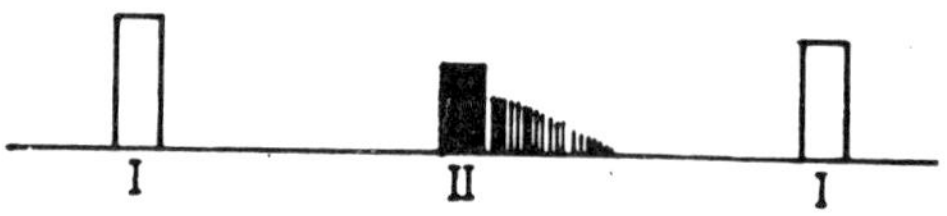

Fig. 12.13a

(b) **Due to pulmonary incompetene (PI) :** It has similar characteristics as that of the murmur of aortic incompetence. It is usually restricted to the left second and third space. More commonly the cause of this murmur is functional, being secondary to pulmonary hypertension (Graham Steel murmur). (Differentiation between the murmurs of AI and PI may be impossible on auscultation alone.)

The most important differentiating point is the presence or absence of peripheral signs of aortic incompetence. The loud pulmonary component of second sound in pulmonary hypertension is the other differentiating point.

(2) **Mid-diastolic :** (a) **Due to mitral stenosis:** (Fig. 12.13b) This is a long mid-diastolic murmur which is the characteristic murmur of mitral stenosis. (Not the presystolic accentuation which may or may not be associated with it.) It is a loud and rumbling murmur which may be preceded by the opening snap of the mitral valve. It is a well localised murmur and may be heard only just inside the apex. It is better heard when the patient is lying on the left side. The length of the murmur is proportional to the severity of stenosis. The longer the mid-diastolic murmur, the more severe is the stenosis. However, the intensity of the murmur is not proportional to the degree of stenosis. For, it

is influenced by other factors like cardiac failure. In the presence of failure the murmur is softer in intensity.

The murmur becomes prominent when the patient is given exercise.

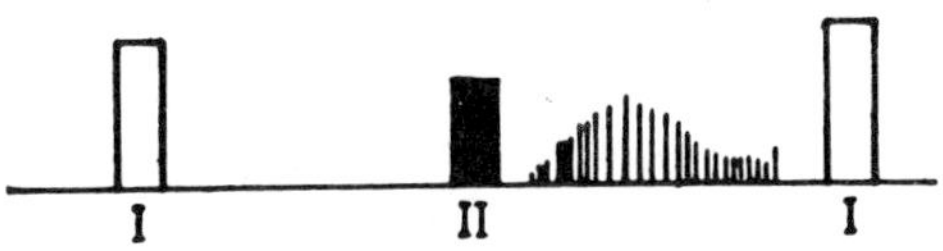

Fig. 12.13b

(b) **Due to increased flow across the mitral valve:** (Functional apical mid-diastolic murmur): Usually this murmur is associated with mitral incompetence, ventricular septal defect (VSD), patent ductus arteriosus (PDA) and atrial septal defect but may occasionally be present in any hyperdynamic state of circulation like thyrotoxicosis mand anaemia. The murmur is usually short mid-diastolic best heard by the apex.

(c) **Due to AV valve inflammation:** (Carey Coombs murmur) : (Fig. 12.13c). It is a short, low pitched mid-diastolic murmur present in acute rheumatic carditis leading to mitral valvulitis. It has a peculiar cooing character and murmur may disappear and re-appear. It is never accompanied by a thrill. It is best heard by the bell end of the stethoscope when the patient is lyng on the left lateral position. The heart sounds are muffled due to myocarditis and murmur has a changing character.

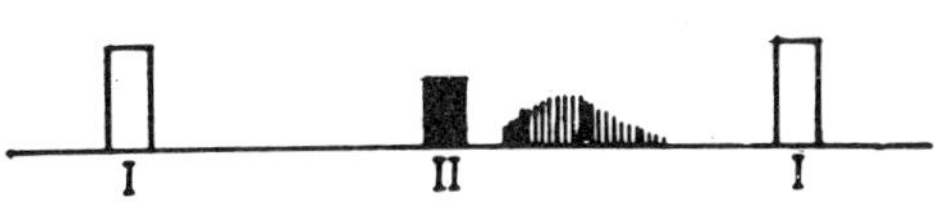

Fig. 12.13 c

3. **Presystolic or late diastolic (a) Due to mitral stenosis:** (Fig. 12.13 d). This is an accentuation of the mid-diastolic murmur by more forceful passage of the blood during atrial contraction. It has a typical crescendo character and the murmur ends in the sharp first sound.

It is usually accompanied by a thrill and is best heard by the bell piece of the stethoscope. It is heard usually over a small area internal to the apex. It disappears when atrial fibrillation sets in (which is a common accompaniment of mitral stenosis) as then the forcible atrial contractions causing this murmur are absent.

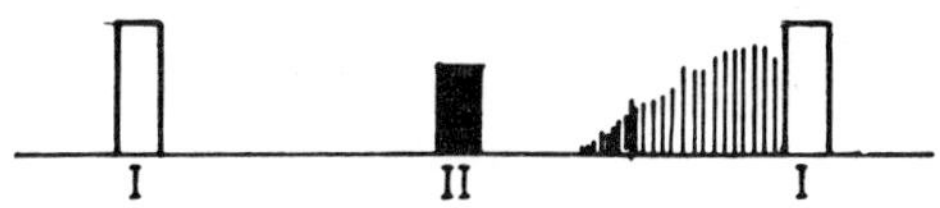

Fig. 12.13 d

(b) **Austin Flint murmur:** It is a presystolic murmur heard at the apex associated with aortic incompetence. There is no associated mitral valve disease. It is due to vibrations of the anterior cusp of the mitral valve by the regurgitant flow of blood which is directed on it.

Differentiation of this murmur from that of an associated mitral stenosis is very difficult. Presence of an opening snap and loud first sound at mitral area show presence of associated stenosis. Fig. 12.13e

4. **Due to tricuspid stenosis:** The murmur has the same characteristics as that of murmur of mitral stenosis but is best heard over the tricuspid area. It is better heard during inspiration.

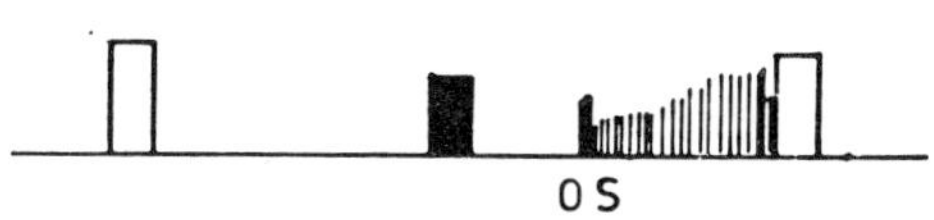

Fig. 12.13e

Continuous murmurs:

1. **Innocent continuous murmurs :** Venous hum: (a) **Jugular Venous hum :** It is a continous murmur due to flow of blood from the jugular vein

into the superior vena cava. It is better heard in the second right interspace and disappears on compression of the jugular vein or when the patient is lying down. This murmur is common in children.

(b) **Anomalous pulmonary Venous drainage:** May give rise to a similar hum which is best heard in the anterior axillary line.

Other innocent, continuous murmurs are the souffle heard over the internal mammary artery during pregnancy or lactation. Sometimes a uterine souffle can be heard over the abdomen in the last trimester of pregnancy.

2. **Due to communication between the left and right side of the heart : (a) Due to patent (persistent) ductus arteriosus (PDA)** (Fig. 12.14) : Classically described as a machinery murmur (also known as Gibson's murmur who described it first), it is practically diagnostic of PDA.

It is a continuous loud murmur, almost always associated with thrill and best heard over the second left interspace in the parasternal area. The murmur has a waxing quality and it waxes in late systole and early diastole, i.e., it is loudest near the second sound.

A similar murmur is heard in aorta-pulmonary window.

3. **Murmurs simulating continuous murmurs :** Any combination of a systolic and diastolic murmur may simulate a continuous or to-and-fro murmur.

However, of the few combinations which mimic it, the closest are :

(a) Ventricular septal defect with aortic incompetence
(b) Mitral and aortic incompetence
(c) Mitral stenosis and incompetence
(d) Aortic stenosis and incompetence

Pericardial rub : Also known as friction rub, it is pathognomonic of pericarditis. It is a harsh grating sound best heard in the left parasternal area (but can be heard anywhere over the precordium). It is heard both during systole and diastole and hence has a to-and-fro nature. It is usually localised to a small area. It is better heard by increasing the pressure of the chest piece of the stethosope on the chest wall and may be better heard when the patient is standing up than when lying down. It is sometimes palpable. Pericardial rubs may disappear from time to time and then re-appear.

Fig. 12.14
Continuous mumur

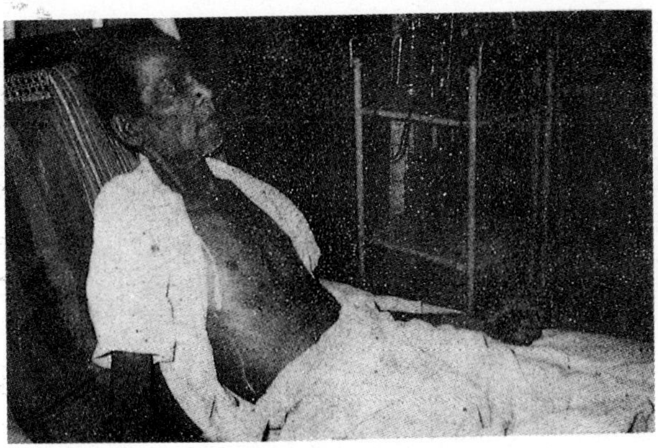

Pl. 11.1 Orthopnea

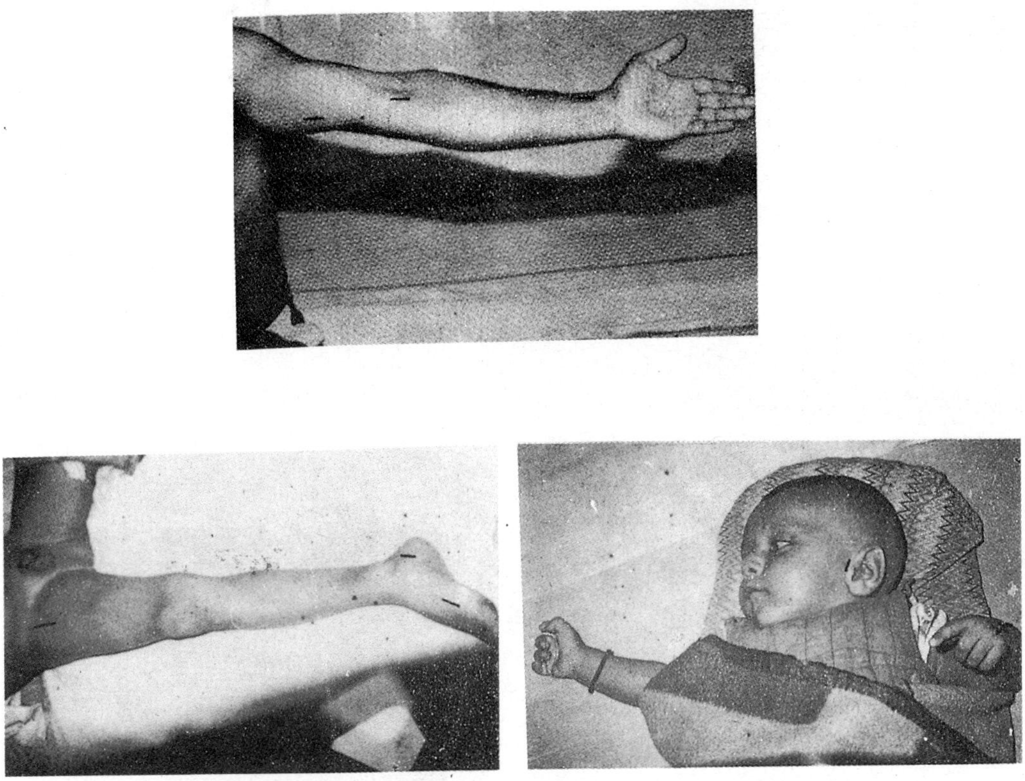

Pl. 12.1 Sites where to palpate various arteries. Temporal artery - in front of pinna of ear. Radial - lateral lower anterior aspect of forearm just above the wrist. Brachial - medial to tendon of biceps. Axillary - medial aspect of middle 1/3 of arm. It should be palpated from medial aspect against the bone. Femoral - at mid inguinal point - i.e. mid way between ant. superior iliac spine and pubic symphysis. popliteal - posteriorly in middle of popliteal fossa. Posterior tibial A - mid way between medial malleolus. and heel. Dorsal pedis - on dorsum of foot at base of 1st metatarsal.

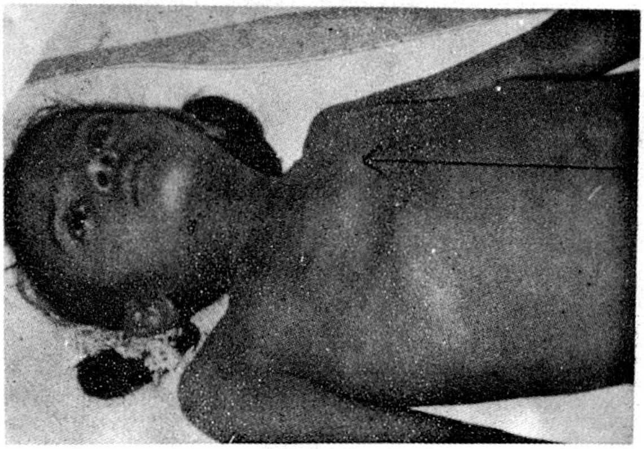

Pl. 12.2 Bulging precordium.

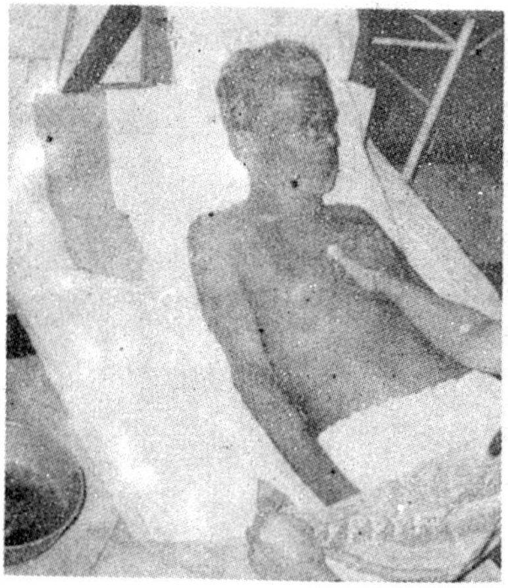

Pl. 12.3 Dressler's method.

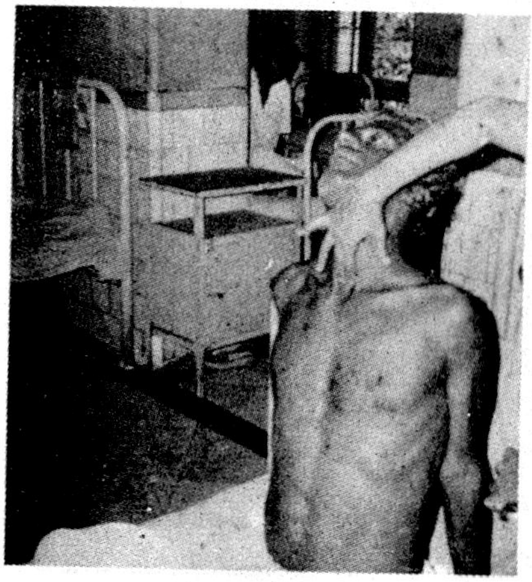

Pl. 12.4 Tracheal tag.

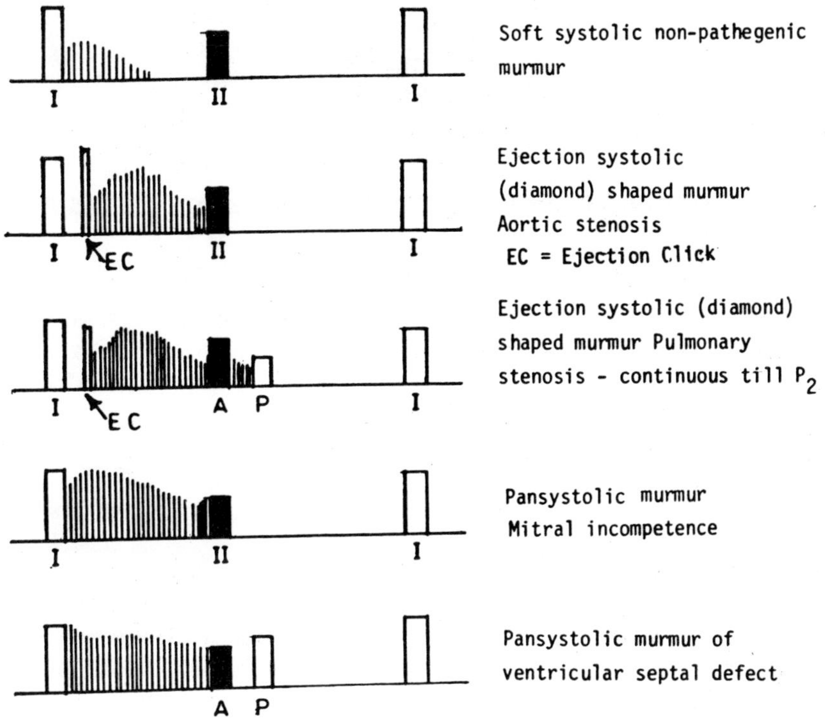

Fig. 12.12

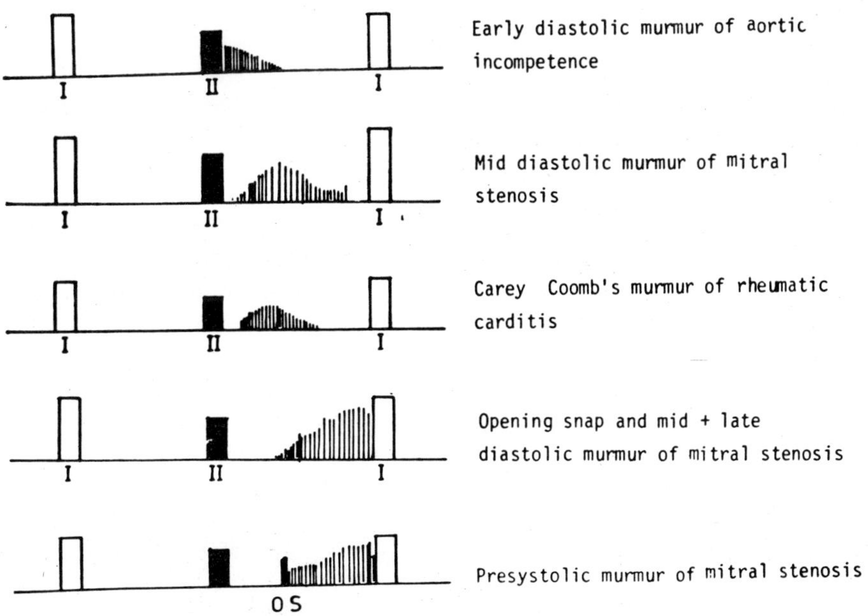

Fig. 12.13

13. Cardiovascular System — Common Disorders Encountered

I. Heart failure:

This term covers a variety of diseases and no single definition may apply to all of them.

The simplest possible definition of heart failure is a condition where the heart is unable to maintain an adequate output despite adequate venous return.

However, this definition does not cover the conditions like shock, etc., where the cardiac failure is due to poor venous return to the heart.

Classification: Various classifications at heart failure are possible :

I. It can be classified according to the output.

High output failure	**Low output failure**
Those conditions with hyperdynamic circulation	with diminished cardiac output
1. Anaemia	1. Secondary to coronary artery disease
2. Beriberi	2. Valvular diseases e.g., mitral stenosis
3. Thyrotoxicosis	3. Congenital heart disease, e.g., VSD
4. Paget's disease of the bone	4. Hypertension
5. Cor pulmonale	5. Myocarditis
6. A. V. fistula	6. Pericardial disease
	7. Endocardial disease (Infective endocarditis)

II. **Right sided failure** (RVF)	**Left sided failure** (LVF)
Caused by purely right sided lesions, such as:	Caused by purely left sided lesions, such as :
1. Pulmonary valve diseases	1. Mitral valve diseases
2. Tricuspid valve diseases	2. Aortic valve diseases
	3. Systemic hypertension

Congestive cardiac failure is the failure of both sides of the heart. This may be due to the right ventricular failure following left sided failure or when both the chambers fail simultaneously.

III. Backward heart failure	**Forward heart failure**
During the failure of one or both ventricles there is rise in back pressure due to elevation of the end diastolic volume in that chamber. This rise of pressure is reflected in the pressures and volumes of atrial chambers and retrograde venous system. The rise of pressure at the capillary end of the venous system is responsible for exudation of fluid out of the circulation and into the interstitial spaces causing edema.	All the symptoms of heart failure are due to inadequate output. Due to reduced output there is a decreased flow in the arterial circulation. Hence there is diminished renal perfusion which causes a retention of salt and water.

The increased renal tubular reabsorption of sodium caused by an increased renal venous pressure contributes towards the water logging.

Both the mechanisms operate together in most patients with heart failure and a distinction between the two cannot be made.

Left sided failure:

Definition: Failure of the left ventricle mainly but sometimes that of left atrium with a normal output of right ventricle.

Etiology:

1. Due to primary myocardial affection of the left ventricle.
   i. Myocardial ischaemia due to ischaemic heart disease.
   ii. Myocarditis
   iii. Cardiomyopathy
2. Obstruction or resistance to the left ventricular outflow (Systolic overload):
   i. Aortic stenosis
   ii. Systemic hypertension
3. Insufficient output due to regurgitant lesions (diastolic overload):
   i. Aortic incompetence
   ii. Mitral incompetence
   iii. Ventricular septal defect
   iv. Patent ductus arteriosus.
4. Left atrial failure — commonest causes are:
   i. Mitral stenosis and acute mitral regurgitation
   ii. The latter condition follows MVP or acute myocardial infarction.
5. Restriction of left ventricular filling or contraction :
   i. Localised constrictive pericarditis
   ii. Endomyocardial fibrosis.

Clinical symptoms:

(1) **Dyspnea:** (a) On exertion, (b) At rest, (c) Paroxysmal nocturnal dyspnea (cardiac asthma), (d) Orthopnea, (e) Attacks of acute pulmonary edema.

(2) **Cough:** (a) Dry or with scanty expectoration, (b) Paroxysms of cough only on exertion.

(3) **Haemoptysis:** (a) Scanty (blood stained sputum), (b) Rarely massive (due to pulmonary infarction).

(4) Profuse sweating.

(5) Fatigue, weakness, insomnia, oliguria (these symptoms are due to reduction in forward flow).

Signs:

(1) **Pulse:** (i) Tachycardia, (ii) Pulsus alternans, (iii) Presence of extrasystoles (though not a characteristic feature, it is very commonly associated).

(2) **Blood pressure:** (i) May reflect the causative disease like systemic hypertension or aortic incompetence, (ii) May fall during attacks of severe left ventricular failure.

(3) **Respiration:** (i) Orthopnea, (ii) Cheyne-stokes respiration.

(4) **Examination of the C.V.S.:** Left ventricular hypertrophy : (i) Apex impulse shifted downwards and outwards, (ii) May be heaving or hyperdynamic on palpation, (iii) Cardiac border on left side is beyond normal limit, (iv) First heart sound may be muffled (tictac rhythm or embryocardia), (v) Gallop rhythm (presystolic, protodiastolic or summation type), (vi) Mid-systolic murmur due to left ventricular hypertrophy or dilatation.

(5) **Examination of the respiratory system:** (i) Prolonged expiration causing bronchovesicular breathing, (ii) Crepitations heard at the bases of the lungs (especially posteriorly), (iii) Coarse generalised rales due to pulmonary edema, (iv) Cheyne-Stokes respiration, (v) Pleural fluid (hydrothorax).

Investigations:

Radiological investigations: X-ray : (a) Hilar congestion, (b) Radiating opaque shadows from the hilum (butterfly wings or bat's wings shadows), (c) Ground glass appearance in interstitial pulmonary edema, (d) Pleural effusions with inter lobar effusions called vanishing tumors of lung, (e) Left ventricular hypertrophy or dilatation.

Electrocardiogram: (a) Left ventricular (L.V.) hypertrophy, (b) L. V. hypertrophy with strain, (c) Myocardial ischemia or infarction, (d) Left atrial hypertrophy

Treatment:

(1) Rest in bed. Preferably with back rest in propped up position (2) Liquid diet in the acute phase. Principles: Low calories diet with restriction of salt (3) Oxygen (4) Sedation (5) Diuretics (6) Bronchodilator (7) Digitalisation (8) Tranquillizer:

II. **Congestive cardiac failure:**

Causes: 1. Right ventricular failure secondary to left sided failure. 2. Cor pulmonale. 3. Pulmonary stenosis or pulmonary hypertension. 4. Tricuspid incompetence of tricuspid stenosis. 5. Localised constrictive pericarditis and endomyocardial fibrosis.

Symptoms: 1. Symptoms of left sided failure: However, attacks of pulmonary edema are absent as the failure of right ventricle prevents the excessive congestion of the lungs. Similarly orthopnea is a late or absent feature. 2. **Edema of the feet or dependent parts :** Earliest around the ankles and may increase after exertion. Later on may become generalised. 3. **Pain in the right hypochondrium :** Congestion of the liver because of stretching of the hepatic capsule can cause acute pain. Seen in acute or recent failures as repeated or continuous stretching of the hepatic capsule makes the pain endings less sensitive to pain. Hence, the pain in right hypochondrium is absent in chronic congestive cardiac failure. 4. **Symptoms due to systemic congestion:** C.N.S.-Restlessness. Lack of concentration, irritability, mental confusion. **A.S.**-Anorexia, nausea, vomiting. **Renal :** Oliguria, nocturia.

Signs: Pulse: Thready and rapid due to congestive failure. Blood pressure : May reflect the abnormality as the causative lesion. J.V. pressure-raised. Hepatojugular reflux present. C.V.S. : 1. Signs of enlarged right ventricle or enlarged both ventricles. 2. Tachycardia. 3. Gallop rhythm (right ventricular). 4. Functional tricuspid incompetence causing a pansystolic murmur. 5. Signs of the causative lesion, e.g. mitral stenosis. **Other associated signs :** 1. Edema of the dependent parts. If the patient is bedridden for a long time the edema will be seen on sacrum. (As much as 5 to 6 litres of fluid may accumulate in the body before edema is detected clinically). 2. Palpable enlarged tender liver with smooth surface. Pulsations may be felt if associated with tricuspid incompetence. (In chronic congestive failure of long duration, liver will develop changes of cardiac cirrhosis. Then it will be nodular. Spleen may be palpable and ascites may be present). 3. Congestion at the lung bases. Rales more easily heard posteriorly. 4. Peripheral cyanosis : Due to sluggish circulation. 5. Hydrothorax. 6. Cardiac cachexia : May be apparent only after diuretic therapy.

Investigations:

Radiology: X-ray chest : May show a diffuse cardiac enlargement. E.S.R.: Reduced in congestive cardiac failure. (Important feature in cases of C.C.F. due to active rheumatic carditis).

Treatment: 1. Rest in bed : Anxiety should be alleviated by the use of tranquillisers. 2. Diet : Low calorie. Salt restricted diet. 3. Digitalisation. 4. Diuretics.

III. **Mitral stenosis:**

Etiology: 1. Due to rheumatic fever in most of the cases. 2. Congenital. 3. Lutembacher's syndrome (associated with A.S.D.). 4. Hurler's syndrome (Gargoylism). 5. Rarely due to endomyocardial fibrosis.

Other diseases which may simulate mitral stenosis: 1. Ball valve thrombus of the left atrium. 2. Left atrial tumours (like myxoma). 3. Cor triatriatum. 4. Austin Flint murmur (due to aortic incompetence).

Mitral stenosis is more common in females than in males and manifests a few years after the attack of rheumatic fever.

Haemodynamics:

The orifice of the normal mitral valve is 4-6 sq cms in area and the normal pressure in the left atrium at rest 6 mm Hg. Due to the stenosis (in a mild case the orifice of the mitral valve is 2 x 1 cm, in an average stenosis 1 x 0.5 cm and in a severe case it may be as small as 5 x 3 mm) there is an increase in the left atrial pressure and hence in the pulmonary circulation a gradient of about 10 mm of Hg is required between the pulmonary arteries and the veins. Initially as the pressure in the pulmonary veins rises, the pressure in the pulmonary arteries also rises passively in order to maintain the pulmonary blood flow. This is known as passive pulmonary hypertension.

However, when the mean left atrial pressure rises above 20 mm Hg the pulmonary artery pressure rises to very high levels due to pulmonary arteriolar constriction and hence there is an active pulmonary hypertension.

This pulmonary vasoconstriction usually affects the muscular arteries of the lower lobes and finally causes their medial hypertrophy. The upper lobe arteries are usually spared and may even be dilated.

Along with the development of this pulmonary hypertension there is a thickening of the capillary walls, interstitial tissue fluid is drained by the lymphatics.

The increased pressure in the pulmonary arteries increase the work load of the right ventricle which consequently may not be able to maintain its normal output against the increased pulmonary artery resistance and then fails resulting in the rise of systemic venous pressure (right ventricular failure).

Symptoms:

1. No complaints in the stage of complete compensation.

2. Symptoms due to left atrial failure. a. Dyspnea at first on exertion then even at rest. b. Attacks of paroxysmal nocturnal dyspnea or cardiac asthma. c. Orthopnea. d. Attacks of acute pulmonary edema. e. Cough. f. Fainting spells because of diminished blood flow to brain due to reduced left ventricular output. g. Haemoptysis.

Haemoptysis can occur under following situations :

i. Sudden massive pulmonary haemorrhage known as pulmonary apoplexy may occur. It is usually an early symptom in the life history of this disease, and is usually due to rupture of a small intrapulmonary vein, due to sudden rise in the left atrial pressure following sudden exertion or during pregnancy.
ii. Blood stained sputum which is associated with attacks of cardiac asthma.
iii. Pink frothy sputum due to acute pulmonary edema.
iv. Due to supervening bronchitis, also called winter bronchitis.
v. Frank red haemoptysis associated with pulmonary infarction.

3. **Symptoms due to left atrial dilatation:** a. Compression of left recurrent laryngeal nerve can produce hoarseness of voice (Ortner's, syndrome). b. Compression of oesophagus can produce dysphagia.

4. **Cardiac pain:** Anginal pains due to limitation of cardiac output.

5. **Palpitations:** a. Due to hypertrophy of the chambers. b. Due to atrial fibrillation.

6. **Symptoms of embolism:** a. Due to obstruction of the blood flow and dislodgement of small thrombi from a ball valve thrombus. b. More common with atrial fibrillaiton. c. Infected emboli when infective endocarditis supervenes.

7. **Symptoms of congestive cardiac failure:** a. edema, b. Pain over the hepatic area due to right ventricular failure. (Usually in long standing cases with severe pulmonary hypertension).

Signs:

General examination: a. Mitral facies and peripheral cyanosis: Peripheral cyanosis is due to a low cardiac output causing peripheral vasoconstriction. More common in patients having severe pulmonary hypertension.

b. Pulse : i. Usually well felt (but low in force, tension and volume). ii. Irregularly irregular if there is atrial fibrillation.

c. J.V.P.: i. Absence of "a" waves when atrial fibrillation is present. ii. Giant "a" waves seen when there is severe pulmonary hypertension.

Cardiac examination:

Inspection and palpation: 1. Apex impulse may be shifted outwards, well felt, tapping in character and may show apical retraction when associated with marked right ventricular hypertrophy. 2. Left parasternal pulsations seen and right ventricular heave felt. 3. Pulmonary second sound felt as a diastolic shock. 4. Diastolic thrill felt in mitral area, more prominent when the patient is turned in the left lateral position.

Auscultation: 1. First sound is accentuated, can be best described as a loud sharp sound (also known as closing snap). 2. A mid-diastolic murmur heard best at the apex. It is localised to an area just inside the apex impulse. (Best heard in the left lateral position). This murmur is more characteristic of mitral stenosis as the presystolic accentuation may disappear when atrial fibrillation sets in. When the stenosis is severe this murmur is softer and longer in duration. 3. Presystolic accentuation of the diastolic murmur (described first by Fauvelin in 1843). 4. Opening snap (O.S.) of the mitral valve (first described by Potain) is heard immediately after the second sound. In severe stenosis, the distance between the second sound and the opening snap is shorter. The sound is produced by the sudden flapping open of the cusps of the mitral valve (mainly the aortic cusps). The fibrosed valves open suddenly due to high left atrial pressure. Opening snap is absent when the valves are calcified. 5. Loud pulmonary component of the second sound best heard over the pulmonary area. 6. Graham Steel murmur : Early diastolic murmur in the pulmonary area and third left parasternal area.

Common investigations: 1. **Radiology:** a. Typical mitralisation of the heart. i. Prominent and convex pulmonary segment. ii. Left border of the heart normal. iii. Typical bulging of the right border due to left atrial enlargement in extreme cases. b. Barium swallow of the oesophagus in the right oblique view shows a typical indentation and pressure on the oesophagus due to the enlarged left atrium. c. Fan shaped mottling of the hilar regions due to pulmonary venous congestion. d. Horizontal linear markings near the hilum (Kerley's Lines). e. Diffuse nodular markings due to hemosiderosis. f. Calcification of mitral ring in advanced cases (especially, if looked for by a penertrating view). g. Acute pulmonary edema seen as a diffuse opacity.

2. **E.C.G.:** a. Right axis deviation. b. P 'Mitrale' broad and notched P wave longer in duration than 0-1 seconds. P wave absent when fibrillation sets in. c. Right ventricular hypertrophy (due to secondary pulmonary hypertension).

3. **Cardiac catheterisation:** a. Used for measuring the degree of stenosis. b. To exclude the presence of associated incompetence.

4. **Echocardiography** to evaluate i. the size of mitral valve, ii. condition and pliability of mitral valve, iii. size of chambers LA, RV, iv. endocarditis.

Complications: 1. Acute pulmonary edema. 2. Haemoptysis. 3. Systemic embolisation. 4. Atrial fibrillation. 5. Pulmonary hypertension with pulmonary incompetence. 6. Tricuspid incompetence. 7. Pulmonary embolism. 8. Infective endocarditis. 9. Massive thrombosis of the left atrium. 10. Recurrent laryngeal nerve paralysis. 11. Dysphagia.

Treatment: a. Restriction of activities (live with the cardiac reserve). b. Diuretics. c. Diuretics with digitalisation. d. Prevention of recurrence of rheumatic activity. e. Prevention of embolism by long-term antiocoagulant therapy when there is a history of embolism. f. Selection for surgery.

Every established case of mitral stenosis with pulmonary hypertension should be considered.

The indications for operation can be enumerated as follows:

1. Exertional dyspnea, Grade III or over. 2. Attacks of acute pulmonary edema. 3. History of embolisation. 4. Long mid-diastolic murmur. 5. Opening snap closer to second sound. 6. Calcified

mitral valve. 7. High left atrial pressure. 8. Severe pulmonary hypertension. 9. Size of mitral valve 1.5 sq cm as detected by echocardiography.

Contraindications for mitral valvotomy: 1. Age group in which recurrence of rheumatic carditis is possible (below 20). 2. After the age of 60. 3. Associated other valvular lesions. 4. Presence of atrial fibrillation. (All these are not absolute contraindications).

Surgical treatment: 1. Closed valvotomy : i. Transatrial approach. ii. Transventricular approach. 2. Replacement with prosthesis - in mitral stenosis and mitral stenosis + mitral incompetence.

IV. **Mitral incompetence:**

Etiology: Organic mitral incompetence: a. Rheumatic fever, b. infective endocarditis, c. incompetence due to papillary muscle dysfunction or rupture, d. mitral valve prolapse, e. congenital (when it is associated with ostium primum defect), f. hypertrophic obstructive cardiomyopathy, g. associated with ankylosing spondylitis, h. with systemic lupus erythematosus (Libman Sacks syndrome), i. endomyocardial fibrosis. (Clinically the first two are the most commonly encountered.)

Functional mitral incompetence: Any condition which causes dilatation of left ventricle may give rise to functional mitral incompetence. Unlike mitral stenosis, mitral incompetence is slightly more common in males than in females.

Haemodynamics: Due to the incompetence, the blood leaks back into the left atrium during left ventricular systole. During diastole, due to the incompetence of the valve, the blood immediately fills the ventricle as there is no obstruction (even in early diastole). Hence, though the left atrial pressure is very high during systole, there is a rapid fall during diastole and hence the mean left atrial pressure is not very high. Left atria] pressure is high only when acute mitral regurgitation occurs, e.g., as in MVP, such sudden rise in atrial pressure may lead to even pulmonary edema.

The pulmonary hypertension is mild and never as severe as in patients with mitral stenosis.

Symptoms: 1-. Symptoms of left ventricular failure may occur but relatively less frequently in the following order: a. Exertional dyspnea, b. paroxysmal nocturnal dyspnea, c. acute pulmonary edema.

2. Symptoms due to congestive cardiac failure. a. Edema of dependent parts, b. pain over the right hypochondrium.

3. Systemic embolisation can occur but much less common than in patients with mitral stenosis.

Signs: General Examination: a. Pulse: Hyperdynamic. b. J.V.pulse — nothing particular.

Cardiac Examination:

Inspection and palpation: 1. Apex impulse may be shifted downwards and outwards. It is forceful and hyperdynamic in character. 2. May be associated with left parasternal retraction. 3. A systolic thrill in the mitral area.

Auscultation: 1. First heart sound well heard in the mitral area (but neither loud nor sharp). 2. Second sound in pulmonary area may widely split as the aortic valve closes early due to short ejection time. 3. Pansystolic murmur begins with the first heart sound and embraces the second heart sound. This murmur is usually uniform in intensity, has high frequency and hence better heard by the diaphragm of the stethoscope. It is well conducted to the axilla from the apex where it is best heard. 4. An audible low pitched third heart, sound due to rapid ventricular filling is present and indicates severe mitral incompetence and shows that there is no associated significant mitral stenosis. 5. When associated with mitral stenosis, presence of third heart sound shows significant incompetence. 6. Absent third heart sound in mitral incompetence shows significant mitral stenosis.

Investigations: 1. Radiology: X-ray chest shows enlarged left ventricle and left atrium which may be aneurysmal. Hilar congestion may be present. 2. E.C.G.: May show a P mitrale with left ventricular hypertrophy. 3. ECHO-LA showing increased pulsation, hyperdynamic LV, ruptured chordae tendinae, and abnormal movements of mitral leaflets.

Complications: 1. Pulmonary edema, 2. hacmoptysis, 3. angina pectoris, 4. systemic embolisation, 5. atrial fibrillation, 6. infective endocarditis.

Treatment: Complete valve replacement after medical line of treatment.

V. **Aortic Stenosis:**

Etiology: I. Rheumatic fever is the most common cause, but some authors believe that rheumatic affection usually produces AS and Al as a combined lesion. 2. Congenital. 3. Calcification of aortic valve. (Supravalvular or valvular stenosis can occur as congenital lesions). Aortic stenosis is more common in males than in females.

Due to the marked resistance to its systolic outflow the left ventricle undergoes a concentric hypertrophy.

In significant aortic stenosis, there is an initial rise in the left ventricular pressure with a steep rise in the isovolumic (isometric) phase and a relatively early rise of the maximum pressure in systole.

The aortic pressure curves show an early steep rise which is interrupted by anacrotic notch and then again a slow rise which reaches its maximum in late systole. The anacrotic notch is earlier in severe cases of stenosis.

Symptoms: 1. Symptoms of left ventricular failure. 2. Symptoms of congestive cardiac failure. 3. Syncope: a. Cardiac syncope is acute and fleeting. When it occurs during exertion it may be due to acute left ventricular failure of due to the fixed low output. When it occurs during rest it can be due to paroxysmal ventricular fibrillation and may result in sudden death. b. Vasomotor syncope is due to the low blood pressure in aortic stenosis which predisposes to vasomotor and orthostatic syncope. 4. Angina pectoris: Due to poor filling of the coronary arteries which occurs as a result of low mean blood pressure and low fixed cardiac output, and increased demand of the hypertrophied left ventricular musculature.

Signs: General examination: 1. Appearance: Pale pink complexion. 2. Pulse: Low volume and sustained (*Pulsus parvus et tardus*).

Cardiac examination:

Inspection and palpation: (1) Apex impulse may be shifted downwards and outwards. It is forceful, well sustained and heaving in character. (2) May be associated with retraction of the left parasternal area. (3) A systolic thrill well felt over the aortic area. Best palpated with the patient leaning forward in full expiration. May be well felt over the neck vessels.

Auscultation : (1) Abnormal or slightly loud first sound. (2) The aortic component of the second sound is delayed and may be fceble or absent. (3) A harsh, ejection systolic murmur usually best heard in the aortic area and well conducted in the neck vessels. Starts well after the first sound and ends before the second sound. May be best heard over the apex. However, its timing and character is to be differentiated from the mitral incompetence murmur by presence of systolic thrill at the base. (4) An aortic ejection click may precede the murmur. (5) Functional mitral incompetence murmur in long standing cases.

Investigations: Radiography: X-Ray chest shows a concentric hypertrophy with a rounded and prominent border of the left ventricle. A calcification of the aortic valve may be seen. A post-stenotic dilatation of the aorta is very common. **E.C.G.:** Always shows a left ventricular hypertrophy with very high voltage of R waves in chest leads.

ECHO cardiography: Confirms and gives size of aortic valve.

Treatment : (1) Symptomatic (2) Surgical.

VI. **Aortic incompetence:**

Etiology:

Common:

(1) Rheumatic,
(2) Syphilitic,
(3) Atherosclerotic,
(4) Traumatic,
(5) Congenital bicuspid or quadricuspid aortic valve,
(6) Infective endocarditis,
(7) Dissection of aorta,
(8) Congenital hypoplasia of the aorta associated with dilatation of the ascending aorta,

(9) Associated with Marfan's syndrome,

Less Common:

(10) Associated with ankylosing spondylitis,

(11) Reiter's syndrome,

(12) Rarely systemic lupus erythromatosus.

The most common causes encountered are rheumatic and syphilitic. Males are more frequently affected than females.

Haemodynamics: Due to the incompetence, the blood from the aorta regurgitates back in the left ventricle during diastole and hence the stroke volume of left ventricle is increased. This causes a stretching of the muscle of the left ventricle and hence the force of its contraction increases. The ejection phase is shortened, and pressure falls rapidly during the late systole. Hence, large quantity of blood is quickly forced into the systemic circulation under a great force. This causes a sudden percussion wave followed by a collapse of the vessels. There is peripheral vasodilatation in these patients to compensate for the defect. This low peripheral resistance encourages forward flow in vasodilatation and is responsible for the peripheral signs. The low diastolic pressure is due to backward reflux as well as due to the peripheral vasodilatation.

Symptoms: (1) Symptoms of left ventricular failure, (2) palpitations (due to forceful ventricular contraction), (3) anginal pains (more common in syphilitic aortic incompetence as the openings of the coronary arteries may be narrowed due to accompanying aortitis). Other factors: (a) Low mean coronary artery filling pressure. (b) Increased demand of the hypertrophied left ventricle. (4) Syncopal attacks: Due to cerebral anoxia.

Signs: General examination: (Peripheral signs). **Pulse:** (1) Water hammer pulse (Corrigan's pulse). (2) Visible pulsations : In the neck: Dancing carotids (Corrigan in 1832 first described these pulsations. Though water hammer pulse and Corrigan's pulse are now used synonymously it is more correct to call the carotid pulsations the Corrigan's sign). In the arm: Dancing Brachials. (3) Nodding of the head due to forcible carotid pulsations (De Musset's sign). (4) Capillary pulsations: Can be seen by gentle pressure on a nail bed or by a slide pressed on the tip of the nail. Also by observing the alternate reddening and blanching of an area on the forehead after previous vigorous rubbing. By gentle pressure on the fingers (Quincke's sign). (5) Loud sound both palpable and audible over the femoral arteries (Traube's sound or pistol shot sound. (6) Duroziez murmurs (first described in 1861). When the stethoscope is pressed over the artery and the artery is pressed proximal to the stethoscope, a systolic murmur is heard (due to obstruction to the forward flow). When the artery is pressed distal to the stethoscope a diastolic murmur is heard (due to the regurgilant flow), If femoral artery is tightly compressed with stethoscope to-and-fro murmur is heard. (7) Blood pressure: The systolic pressure is raised with a very low diastolic pressure (at times even 0 in a very free and severe incompetence). Blood pressure in the inferior extremities is higher than that in the superior extremities (normal difference is about 20 mm). This is also known as Hill's sign which is supposed to be due to a compensatory mechanism which diverts the blood supply to the vital organs.

Peripheral signs are more marked in A.I. of syphilitic origin than that of rheumatic origin.

Cardiac Signs:

Inspection and palpation: (1) Apex impulse shifted downwards and outwards. Forceful and hyperdynamic in nature. (2) Associated left parasternal retraction in severe L.V. hypertrophy.

Auscultation: (1) Characteristic early diastolic murmur. Best heard not in aortic, but in the third and fourth left space lateral to the sternal margin. It can be heard at the apex. Starts immediately after the second sound and is decrescendo in character. Better heard with the patient leaning forward and in full expiration. Better heard by the diaphragm of the stethoscope. Length of the murmur is usually proportional to the degree of incompetence. Rarely associated with a thrill (more common with ruptured aortic cusp). (2) Systolic ejection murmur over the aortic area. (3) Austin Flint murmur at mitral area — mid-diastolic murmur with presystolic accentuation. (4) Systolic murmur at the apex. Due to stretching of' the initral ring as a result of' hypertrophy and dilatation of the left ventricle. (5) Second sound may be feeble or absent due to incomplete closure of the aortic valves.

Investigations: (1) Radiology : Dilated left ventricle produces a boat-shaped enlargement. Pulmonary venous congestion. E.C.C;. shows a left ventricular hypertrophy. (3) ECHO (echo cardiography) to see the amount of regurgitation and presence of associated stenosis.

Treatment: (1) Symptomatic. (2) Surgical.

VII. **Rheumatic Fever**

Definition: It is a specific inflammatory response, most probably allergic or autoimmune following an infection by beta hemolytic streptococci of Lance field group A.

Its main features are fever, polyarthritis, pancarditis, chorea, subcutaneous nodules and erythema marginatum.

Etiology: (1) Infection due to Group A beta hemolytic streptococci. (2) Common infections: (a) Upper respiratory tract infection, (b) otitis media, (c) scarlet fever. (3) Age and sex: Rare before the age of 5 years. Common age group 5 to 15 years. (4) Socio-econoinic factors: More common in poorer communities, overcrowding, unhygienic and damp surroundings.

Diagnosis: The diagnosis of rheumatic fever can now be confirmed by clinical criteria and other laboratory evidence. The criteria described by Ducket Jones (Jones criteria) provide a basic guideline.

Modified Jones Criteria

Major manifestations	**Minor manifestations**
Carditis	Fever
Polyarthritis	Arthralgia
Chorea	Previous rheumatic fever or rheumatic heart disease
Erythema marginatum	Increased E. S R. c.reactive protein, leukocytosis
Subcutaneous nodules	Prolonged P.R. interval in E.C.G.

The diagnosis of rheumatic fever is established when minimum one major and three minor or when minimum two major and two minor manifestations are present.

Clinical peculiarities of rheumatic polyarthritis: 1. Usually major joints involved in children (Knees, ankle, wrist and elbow in order of frequency). 2. Painful, swollen, hot and tender with marked reddening. 3. May be associated with sterile effusions. 4, Fleeting or migration of pain from one joint to the other is a characteristic feature. 5. Small joints involved more commonly in adults. 6. Inflammatory process subsides completely leaving no sequelae. 7. Sometimes present as growing pains when the mild pain is complained of in hips, knees or ankles. 8. A history of sore throat 1 to 3 weeks preceding the arthritis is usually available. 9. The joint swellings are usually associated with fever.

Clinical manifestations of rheumatic pancarditis: Rheumatic fever may affect the endocardium, myocardium with its conducting tissues and pericardium (hence known as pancarditis). The chief manifestion is high sleeping pulse rate.

1. **Endocardial affection or valvulitis:** Mitral valve is the most commonly affected either with or without affection of aortic or tricuspid valve. Aortic valve can be affected alone but tricuspid valve is never involved without the involvement of mitral valve. (Diagnosis of endocarditis may be difficult in the presence of myocarditis.)

a. Affection of mitral valve: Classic sign is Carey Coombs murmur (soft, low pitched and short, and heard best by the bell of the stetho-scope) mid-diastolic which may disappear completely or remain until a classic mitral stenosis is established (after a period of years). Mitral in- competence starts from the outset manifesting as a pansystolic murmur.

b. Affection of aortic valve: Inflammation of this valve may start as incompetence from the very beginning and this produces the typical early diastolic murmur. An aortic systolic ejection murmur, is not characteristic of aortic valvulitis.

2. **Myocarditis:** a. Tachycardia. b. Feeble first heart sound. c. Gallop rhythm. d. Cardiac dilatation. e. Appearance of C.C.F. during the phase of acute rheumatic fever. f. Systolic ejection murmur at the apex. g. Muffled heart sounds. h. Affection of the conducting tissue is best diagnosed by the prolonged P.R.interval in the electrocardiogram.

3. **Pericarditis:** a. Occurs in about 10% of the cases. b. Leaves no sequelae. c. Usually presents as a transient pericardial rub. d. May present with severe pain and other inflammatory signs. e. There may be a rapid accumulation of pericardial effusion which later on gets absorbed completely leaving no sequelae.

Other clinical manifestations of rheumatic fever:

1. **Subcutaneous nodules:** Their presence means rheumatic activity. They vary in size from very small to about 1 cm in diameter. They recur in crops and each nodule may persist for a few weeks. They arc tender and skin can be moved over them. They are usually seen over bony prominences as on the knuckles, occiput or on the elbows and knees, spinous processes, shins of tibiae in short over dorsal surfaces.

2. **Erythema marginatum:** This manifests as a pale pink irregular serpentine linear rash forming curved lines or circles. It is usually transient migratory and rarely if ever affects the face.

3. **Rheumatic pneumonia and pleurisy:** These are very rare manifestations of rheumatic fever; pneumonia is transitory and the effusion is completely absorbed without fibrosis.

4. **Mild clubbing of nails:** May be present in rheumatic fever.

5. **Chorea:** Presents with jerky irregular involuntary movements increased under stress and disappear during sleep (described in C.N.S).

Investigations: 1. Evidence of inflammation; a. Leucocytosis: Usually polymorphonuclear (up to 20000/cu.mm). b. Normocytic normochromic anaemia. (c) E.S.R. raised. (Except in uncomplicated chorea and in presence of C.C.F.). d. C. reactive protein. A positive test in serum if available provides an indication of rheumatic activity. May be positive in other infections and collagen disease. e. ASO titre — Antistreptolysin O titre is most commonly used test. Levels above 250 Todd units in adults & above 333 Todd units in children are suggestive in rheumatic activity. It indicates recent infection with group A beta hemolytic streptococci. Titres mentioned above are of diagnostic value. f. Streptozyme test (STZ) is positive even when ASO titre may not be diagnostic. g. Throat swab culture showing the growth of beta hemolytic streptococci is very strong evidence that the disease process is rheumatic. 2. E.C.G.: a. Prolongation of P.R. interval. b. Evidence of inyocarditis. c. Low voltage when pericardial effusion is present. 3. X-ray chest : May show enlargement in cardiac size. 4. Echocardiography — generalised dilatation of the heart with vegetations.

Treatment: 1. Rest in bed: Complete bed rest either in lying down position or semi-recumbent position is essential. Incidence of chronic valvular disease is very high in patients who are unable to follow this. This should be continued until the signs of rheumatic activity subside.

Criteria for cessation of rheurtiatic activity are:

a. Normal sleeping pulse rate. b. Normal temperature. c. Normal E.S.R. d. E.C.G. returning to normal. e. Rise in haemoglobin level--anaemia is corrected. f. Weight gain.

2. Diet : Light diet.

3. Drugs : Penicillin and antirheumatic group of drugs.

Other measures: (a) Protection of inflamed joints. (b) Digitalisation for cardiac failure.

Prophylaxis: a. Continued penicillin therapy. b. Tonsillectomy if they are infected and are thought to be the source of streptococcal infection.

VIII. Infective endocarditis:

Definition: Infective endocarditis means microbial infection of the heart valves or endocardium in proximity of congenital or acquired cardiac defects or surgically replaced valves.

More cases of infective endocarditis , are seen as surgery has become a common mode of treatment in congenital and acquired heart disease.

Types: The two main types recognised are:

a. Acute infective endocarditis(caused by organisms of high pathogenicity).
b. Subacute infective endocarditis (caused by organisms of low pathogenicity).

Nowadays the distinction between the two is thought to be less precise than what it was previously.

However, acute infective endocarditis is usually a part of a generalised systemic infection and may affect normal healthy valves while subacute infective endocarditis is usually caused by organisms of low virulence and always affects previously diseased or congenital malformed valves or surgically replaced valves.

Subacute infective endocarditis: Affects a previously abnormal valve or structure.

In the acquired defects, old rheumatic valve lesions are affected most commonly (about 80%) mitral, aortic, tricuspid and pulmonary in order of frequency.

In the congenital defects, P.D.A. biscuspid aortic valve, V.S.D. and coarctation of aorta are the lesions which are most commonly involved. Curiously atrial septal defect is very rarely affected by infective endocarditis.

The leftsided cardiac defects are more commonly involved than the rightsided ones. Prosthetic valves predispose to endocarditis.

The organisms enter the body from the upper respiratory tract, teeth and gums. A history of teeth extraction, tonsillectomy, surgery or child birth is very frequently present. It can follow catheterisation, abdominal operation procedures like cystoscopy, or bowel operations and even intravenous infusions.

Bacteria destroy the surface of the normal to deformed valves and cause superficial lesions. The lesions are finely granular and form friable vegetations on the surface. They are easily detached and are the cause of multiple embolisation. These vegetations can spread over the mural endocardium (walls of atria and ventricles). Their direction of spread is always in the direction of the blood flow.

Clinical Features: Age: Common in young adults. Sex incidence: equal.

The initial presentation may be varied and hence the diagnosis is missed at the onset in a fair proportion of patients. These patients may present with prolonged higher grade fever and anaemia, fatiguability without any apparent cause. The presentation may be due to one of the embolic manifestations and the initial picture may be that of meningitis, cerebral abscess, peripheral vascular obstruction or uraemia due to renal infarcts, pulmonary infarcts, sudden blindness.

However, if the previous cardiac history is known, the diagnosis can be suspected and confirmed early.

The physical signs can be divided for discussion as follows:

1. Due to infection. 2. Cardiac signs. 3. Signs due to embolisation.

1. **Signs due to infection:** a. Fever : Which may be high or low grade and may be intermittent. b. Anaemia: Normocytic normochromic anaemia which gives a peculiar yellow discolouration of the skin. Anaemia is gradually progressive if the infection is not controlled in time, c. Clubbing: Clubbing of both fingers and toes is present and takes about 3 to 6 weeks to develop. It disappears when the patient is cured. d. Enlargement of the spleen: Mild to moderate degree of splenomegaly is present due to infection. A sudden enlargement of spleen associated with a rub over its surface is due to splenic infarction.

2. **Cardiac signs:** a. Usually the cardiac signs of the underlying diseases are present. Initially they may be absent as in case of congenital bicuspid aortic valve when the diagnosis is extremely difficult. b. Appearance of a murmur which was not present previously is a very good evidence of infective endocarditis. c. Changing intensity of murmurs is another indication of infective endocarditis. d. Toxic myocarditis causing

congestive cardiac failure is a rare manifestation.

3. **Signs of embolisation:** a. Petechiae: Common and appear in crops. Common sites are below the nails, in the fundii, in the conjunctiva or anywhere in the mucous membranes or skin. Below the nails they appear as splinter haemorrhages. Petechiae may not be embolic and they could be due to anaemia and toxic damage to capillary wall leading to vasculitis. b. Retinal petechial haemorrhages may have a pale centre and they may be shaped like a canoe when they are known as Roth's spots. c. Osler's nodes : They are raised, palpable and tender, painful nodes found in nail beds, finger and palms. They are due to cutaneous emboli and the causative organisms may be cultured from them — may be due to immune complex deposits. d. Large non-tender muscles are seen commonly. c. Janeway's lesions — swellings which are very large in size may occur in the palms of hands or soles of feet. The lesions are maculopapular and may ulcerate. Bacteria may be cultured from these lesions (bacteria identical to those found in blood). f. Emboli in the other vessels: i. Cerebral embolism may produce hemiplegia by blocking.of a main vessel or by rupture of a mycotic aneurysm in the wall of the blood vessel. ii. Peripheral vessels of limbs may get blocked. They may manifest only as absent pulses of limbs or as peripheral gangrene because of occlusion of a blood vessel. iii. Pulmonary artery embolism may result in pulmonary infarction. iv. Retinal artery involvement may cause sudden blindness. v. Renal emboli may give rise to (a) sudden renal colic with microscopic or frank haematuria. b. Rarely associated with acute glomerulonephritis due to the streptococcal lesion. vi. Mesenteric artery embolism may give rise to acute abdominal colic with malena. vii. Splenic artery embolism will cause severe local pain with palpable rub.

Investigations: 1. **Blood culture:** Should be taken before any antibiotic therapy is started. Repeated cultures may be necessary and both aerobic and anaerobic culture media should be used. If venous, blood cultures are negative, either arterial blood cultures or bone marrow cultures may be indicated. 2. **Urine:** Microscopic haematuria may provide the diagnostic clue. 3. **Blood count:** There is usually normocytic normochromic anaemia. Leucocytosis may or may not be present but usually present. E.S.R. may be moderately raised. However, a normal E.S.R. does not rule out the diagnosis of infective endocarditis. 4. **Echocardiography:** To detect large vegetations and to identify high risk patients.

Management: Prophylactic: 1. Correction of congenital or rheumatic valvular defects which predispose to endocarditis. 2. Dental care and adequate antibiotic cover after upper respiratory operations like tonsillectomy. 3. Surgical operations of the lower genitourinary tract and rectum should be covered by broad spectrum antibiotics.

Curative: Early use of suitable antibiotics prevents the growth of vegetations and minimises the danger of embolisation. Hence, the therapy should be started immediately after the blood samples are collected and in obvious cases before their results are available.

Follow up: After the apparent recovery the patient should be frequently checked for evidence of relapse. Relapses are common in the first two months. Any rise in temperature should be looked for and repeated blood cultures for a period of two months may be advisable. Cardiac surgery may have to be considered in those patients in whom the defect is worse due to infection.

IX. Ischaemic Heart Disease:

Definition : Ischaemic Heart Disease (IHD) is a condition resulting from inadequate blood supply to myocardium.

Terminology: 1. Atherosclerotic heart disease. 2. Coronary heart disease. 3. Coronary artery disease.

Causes: Though atherosclerosis of coronary arteries is the most common cause of ischaemia, heart can be rendered ischaemic by arteritis, embolism of coronary arteries, aortic valve disease and/or in association with hypotension or anaemia.

Ischaemia develops depending on involvement of the coronary arteries and development of collateral circulation.

Spectrum of IHD: Asymptomatic, angina pectoris, acute coronary insufficiency, myocardial infarction.

Predisposing causes: Obesity, hypertension, diabetes millitus, hypercholesterolemia, tobacco consumption, heredity, sedentary habits, psychological tension.

Biochemical changes: Acidosis, accumulation of lactic acid, SGOT increased, LDH increased.

ECG changes: ST segment changes.

Angina Decubitus: Sudden attack of pain in the chest during recumbent posture or during sleep. Attack resembles that of paroxysmal nocturnal dyspnea. Dyspnea is an accompaniment. Hypertension and dreaming episode might be precipitating factors.

On examination: Hypertension, enlarged heart, mitral systolic murmur like regurgitation due to dysfunction of papillary muscles.

Investigations: ECG changes: The changes prove the diagnosis but normal ECG does not rule out angina.

Biochemical changes: Enzymes are normal. **Stress test :** Basis — inability of coronary blood flow to increase in proportion to the metabolic demands.

Aim of stress test is to detect IHD, to estimate extent of IHD and to evaluate left ventricular function.

Tests: 1. Master's two-step test: This is standardised for height, weight. It is rough test. 2. Graded treadmill and bicycle test impose graded and calculated exercise and thus greater demand on coronary circulation. So they are of more value in assessing left ventricular function. With proper selection of cases, and proper precautions the results are interpreted by taking into consideration:

1. duration and severity of exercise imposed,
2. extent of tachycaidia,
3. extent of ST depression and T inversion,
4. subjective symptoms of angina. If ST depression is more than 1 mv and is more than 0.08 sec in duration, it is significant.

Sequelae of ischaemia: 1. Contractability of ventricle impaired. Hence, contraction is inefficient. 2. Infarcted or ischaemic portion of heart bulges during contraction adding to inefficient ventricular contraction. All these changes lead to increased left ventricular filling pressure (i.e. chamber is not empty after systole so there is diastolic overload). 3. Ischaemia leads to myocardial irritability which in turn leads to extrasystoles, tachy-cardia and fibrillation.

Treatment depends on the diagnosis, i.e., angina, acute coronary insufficiency and myocardial infarction.

1. **Angina :** It is a clinical syndrome characterised by transient chest pain on exertion, or on emotional upset or excitement and relieved by rest; duration of pain is 1-2 minutes.

Types of pain : Heaviness in chest, choking sensation, squeezing in chest, tightness in chest, sometimes knife like cutting pain. Site of pain: substernal, arms and shoulders, neck, jaw, throat.

Precipitating factors : exertion, excitement, emotional upset, anger or fright.

Coronary arteriography is indicated in all patients to evaluate the status of patient whether surgery would be helpful.

Usually patients with persistent angina for 3 months not controlled by medical therapy are subjected to coronary angiography.

Catheter is introduced through femoral artery directly into orifice of coronary artery and radio opaque material injected.

Management : General measures to prevent or minimise attacks of ischaemia are :

a. atherosclerosis,
b. hypertension,
c. hyperlipaemia,
d. obesity.

These are the predisposing causes of angina and as the lesions produced by these first three factors cannot be regressed, their progress should be checked by the following: a. reduction of weight, b. reduction of animal fats content in diet, c. graded exercise, d. maintenance of blood pressure, e. control of diabetes, f. reduction of emotional stress, may even involve change of job, g. discontinuation of tobacco consumption.

Specific: a. Patient must learn to live within

his physical limits. b. Drugs — anti anginal drugs.

Bypass Surgery: Does not alter the natural history of the disease.

Principle: Piece of saphenous vein is used to form a connection between aorta and coronary artery distal to the obstruction.

Advantages: Immediate relief of symptoms, factors which decide the necessity of bypass surgery are symptomatic status, coronary anatomy, coronary arteriograph, ventricular function.

Ideal patient is one who has 80% or more obstruction in proximal portions of 2-3 major arteries.

2. **Myocardial infarction:** Presenting symptoms:a. pain not relieved by rest, b. sinking feeling, c. sweating, d. nausea, vomiting, e. gid-diness, f. profound restlessness, g. sudden unconsciousness, h. unexplained low BP.

Predisposing and precipitating factors are the same as those for angina. Though pain is the most common symptom, few cases may have silent painless infarcts, especially in elders and diabetics.

Clinical findings: Shock, cyanosis, severe pallor, hypotension, atrial gallop rhythm, apical systolic mitral murmur, pericardial rub may be present.

Laboratory findings: a. Biochemical changes : SGOT and CPK: rise and fall rapidly and/or rise during first 24 hours and fall within 3-4 days.

LDH — Rises later and stays higher longer, starts rising on 1st day, peak levels on 3rd-4th day, falls to normal by 14th day.

b. **Nonspecific changes:** Leucocytosis, ESR-slow rise — peak during 1st week — elevated for several weeks.

c. ECG : QS wave makes appearance, R wave disappears, ST high take off, T inversion in leads, depending on site of infarct.

Complications:

1. **Early:** CCF, pulmonary edema, shock, cardiac dilatation, cardiac arrhythmias — a. Tachyrrhythmias — Tachycardia — i. supraventricular, ii. ventricular, extrasystoles, atrial fibrillation and flutter, venlricular fibrillation, ventricular tachycardia, extrasystoles and fibrillation are most serious complications. b. Bradyrrhythmias — bundle branch block, nodal rhythm, complete heart block are also serious complications. The last being the most serious one.

2. **Late :** Aneurysm, resistant CCF.

Management : As arrhythmias lead to death, management is directed towards prevention of arrhythmias. Hospitalisation, preferably in ICCU is necessary.

Treatment of arrhythmias: With suitable drugs.

3. **Intermediate syndromes :** In angina there is no death of myocardial tissue while at the other end, in myocardial infarction there is death of myocardial tissue as evidenced by ECG changes and raised serum enzymes levels. Several cases fall in 'inbetween' categories such as acute coronary insufficiency, unstable angina and crescendo angina.

Acute coronary insufficiency: Pain starts with exertion which does not get relieved by rest and lasts few minutes, ST changes usually present, Q wave absent, conduction disturbances may be present serum enzymes normal. Angiography may show narrowing of arteries — ideal patient for surgery.

Management: Admit in specialised unit. Treat as infarction with suitable schedules. Management should be directed to rehabilitate the patient to his normal routine.

Different Types of Murmurs at a Glance

Patho-genic murmur	Timing	Site where murmur is heard	Causes	Associated thrill	Intensity and character	Conduction	Diagrammatic representation
Diastolic	Early	— Aortic area — Left parasternal border — Apex	A.I.	+	High pitched diminuendo soft blowing	Along left border of sternum to apex	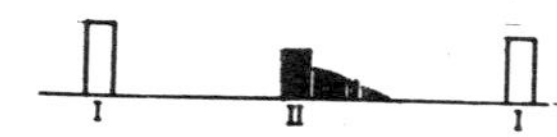
		Pulmonary area	Dissecting Aneurysm or Dissection of aorta Congenital dilatation of aortic ring		”	—	
			Pulmonary incompetence (functional) Pulmonary hypertension primary or secondary	+	Graham steel murmur	May be conducted to apex	
			Pulmonary aneurysm				
	Mid	Mitral area	M. S.	+	Rumbling with opening snap	Not conducted	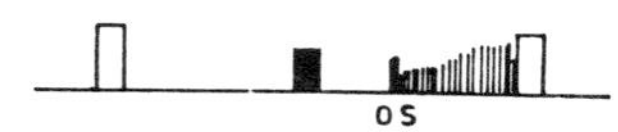
			Ball valve obstruction at A-V valves		Gr. III-V (M_1)		

Al = Aortic incompetence; MS = Mitral stenosis; A-V = Atrio ventricular; L R shunt = Left to right shunt, PA dilatation = Pulmonary artery dilatation
VSD = Ventricular septal defect; ASD = Atrial septal defect; PDA = Patent ductus arteriosus.

Patho-genic murmur	Timing	Site where murmur is heard	Causes	Associated thrill	Intensity and character	Conduction	Diagrammatic representation
	Mid diastole	Mitral area	Functional in M.I. because of increased flow across AV valve which has resulted from large volume of blood regurgited in LA in systole		Gr. II-III (M_1 not loud)	Not conducted	
			Carey Coomb's murmur (Rheumatic carditis)		Cooing character Gr. II. changing character not loud	Not conducted	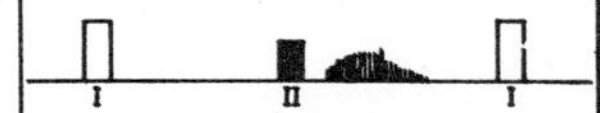
		Tricuspid area	Tricuspid stenosis	+	Rumbling Gr. III-IV	Not conducted	
	Late diastolic (Pre-systolic)	Mitral area	M.S. Austin Flint	+ ●	Crescendo (M_1) loud and sharp Crescendo M_1 not loud	Not conducted Not conducted	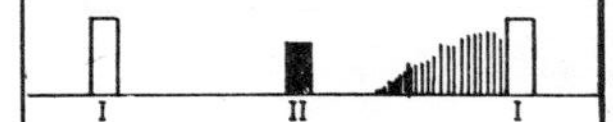
		Tricuspid area	Tricuspid stenosis	+	Crescendo better heard during, inspiration	Not conducted	
Systolic	Early	Aortic area	1) Stenosis	Usually present	Harsh Gr. III-IV Ej-Click	Well conducted into carotids	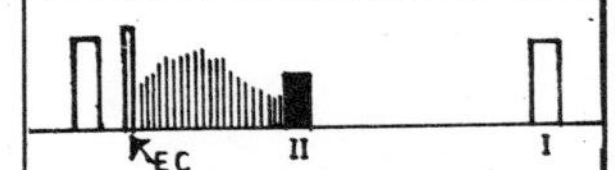
			2) Dilatation of aortic chamber	+	Harsh Gr. III-IV		
			3) Syphilitic aortitis				

Al = Aortic incompetence; MS = Mitral stenosis; A-V = Atrio ventricular; L R shunt = Left to right shunt, PA dilatation = Pulmonary artery dilatation
VSD = Ventricular septal defect; ASD = Atrial septal defect; PDA = Patent ductus arteriosus.

	Timing	Site where murmur is heard	Causes	Associated thrill	Intensity and character	Conduction	Diagrammatic representation
Systolic	Early (Due to forward flow-Ejection)	Aortic area	4) Coarctation of aorta	+	Harsh Gr. III-IV	Interscapular region	
			5) Aortic incompetence	thrill ±	Harsh Gr. III-IV Ejection click may not be present	Transmitted to carotids	
			6) (Rare) complete heart block	+	Gr. II-III	Not conducted	
	Early (Due to forward flow-Ejection)	Pulmonary area	— L. R. Shunt) 1) V S D, A S D)		Gr. II-III (ASD)	Not conducted Left 2nd-3rd space	
			2) Pulmonary	+	Harsh Gr. III-IV	Heard in left parasternal line	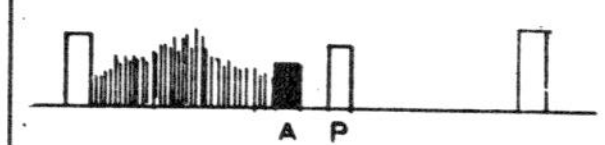
			3) Pulmonary stenosis	+	Harsh Gr. . III-IV	—	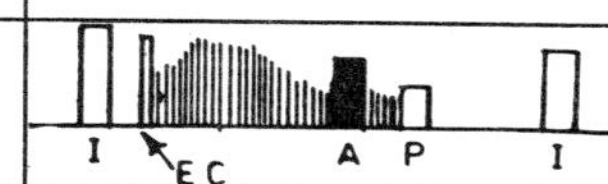
			4) P A dilatation	+	Harsh Gr. . III-IV	—	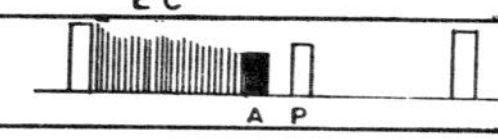
	Pan systolic (Due to regurgi-tation)	Mitral area	Mitral incompetence (pathological or functional)	Thrill +	Pansystolic loud and harsh	into axilla	
		Tricuspid	Tricuspid incompetence (pathological or functional	”	”	May be into axilla	

Al = Aortic incompetence; MS = Mitral stenosis; A-V = Atrio ventricular; L R shunt = Left to right shunt, PA dilatation = Pulmonary artery dilatation VSD = Ventricular septal defect; ASD = Atrial septal defect; PDA = Patent ductus arteriosus.

Patho-genic murmur	Timing	Site where murmur is heard	Causes	Associated thrill	Intensity and character	Conduction	Diagrammatic representation
Systolic	line	Left parasternal	V S D	+	Pansystolic Harsh	—	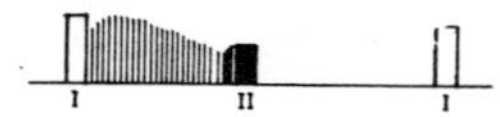
		Pulmonary area or below (L) clavicle	Early stages of 'P D A	+	+	Conducted from pulmonary area to left sub-clavicular area or heard in left subclavicular area	
Innocent Continous Murmurs—Venous Hum—2nd (R) Space--changes in respiratory phase and by changing posture							
Continu-ous murmur		Left right - shunt	— P D A — Aorto pulmonary window — A - V fistula — Anomalous pulmonary venous drainage	+	Harsh Gr. III-IV (Gibson's murmur)	Conducted to subclavicular region	
		Simulating continuous murmur	— V S D - AI — M S - M I — A S - A I	+ + +	as original lesion " "	Depending on dominant lesion	

AI = Aortic incompetence; MS = Mitral stenosis; A-V = Atrio ventricular; L R shunt = Left to right shunt, PA dilatation = Pulmonary artery dilatation
VSD = Ventricular septal defect; ASD = Atrial septal defect; PDA = Patent ductus arteriosus.

		Timing	Site	Accompanying thrill	Intensity Or Grade	Effect of change in posture, etc.	Conditions in which murmur is present
Non pathogenic murmurs	1) Innocent	Systolic	Pulmonary Left parasternal	Usually absent	Gr. I to II	—Changes with respiration or change of posture — No effect of Valsalva's manoeuvre	No structural change in heart or nerve
	2) Flow	Systolic	Rarely at apex	Absent	Gr. I to 11	— Changes with respiration or change of posture — No effect of Valsalva's manoeuvre	Hyperdynamic circulation as anaemia thyrotoxicosis

Al = Aortic incompetence; MS = Mitral stenosis; A-V = Atrio ventricular; L R shunt = Left to right shunt, PA dilatation = Pulmonary artery dilatation VSD = Ventricular septal defect; ASD = Atrial septal defect; PDA = Patent ductus arteriosus.

Section V : Central Nervous System

14. Central Nervous System: Symptomatology and History Taking

History-taking in CNS:

It will not be out of place to state that history-taking is one of the most important aspects when approaching a neurological problem. The reason for this is that unlike other systems the central nervous system cannot be examined directly (except for the fundus of the optic nerve). The same physical signs may be present in various conditions due to different causes, e.g., hemiplegia may be caused either by embolic, haemorrhagic, thrombotic or space-occupying lesions. It is only the natural history as narrated by the patient which will point towards the probable cause.

The narration of the history is hardly ever spontaneous by the patient. The ailing patient is naturally engrossed in presenting his complaint. To find out the important points which will help in diagnosis, the exaniner must not only have a complete knowledge of the various causes but must also be prepared to patiently ask him the relevant questions and to interpret the answers correctly. An attempt has been made in the following pages to streamline the wide variety of questions which one may have to ask during examination of a neurological case.

Medicine, though primarily a science, is really an art. Any attempt to rigidly categorise it will fail in more than one way. At the end of history-taking and examination one must be prepared to answer the cardinal questions :

"What is the lesion?"
"Where is the lesion?"
"What is the extent of the lesion?"
"What is the cause of the lesion?"
"Is it a single lesion or multiple?"

Before taking the history of the patient it is important to find out whether the patient is right handed or left handed.

Method : A patient with neurological deficit will usually come with complaints relating to :

I Motor system.
II Higher functions: (1) Changes in state of consciousness, (2) Mental changes, (3) Memory defect, (4) Speech defect, and (5) Convulsions.
III Sensory system.
IV Sphincter Control
V Cranial Nerves
VI Past history like H/o. diabetes, hypertension, syphilis, tuberculosis, trauma, fever, rheumatic heart disease, etc., will establish the cause of the lesion which forms the last item in the list of complaints.

So a detailed history and also a correct interpretation of the complaints will lead the examiner to make an intelligent guess to answer the cardinal questions.

Details of all components of CNS (I to VI) must be inquired into so as to arrive at the correct diagnosis.

Before discussing the detailed analysis of this symptomatology following points must be remembered:

(I) The presenting symptoms should be analysed first in detail. The component of the nervous system which is affected should be noted. If there are more than one presenting symptoms They should be analysed either in chronological order, if they have appeared simultaneously or as per their clinical importance.

(2) According to the presenting complaint, the

examiner should first determine as to which component of the central nervous system is affected. Then the history regarding the other deficits which may be the result of the affection of the same component should be asked for. A negative or positive answer should be recorded.

For example, if the patient complains of weakness, this would be due to affection of the motor system. He must be questioned regarding the nutrition of his muscles or any involuntary movements, etc., which constitutes the other aspects of the motor system. (A detailed description of each component will follow later.) Quite often the patient may not volunteer to mention some minor or unimportant details, which can really be of paramount importance in the differential diagnosis, i.e., if the paralysis or weakness is accompanied by even a minor wasting of the affected muscles, the lesion may be in the peripheral nerve and if it is accompanied by fasciculations, most probably the site of lesion is in the anterior horn cells. The patient may fail to mention this unless asked.

Absence of these will mean that the lesion is in the upper motor neuron.

(3) Even if the patient does not volunteer any complaints relating to other components, those should be inquired into and recorded as either positive or negative points.

This may be of great importance in determining the disease process. The same neurological deficit may be caused by different. disease processes, and either a positive or negative history of these other points may help the diagnosis, e.g., in a patient, weakness and wasting of legs may be due to poliomyelitis without associated complaints of sensory system or sphincter disturbances. While, weakness and wasting of legs due to spinal cord compression, will be associated with sensory and sphincter disturbances.

(4) History pertaining to cranial nerve paralysis may have to be specifically asked for.

Certain cranial nerves are specifically or commonly affected along with certain diseases of the nervous system and to ask for a specific history a knowledge of these diseases is essential. For instance, in infective polyneuritis facial and oculomotor nerves are involved along with the paralysis of limbs and hence questioning about their affection is essential.

(5) After recording the history as above, the examiner should ask the patient certain questions which may determine the cause of the lesion. Detailed history recording should be done as follows :

1. **Motor System :** The complaints of the patient due to affection of the motor system can be as follows :

(1) weakness or paralysis,
(2) stiffness or difficulty in movement,
(3) abnormality of coordination,
(4) wasting rarely hypertrophy of muscles,
(5) involuntary movements.

Initially it may be difficult to understand as to how all these symptoms are included under the heading of motor system complaints. It should be remembered that the integrity of the motor system is necessary not only for maintenance of normal power, but also to preserve normal tone, coordination, nutrition and prevention of involuntary movements.

For a proper analysis of the defect producing weakness in the motor system, the inquiry should be conducted as follows :

(a) Which parts of the body are affected?
Hemiplegia : weakness of one side of the body and face,
Monoplegia : weakness of one limb,
Paraplegia : weakness of both lower limbs,
Quadriplegia: weakness of all four limbs,
Double hemiplegia: weakness of all four limbs and both sides of the face — upper motor neuron.
(b) Or is the weakness limited to an individual muscle or part of a limb, i.e., a group of muscles.
(c) When did it start?
(d) Was the onset sudden or gradual?

The interpretation of these questions is given in Table 14.1.

Table 14.1

Onset	Cause
i. Instantaneous	: Cerebral Embolism
ii. Fairly sudden (over a period of few hours)	: Cause is likely to be : Cerebral haemorrhage
iii. Gradual symptoms (developed for over a period of 1-2 days)	: Cerebral thrombosis
iv. Very gradual symptoms (developing for a period of few days to weeks)	: Space occupying lesion (SOL), subdural hematoma or cerebral abscess. or tuberculoma.

(e) Has the weakness remained confined to the originally affected parts or muscles or has it spread to any other parts? When patient narrates the history that weakness has occurred first in the legs, then the arms and then the face, this sequence points towards the way in which the lesion has progressed. If so, how has it spread? (Anatomical: i.e., first one leg then the other).

(f) Degree of weakness: Is it total or partial?

g) Has the weakness progressed gradually, suddenly or is it stable?

(h) Has the patient noticed any return of strength (improvement) since the onset?

Vascular lesion like thrombosis or embolism will show some degree of improvement in the weakness after a few days, while the weakness due to SOL will worsen day by day.

The answer to these questions can lead to the localisation of the lesion in the CNS and sometimes may indicate the nature of the underlying disease process.

As stressed before in the discussion of the method of history-taking whatever may be the presenting symptoms, a history of the remaining components of the motor system should be inquired into.

Hence, even if the complaint is that of motor weakness an inquiry should be made regarding the nutrition of the muscles or the presence of any involuntary movements as follows:

(1) Has the patient noticed any wasting of the parts affected or is there any increase in the muscles mass even though there is weakness of the affected muscles?

(2) Are there any involuntary movements, i.e., tremors or any other uncontrollable movements?

(3) Does he complain of any marked unsteadiness or inco-ordination of limbs disproportionate to the loss of power?

(4) Does he experience any severe stiffness of the affected parts?

Abnormalities of tone, co-ordination, nutrition and abnormalities of voluntary movements are given in Table 14.2

Table 14.2

	Manifestations	Cause
Abnormalities of tone:	Stiffness of movement or difficulty in movements.	increased tone or rigidity due to pyramidal or extra-pyramidal overtone.
	Limp-limbs (flaccidity)	Atonia due to lower motor neurone involvement
Abnormality of co-ordaination :	Inability to walk steadily, inability to stand, inability to carry out finer movements like buttoning of shirt or threading a needle, change in handwriting.	Inco-ordination due to cerebellar disease or chorea
Abnormality of nutrition :	1. Wasting of muscles that is either his hands or feet or some other specific muscle mass getting smaller in size.	Atrophy due to LMN lesion or myopathies. (L.M.N. means lower motor neuron).
	2. Rarely abnormal increase in the size of the muscles like calf muscles or gluteal muscles.	Pseudohypertrophic muscular dystrophies.
Abnormality of voluntary movements or involuntary movements:	Tremors, choreiform movements, athetoid movements, convulsions etc., (uncontrollable movements of hands and/or feet).	lesions at various sites in CNS or may be due to other systemic diseases. May be extrapyramidal or cerebellar syndrome.

11. **Higher Functions :** Points to be asked are as follows :
    1. Change in state of consciousness,
    2. Change in behaviour or/and mental state,
    3. Loss of memory,
    4. Loss of speech or speech defect or defect in power of expression,
    5. H/o. convulsions.

1. **Change in state of consciousness :** H/o. unconsciousness is important in neurological examination. Coma can either be due to CNS diseases or due to various other systemic diseases. Unconsciousness due to cerebral causes can be inquired into as follows:

(a) H/o of sudden unconsciousness:
   i. cerebral catastrophe,
   ii. epilepsy.

(b) H/o. rapid loss of consciousness (over a period of few hours) :
   i. some cases of slow intracranial haemorrhage,
   ii. cerebral thrombosis,
   iii. toxic (poisoning — internal or external),
   iv. infective (encephalitis, meningitis, etc.).

2. **Change in behaviour or/and mental state:** Occurs in cerebral involvement :

(a) The patient himself/herself may not be aware of the change in behaviour. But the near relatives, colleagues at work may state or notice distinct change in his/her behaviour. Such change in are indicative of frontal lobe involvement.

(b) Slow deterioration of mental function associated with episodes of behavioural changes are indicative of temporal lobe involvement.

(c) Mental deterioration along with speech defects occurs in parietal lobe involvement in dominant lobe (i.e. left parietal lobe involvement in right handed person).

(d) Lesions affecting non-dominant parietal lobe cause no speech defects but lead to unusual deficits like difficulty in dressing, disorientation and the patient may not be aware of them. Such history is obtained from near relatives or friends, i.e., if left hemisphere is dominant and lesion is in right hemisphere. Patient forgets to put on the left shoes, the left sleeve of shirt, etc.

(e) Lesions affecting parietal lobe also will cause sensory disability.

3. **Loss of memory :** Patient may lose memory along with mental disorientation. He may give this complaint or his relatives may give such a history. This symptom usually indicates cerebral, especially frontal lobe involvement. Loss of memory of recent events is indicative of Korsakoff's psychosis due to alcoholism. Patient may not remember what day it is, what he had for breakfast, etc.

4. **Speech defects :** Defect in expression of thoughts may be total or altered and only near relatives or office colleagues may give such a history. Details of speech defects usually are to be found only on examination. From history one can have only H/o. speech defect present.

5. **H/o. convulsions :** H/o. convulsions should be always inquired into. Convulsions can either be the cause of neurological deficit or they may be produced due to the lesion itself. Often they will lead the examiner to the site of the lesion, for example, if the aura is typical like in uncinate fits, the lesion will be in the opposite temporal lobe or if the convulsions are Jacksonian, the lesion can be placed in the opposite motor area of the cerebrum.

(A) H/o. convulsions should be inquired into in generalised convulsions as follows:

(a) **Aura :** Whether the patient has any premonitory warning which could either be: Motor or sensory

Motor : Twitching of a group of muscles.

Sensory : i. Related to sensory system, paraesthesiac like tingling and numbness.

ii. Related to special senses: olfactory, visual, auditory rarely hallucinations of taste.

iii. Vague symptoms : Patient knows that he is going to get the attack. Sensation of sinking in the pit of the stomach.

(b) Sudden onset of unconsciousness :

i. Sometimes preceded by the epileptic cry.

ii. Whether there is any injury during this phase (hysterical patients usually will avoid any serious injury).

(c) Tonic phase followed by clonic phase.

(d) H/o. frothing, biting of tongue and/or incontinence of bladder and bowels.

(e) Duration of the attack (usually one epileptic attack will last for few minutes but hysterical convulsions may go on for a long period).

(f) Post-epileptic phenomenon:

i. Usually headache and confusion followed by a period of sleep.

ii. Post-epileptic automatism or behaviour disorders.

(g) H/o. previous convulsions (repeated) or history of febrile convulsions during early childhood.

(h) Family history of convulsions,

(B) H/o. focal convulsion: A focal convulsion (Jacksonian convulsion) will usually start with clonic twitchings at one of the following sites: (a) angle of the mouth, (b) thumb, (c) great toe. There is no tonic phase and consciousness is not lost at the onset. The convulsive movements then spread to the affected side of the body and only if they become bilateral, consciousness is lost. The types of attack can be followed by paralysis of the parts which were affected by convulsions. This lasts for a short period and is due to exhaustion of neurons (post-epileptic paralysis of Todd).

III. **Sensory System:** The involvement of sensory system at various levels will produce signs and symptoms as follows :

1. Peripheral nerve
2. Root lesions
3. Spinal cord lesions
4. Thalamic lesions
5. Sensory cortical lesions

1. **Nerve lesions:** Pressure on the sensory nerve or its irritation will produce parasthesiac like tingling or numbness or burning sensation along the distribution of the nerve.

Complete damage to the sensory nerve will produce a loss of all modalities of sensations in its distribution.

2. **Root lesions:** Irritation of the root will produce pain along its course. These root pains have a very classical clinical picture, and are of great help in localising the lesion. The pain is (described as sharp, cutting or burning. It radiates along the distribution of the sensory root usually starting from the vertebral region and spreads along the path of the involved root. It is increased by coughing or sneezing (as these actions increase the intraspinal pressure) and by movements of the vertebral column. The pain is sometimes relieved temporarily by a change of posture.

The root pains in the distribution of T3 to T12 radiate around the chest or abdomen and hence they are known as girdle pains. The importance of root pains is their localising value as their presence points towards the exact level of lesion. Complete destruction of the root will produce a loss of all sensations along its distribution

3. **Spinal cord lesions** can produce various types of sensory loss depending on the type of lesion:

(a) Complete destruction.

(b) Incomplete destruction: (i) Spinal cord compression (extramedullary), (ii) intramedullary lesions (syringomyelia).

(a) **Complete destruction** of spinal cord disrupts the communication in all spinal tracts, e.g., from trauma or transverse myelitis. The result is total loss of all the sensations below the level of lesion. (Other symptoms, i.e., motor symptoms etc, are not described here).

(b) Incomplete destruction:

i. **Spinal cord compression :** If the compression is from outside, initially the loss of pain and temperature starts in the lower extremity on the opposite side. This is due to the fact that the fibres carrying the sensations of pain and temperature from the legs are the outermost in the spinothalamic tracts and hence are affected first.

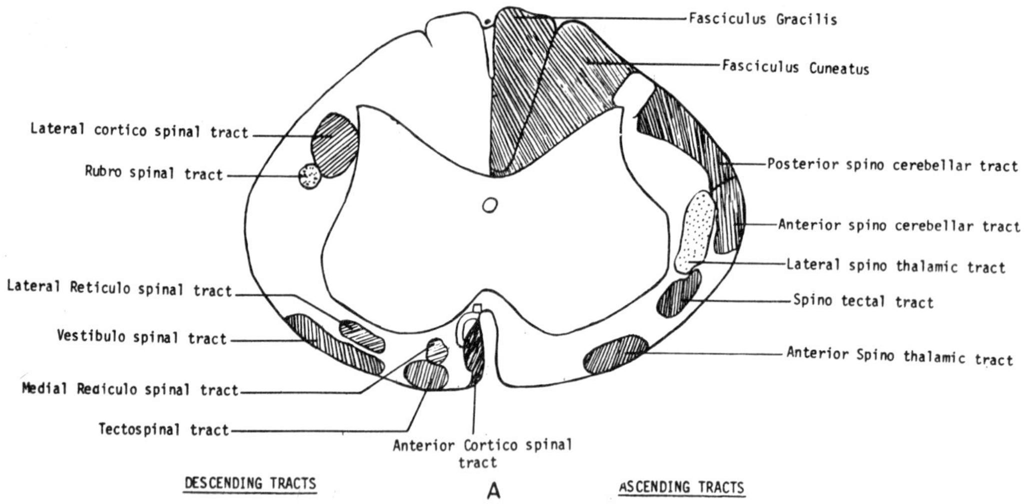

Fig. 14.1
Cross section of spinal cord to show ascending and descending tracts.

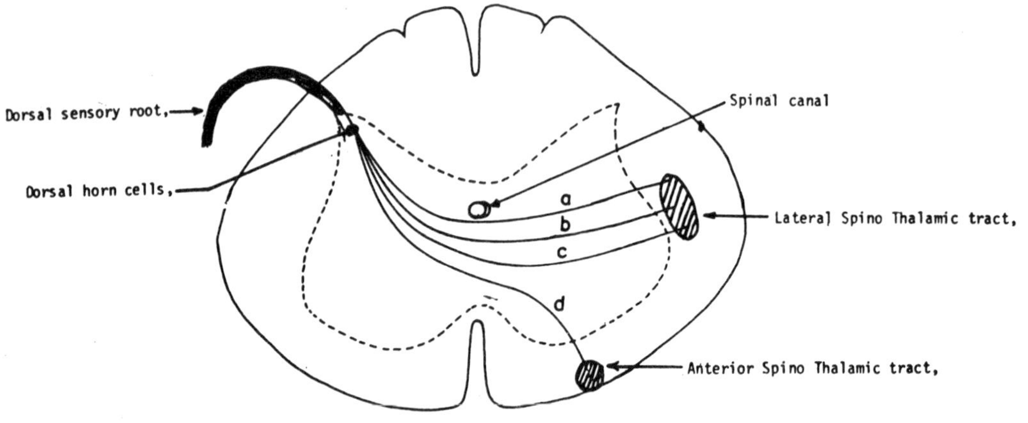

Fig. 14.2
Cross section of spinal cord to show diagramatically the crossing of sensory fibres near the spinal cord. The dissociated sensory loss which occurs in syringomyelia is because of the close proximity of these fibres to the spinal cord. a. Fibres for thermal sensations; b. Fibres for pain sensations; c. Fibres for touch sensations; d. Fibres for light touch sensations. Note that fibres for touch sensations are carried out in both anterior and lateral spinothalmic tracts.

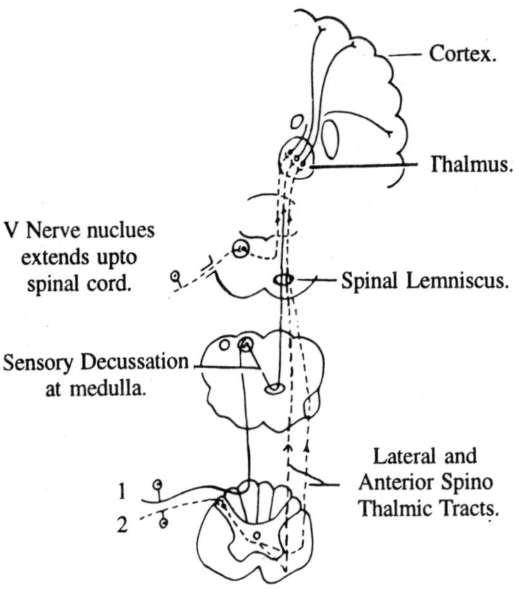

Fig. 14.3
Ascending sensory tracts

1. Sensory fibres carrying proprioceptive impulses tactile discirmination form fasciculus gracilis and fasciculus cameatus.
2. Sensory fibres carrying touch, pain and temperature form spinothalamic tracts.

As the lesion progresses the level of sensory loss goes on ascending, the upper level of this sensory loss does not correspond to the anatomical level of spinal cord damage. This is because the sensory fibres ascend for 2-3 segments before crossing to the opposite side (Fig. 14. 1).

ii. **Intramedullary lesions:** In case of syringomyelia the lesion is near spinal canal so that the fibres carrying temperature and pain get destroyed when crossing to the opposite side, resulting in loss of these sensations, while touch, joint and vibration sensations are preserved. This type of sensory loss is called 'dissociated sensory loss'. This dissociation occurs because of the fact that the fibres carrying sensation of temperature cross closest to the spinal canal, next to them are the fibres carrying sensation of pain; and fibres carrying sensation of touch are comparatively away; hence, the sensation of touch is lost when lesion is advanced (Fig. 14.2).

4. **Thalamic lesions:** As all the sensory tracts namely, spinothalamic tracts, posterior columns (Fasciculus gracilis and Cuneatus), trigeminal lemniscus (fibres carrying sensations from face), relay in thalamus, all the sensory fibres are densely packed in this area (Fig. 14.3).

Thus thalamic lesions produce hemianaesthesia, i.e., loss of touch, pain, temperature, posture and vibrations on the opposite side of the body including the face.

The special feature is associated astereognosis and unpleasant excruciating painful sensations (for the sake of convenience signs of thalamic lesion are included here). Astereognosis is diagnosed by asking patient to localise the affected limb. Patient searches for the limb in air if the eyes are closed. This is called 'thalamic phantom limb'. Painful unpleasant sensations occur on the affected side; the exact reason remains unknown.

Associated symptoms related to vision, hearing, cerebellum may be present because of proximity of these fibres to sensory tracts. Similarly because of proximity of basal ganglia choreo-athetoid form of involuntary movements may also occur.

To summarise, peculiarities of thalamic lesions are as follows :

i. Hemianaesthesia with inclusion of face.
ii. Astereognosis thalamic phantom limb.
iii. Unpleasant excruciating painful sensations.
iv. Vision and hearing may be involved.
v. Involuntary movements may be present.

5. **Sensory loss in cortical lesions:** Following are the peculiar features:

(a) Loss of sensations on the opposite side of the body but the loss is not so total and severe as in case of thalamic lesions. It is the tactile localisation and tactile discrimination which are greatly affected.

(b) Astereognosis - with eyes closed, the patient cannot identify an object given in the affected hand.

(c) Painful unpleasant sensation may be present as in case of thalamic lesion.

(d) Change in the state of consciousness if the lesion is acute.

After analysis of sensory symptoms at various levels following questions should be asked:

1. Does the patient complain of any loss of sensations - anaesthesiae or hypoasthesia?

(a) If so, is the loss total or partial?

(b) Which parts of the body are affected?

(c) Does it correspond to any particular nerve distribution or is it bilaterally symmetrical? (polyneuritis or complete transaction).

(d) Are all the modalities of sensations affected or is the loss restricted to any particular sensation? - syringomyelia

2. Does he complain of abnormal sensory symptoms (parasthesiae)?

(a) Does he have any tingling or numbness? If so, what is its distribution - root lesion or polyneuritis.

(b) Does he have any lightning pains in the calf muscles?

(c) Is there any sensation of band-like constriction around the legs? (Such lightning pains occur in compression or irritation of spinothalamic tracts; and compression of posterior columns produces a sensation of band-like constriction or tingling numbness).

(d) Is there any complaint of sudden, severe, shooting pains starting from a specific area in the vertebral column and radiating along a particular nerve root?

(e) Is there any complaint of burning sensation? Is it restricted to a root distribution or is it bilaterally symmetrical? (root compression or polyneuritis).

(f) Is there any complaint of pain localised over a particular area in the vertebral column? (tuberculous spine or secondary deposits in the spine or trauma to spine). Information derived from these questions will point to anatomical lesions at various sites.

(g) Can the patient assess the position of the affected limb when his eyes are closed? (thalamic phantom limb).

IV. **Sphincter Control:** History-taking in sphincter disturbances: History is more valuable than examination in arriving at diagnosis in the case of neurological disturbances of bladder.

Symptoms related to neurological bladder disturbances:

1. Does the patient feel the fullness of bladder?

2. Can he hold the urine if there is no oppurtunity to evacuate bladder? Does he have to evacuate the bladder as soon as he feels the fullness? (urgency)

3. Does the patient complain of delay in initiating the act of micturition? (hesitancy)

4. Does he complain of retention of urine, if so, does he have the sensation of bladder being full or not?

5. Can he stop passing of urine in midstream at will?

6. Does he evacuate the bladder spontaneously from time to time without any control or sensation? (precipitancy)

7. Does he get a feeling of incomplete evacuation, i.e., feeling of residual urine?

8. Does the patient have dribbling of urine, i.e., passing few drops of urine at a time after the act is over? (incontinence) Is he aware of this dribbling?

9. Is there any associated rectal incontinence or impotency?

10. Is there any numbness in perineal region?

These symptoms point to lesions at various sites in CNS. (Details in Chapter 16, p 252)

V. **Cranial Nerves:** History-taking - H/o. cranial nerve affection should be asked as follows:

Nerve I: Olfactory nerve: Questions: 1. Whether the patient can smell properly. A negative answer does not mean a lesion of the nerve in most of the cases as local nasal conditions like injection, etc., are the most common causes of anosmia. 2. Whether he has any abnormal sensation of smell? That is even a normally pleasant smell evokes an unpleasant sensation. This condition is known as perverted sensation of smell. 3. Whether there are any hallucinations of smell-rarely these may be present in 'uncinate fits'.

Nerve II : Optic nerve: 1. Whether the patient can see normally? 2. Whether his vision for both distant and near objects is normal? This will be affected commonly due to local conditions of lens (i.e., cataract). However in conditions where there is specific paralysis of accommodation the patient will complain of difficulty in reading (near vision) of recent onset. 3. Whether the patient can see normally with both the eyes and is he unable to do so with only one eye? 4. If he is unable to see properly, is the vision slowly getting blurred (as can happen when the patient is developing papilloedema)? 5. Is there a complaint of sudden blindness from which the patient has recovered? If so, was it in both the eyes (as can happen in demyelinating diseases) or only one eye? (embolism of the central retinal artery) 6. If there is a defect in vision, can the patient localise it as being on one side or in one of the quadrants (as happens in field defects)? 7. Can the patient appreciate basic colours?

Nerves III, IV, and VI: Oculomotor, Trochlear, Abducens, complaints relating to these nerves will have to be considered together as their functions are closely interrelated and though isolated palsies are present, the symptomatology can be easily discussed together.

1. Is the patient able to open his eyes properly? Severe ptosis will be seen by the examiner and no questioning may be required on this point.

2. Or does the inability to open the eyes come gradually especially by evening? (myasthenia gravis)

3. Has the patient noticed any squint recently?

4. Is there any diplopia, i.e., double vision?

a. If so whether it is on looking on one side? (VI nerve paralysis)

b. Or is there any diplopia in looking in any direction? (111 nerve paralysis)

c. Or is the diplopia present on looking downwards and inwards? (IV nerve paralysis usually manifests itself when going down the stairs).

5. Does the patient feel that one of his eyes is appearing smaller than the other? (Horner's syndrome)

Nerve V: For Trigeminal nerve, inquiry will have to be made of both components, that is, sensory as well as motor.

Sensory component:

1. Is there any H/o. sudden, shooting, excruciating pain affecting either a part or whole of the face? (one or more divisions of the nerve) If so which part (division) is affected? Is this pain precipitated by irritation of any particular areas? (trigger zones) This history will be positive in patients suffering from trigeminal neuralgia.

2. Is there any anaesthesia or hypoaesthesia over any part of the face? I f so on which side and whether the whole face is affected or only part of it?

Motor component:

Is the patient able to perform the jaw movements properly, i.e., whether he can chew properly and open his mouth normally without any deviation of jaw.

Nerve VII : Facial nerve:

1. Has the patient noticed any asymmetry of the face? If the patient complaints of asymmetry of the face, then the following questions should be asked for finding out whether the whole face or part of it is affected.

2. Is he able to close his eyes properly on the affected side? And is there any excessive lacrimation on that side?

3. Is there any dribbling to liquids or saliva from one side of the mouth?

4. Is there an inability to purse the lips and whistle?

5. Is there any difficulty in uttering certain letters like p., b., etc. (labials).

This questioning will enable the examiner to distinguish between supranuclear and infra-nuclear types of paralysis. In the former, eye closure will be unaffected, while the whole side of the face will be affected in the latter. In supranuclear facial palsy superior part of face escapes.

Nerve VIII: Auditory: The two components of the nerve are auditory and cochlear. Separate inquiry in their functions should be conducted as follows:

Auditory:

1. Can the patient hear normally on both sides? Inability to hear properly is commonly due to local conditions or nerve defect.

2. Is there any tinnitus (ringing, buzzing, hissing or roaring sound) in either ear?

Vestibular:

1. Is there any vertigo?

2. Is it accompanied by any vomiting?

3. If present, is it of sudden onset or gradually getting worse?

Vertigo, non neurological in origin is not discussed here.

Nerves IX, X, XI (cranial part): Glossopharyngeal, vagus, cranial accessory:

1. Is there any sudden severe pain on one side, of the throat which then radiates down the side of the neck in front of the ear and then to the back of the jaw? This rare complaint is present in glossopharyngeal neuralgia.

2. Is there any hoarseness of voice or aphonia or feeble voice? (recurrent laryngeal nerve paralysis - X nerve)

3. Is there any nasal twang to the voice? (palatal paralysis IX, X nerves).

4. Is there any dysphagia with or without nasal regurgitation of food? (pharyngeal and palatal paralysis IX, X, XI nerves)

Spinal XI : Spinal accessory:

1. Is there any difficulty in turning the head o one side? (weakness of sternomastoid on the contralateral side)

2. Can the patient lift the head from the pillow easily? (weakness of both sternomastoids)

3. Is the patient able to 'shrug' shoulders, i.e., to elevate the shoulders properly? (weakness of trapezius).

Nerve XII : Hypoglossal

1. Is the patient able to protrude the tongue properly?

2. Has the patient noticed any unilateral or bilateral wasting of the tongue?

3. If so does he have any fasciculations?

4. Is there any difficulty in speech or swallowing which the patient feels is due to weakness of the tongue?

5. Does he feel his tongue 'heavy'? (pseudobulbar palsy)

VI. History which may indicate the cause of the lesion:

After the above enquiry in history-taking the following points should be asked to determine the cause of the lesion.

Sometimes these may be volunteered by the patient, but quite often the patient may have forgotten them or according to him, they may be of no importance and hence they will be brought out only by direct inquiry.

The causes of neurological condition are as follows and should be enquired in detailed and systematic manner. 1. trauma, 2. infection, 3. vascular, 4. space-occupying lesion, 5. degenerative, 6. demyelination.

1. **Trauma:** H/o. trauma is extremely important as that will enable the examiner to come to the conclusion regarding the cause immediately.

In diseases within the cranium, H/o. direct trauma will point towards:

a. local haemorrhage causing compression,

b. generalised intracerebral haemorrhage due to the rupture of a large vessel,

c. direct penetrating injury causing disruption of the tissue of the brain,

d. depressed fracture of the skull causing compression.

H/o. minor trauma to the skull in the past (even a few months ago) might cause a subdural haematoma with gradually progressive symptoms of compression.

One point of clinical importance should be remembered. If a chronic alcoholic has injured himself his alcoholic stuperose condition, he may have genuinely forgotten about his injury.

In spinal cord lesions, trauma directly to the vertebral column will cause compression at the site of injury. Usually such injuries damage the spinal cord when an element of rotation is present.

However, lifting a heavy weight may suddenly cause rupture and an acute protrusion of the intervertebral disc with sudden onset of symptoms of compression.

Sometimes a fall from a height on the gluteal region may cause injury to the cervical spine by transmission of the shock to the cervical region (transmitted pressure).

History of trauma to head or spine very often precipitates tubeculous meningitis and tubeculous spine.

2. **Infection:** H/o. infection of the meninges which is common cause of affection of the CNS especially of the brain will cause headache, backache, fever and vomiting.

This could be the primary cause in various cranial nerve palsies or hemiplegia (more common in children).

As tuberculosis is one of the most common causes of meningeal infections, H/o. systemic tuberculosis, like history of cervical lympha denopathy or chronic cough with haemoptysis suggestive of pulmonary tuberculosis should be asked for.

H/o. exposure (syphilis) should always be asked as it can give rise to a variety of either cranial or spinal cord lesions.

H/o.fever, back pain and other symptoms like generalised weakness, bodyache, malaise which are the usual features of a viral infection will precede the onset of paraparesis in viral myelitis.

However, H/o.fever with sore throat about 2 weeks prior (which the patient may consider as of no importance) is usually present before the onset of ascending paralysis in infective polyneuritis.

H/o.conjunctivitis in recent past may be of importance in case of myelitis. H/o.infectious diseases as measles mumps, chickenpox may precede myelitis or encephalitis.

H/o.infectious diseases like measles, mumps or chickenpox may precede encephalitis.

Tuberculosis of the spine is an infective process but as it usually causes symptoms due to either compression or vascular complications it will be discussed under those headings.

3. **Vascular:** As vascular lesions are the predominant cause of a lesion in the brain, H/o. those conditions which will cause damage to the arteries should be inquired.

a. H/o. hypertension.

b. H/o. diabetes/either symptomalology-polyuria, polydypsia or polyphagia or history of previous estimation of blood sugar.

c. H/o.syphilis as it may affect the CNS by causing vascular damage (endarteritis obliterans).

d. H/o.rheumatic vascular disease and/or infective endocarditis leading to embolic phenomena (especially in younger age group patients with CNS complaints).

e. Very rarely H/o.haemophilia or any other bleeding disorder may be present in patients with cerebral haemorrhage.

f. Pott's spine may cause sudden paraparesis because of anterior spinal artery thrombosis.

g. Tuberculous meningitis leads to lesions of arteries and veins with subsequent morbidities.

4. **Compression:** (Spinal cord and intracranial): In intracranial compression, H/o. head- ache, vomiting and blurring of vision is the triad of symptoms complained of by the patient. Of course the same type of symptomatology along with fever will be present in patients due to an infective process like meningitis or tuberculoma.

A vertebral disease causing compression may cause a local pain at the site of vertebral disease. H/o. root pains which has already been inquired about is also common feature of vertebral diseases causing compression. H/o. local deformity of the spine (gibbus) may be present in tuberculosis of spine. Tuberculosis of spine can lead to compression of the cord by virtue of cold abscess or prolapse of the vertebral body or by pressure of tuberculous granulation tissue.

5. **Toxic and degenerative diseases:** (a) Progressive bilaterally symmetrical motor deficit is caused by degenerative disorder (e.g., motor neuron disease). (b) H/o.ingestion of kesari dal or TOCP (Tetra orthocresyl phosphate) can cause progressive spastic paraplegia due to toxic degeneration of pyramidal tracts. (c) H/o. anaemia and vague gastric symptoms with or without alcoholism may be a clue pointing towards subacute combined degeneration. (d) Ataxia, papilladema and drousiness may be due to lead poisoning with consequent cerebral swelling. (e) Peripheral neuropathy can result from poisoning due to lead and benzene derivatives.

6. **Causes leading to demyelination:** (a) H/o. optic nerve affection (partial or total) leading to blindness along with paraplegia is again a feature of demyelinating disease. (b) H/o. injections of vaccines, e.g., antirabies serum and sera should be asked as they may lead to demyelination. (c) H/o. previous episodes of neurological deficit from which the patient has made partial or complete recovery may be a feature of demyelinating disorders, e.g., multiple sclerosis.

7. H/o. similar illness in any other member of the family or previous generation. (Myopathies, cerebellar ataxia, epilepsy).

8. H/o. Consanguinity - marriage in blood relation. Heredofamilial disease, eg., epilepsy, cerebellar ataxia.

15. Central Nervous System : Clinical Examination

Important Features in General Examination

Skull & Spine:

I. **Skull:** (a) Size and shape of the skull should be noted, microcephally will be obvious. (b) Sometimes bony bossing may be present over an underlying meningioma. (c) Localised deposits causing irregular local deformities may be seen due to leukaemia or malignant disease. (d) Increased intracranial tension in children may result in separation of the sutures. (e) Head circumference normal (50 cms). Increase in circumference shows hydrocephalus, decrease due to any cause like microcephally or craniostenosis.

II. **Spine:** (a) Local deformity or gibbus is one of the most common abnormalities seen on examining the spine. It is usually caused by tuberculosis of vertebral bodies. (b) Local tenderness over the spine will indicate a tuberculous process, secondary deposit, a primary neoplasm or any local osteitis.

III. **Stance and gait:** If during history-taking it is felt that the patient is well enough then this examination should be conducted initially as it may help the examiner to point out the lesion immediately. If the patient is unable to stand or walk paraplegia can be diagnosed. The patient should be asked to stand. After standing for a few minutes, he should be asked to walk across the room, turn and then come back to the bed.

Even while getting up, patient suffering from myopathy will have a typical method of getting up. He will first turn to one side, then lift himself on his hands and knees and grasp the legs with hands and then slowly climb upwards on his own legs.

Stance itself will give very important information:

1. If the patient is unable to stand with normal strength the cause may be hysterical, or due to a lesion of the cerebellum. 2. If the patient is able to stand with eyes open he should be asked to close his eyes with his feet together. 3. In Rombergism : Posterior columns are affected. The patient will sway from side to side and may fall if not supported. He is unable to stand straight with eyes closed. 4. Hemiplegic stance: The patient usually is slightly bent on the affected side. His arm is flexed at the elbow and internally rotated at the shoulder. The leg is extended and there is foot drop (loss of power of dorsiflexors). 5. Stance in Parkinson syndrome (Pl. 15.1) : There is a mask-like face, and stooping on the affected side. The upper arm is flexed at the elbow and fingers perform the pill rolling movements. The leg is slightly bent at the knee. 6. Lordotic stance: Usually seen in myopathy where the patient assumes this posture to avoid losing his centre of gravity.

Gait:

Hemiplegic gait: The first point which comes to the examiner's attention is dragging of the foot on the affected side. The resultant obstruction to walking is avoided by throwing the whole leg outwards from the hip with bending towards the opposite side (circumduction of the leg to clear the ground). The arm is flexed across the body and does not take part in the normal walking movements.

Gait in bilateral upper motor neuron lesion (Scissors gait): Seen most classically in cerebral diplegia (spastic cerebral palsy) it can also be produced by any bilateral pyramidal damage. The difficulty in walking is mainly due to bilateral adductor spasm and the weakness of dorsiflexors. The patient crosses one leg over the other at every step.

Gait in Parkinson's syndrome: Shuffling gait or festinant gait is seen as series of short small shuffles during which the patient slides rather than lifts one foot after the other. There is no natural swing of the arms. When such a patient is pushed forwards he goes on walking progressively rapidly (propulsion) or if he is pushed backwards, he goes on walking backwards more and more rapidly (retropulsion). These movements usually stop only when the patient falls or bangs into a wall or some obstruction.

Kinesia paradoxa is the term given to the peculiar phenomenon observed in Parkinsonism. The patient with this disease, if in a hurry may be able to run quite fast but when he starts walking he cannot do so normally and has to revert to his shuffling gait.

Ataxic gait: In cerebellar ataxia, the patient's feet are based wide apart and he walks in a zig-zag manner, that is, the patient sways on any side in reeling and staggering fashion. This gait is also seen in patients suffering from Freidrich's ataxia and multiple sclerosis.

In sensory ataxia as in tabes dorsalis the patient walks with a stamping gait. The feet are widely placed. The legs are raised too high and thrown outwards or waved about before bringing them down in a stamping fashion. The heels are brought in contact with the ground first.

High stepping gait: The feet are raised high to overcome foot drop seen commonly in peripheral neuropathy. The patient is not ataxic but wide based and the toes come into contact with the ground first.

Waddling gait: This type of gait is seen commonly in myopathies. The pelvis is rotated excessively and this is accompanied by movements in the opposite direction of the upper trunk. There is also marked lordosis.

This is also seen in congenital dislocation of the hips.

Gait in chorea: In chorea of any etiology, the patient has a wide based, lordotic gait in which he lurches from side to side on his heels and has tendency to fall.

Hysterical gaits: They have no fixed pattern and even vary from time to time. The patient may fall or bang himself without any injury. The gait is usually wide based but otherwise has no other features seen in wide based gaits.

IV. **Trophic changes:** Trophic changes in the nervous system usually follow lesions of the sensory pathways.

Skin: Skin may be abnormally glossy and thin and may lose its natural lustre. It can also become hyperkeratotic with pigmentation. Cutaneous ecchymoses or rarely cyanosis may also occur.

Perforating ulcers are usually features of sensory root damage. The most common example of this is the ulcer of tabes dorsalis and diabetes mellitus.

Nails can become thickened and brittle.

Leprous ulcers on the hands and feet and the face can be ragged and the resulting deformity is the main reason for the social stigma of this disease.

V. **Bones:** Bones may be decalcified and hence become fragile resulting in pathological fractures. Bony growth may be stunted in a case of long-standing poliomyelitis.

VI. **Joints :** Arthropathy presenting as abnormal swelling of the joints which is painless, though commonly seen in knee joints in case of tabes dorsalis, they can be seen in upper extremities in patients suffering from syringomyelia.

VII. **Blood pressure recording:** To confirm the presence or absence of hypertension; also to note postural hypotension (peripheral neuropathies).

VIII. **Palpation of carotid arteries:** It is important to note whether they are equally well felt on both sides. Carotid and other arteries in the neck should also be auscultated for bruit. Left carotid artery may not be well felt in case of right sided hemiplegia.

IX. **Palpation of certain peripheral nerves for thickening and tenderness.** Ulnar nerve in leprosy, diabetic and peripheral neuropathy.

Examination of the Neurological System :

So many volumes have been written on this subject, that it will be impossible to cover the various details of an extremely thorough neurological examination. However, a practical method of examination will be discussed here along with the common abnormalities and their interpretation.

1. **Higher functions:** Examination of the CNS requires a full understanding and co-operation from the patient. Hence, the first and foremost requirement will be to assess his higher functions. A brief resume of them is given in Table 15.1.

In states of altered consciousness, it is impossible to take the history of the patient directly and test for any other functions; in such cases history should be taken from the relatives.

Sometimes due to lack of comprehension following a defect in the receptive areas some problem may be encountered.

2. **Memory:**

(a) For recent events: Elicited by asking him questions about his breakfast, lunch or about his activities on the previous day,

(b) For remote events: Elicited by asking about his date and place of birth, schooling, about his previous jobs or any such past activities or regarding any important news item from newspapers.

Table 15.1

1. **State of consciousness :**
Grades of disturbances of consciousness:

Conscious state :	State of awareness of one self and one's environment.
Confused, dazed state :	Patient is conscious, has fixed gaze and has disturbed orientation of the environment.
Drowsy or lethargic state :	Resembles sleepy state : Person can be aroused easily by stimuli but tends to sleep as soon as stimuli are withdrawn.
Stuporous state :	Resembles state of deep sleep: Person can be aroused with difficulty, and goes back to sleep quickly.
Semi-conscious state :	Person is unaware of surrounding and responds to painful stimuli.
Unconscious state :	Patient is unaware of environment and all the mental activities are suspended. He does not respond to painful stimuli.

In loss of recent memory, usually there is disorientation in time and space also. This is a feature of Korsakoff's psychosis where the memory of recent events is lost. Usual cause of this type of psychosis is alcoholism which leads to lesion in anterior hypothalamic region.

With advancing age, patient forgets recent events - e.g. whether he had bath, breakfast etc; but he remembers clearlly events from his childhood.

3. **Intelligence:**

This will be apparent on usual questions and answers during history-taking. A lack of intelligence and presence or lack of insight will have to be taken into account in interpreting the answers given by the patients during history-taking.

4. **Emotional state:**

The emotional state of the patient should be noted, i.e., whether he is anxious, excited, frightened, depressed, apathetic or euphoric.

Excluding the usual nervous tension causing anxiety which most of the patients experience when they come for interview the following emotional abnormalities could be due to organic diseases.

(a) Euphoria: Common in multiple sclerosis.

(b) Flippant or jovial attitude : In frontal lobe disorders.

(c) Aggressive euphoria: Post-traumatic (after- head injuries in some cases).

(d) Emotional instability: Manifests as sudden crying or laughter in pseudobulbar palsy. (Psychiatric disorders causing changes in the emotional state are not discussed here.)

Speech:

Speech can be defined as the ability of communication through the dual processes of speaking or writing. This itself entails an understanding and interpretation of the spoken or written word. Speech centres are localised in the dominant hemisphere of the brain, i.e., in left hemisphere in a right handed person. As the centres are not localised or defined accurately, they are known as areas rather than centres. The best known area is Broca's area which governs the motor speech (chiefly the spoken word) and it is in the lower and posterior part of the third frontal convolution.

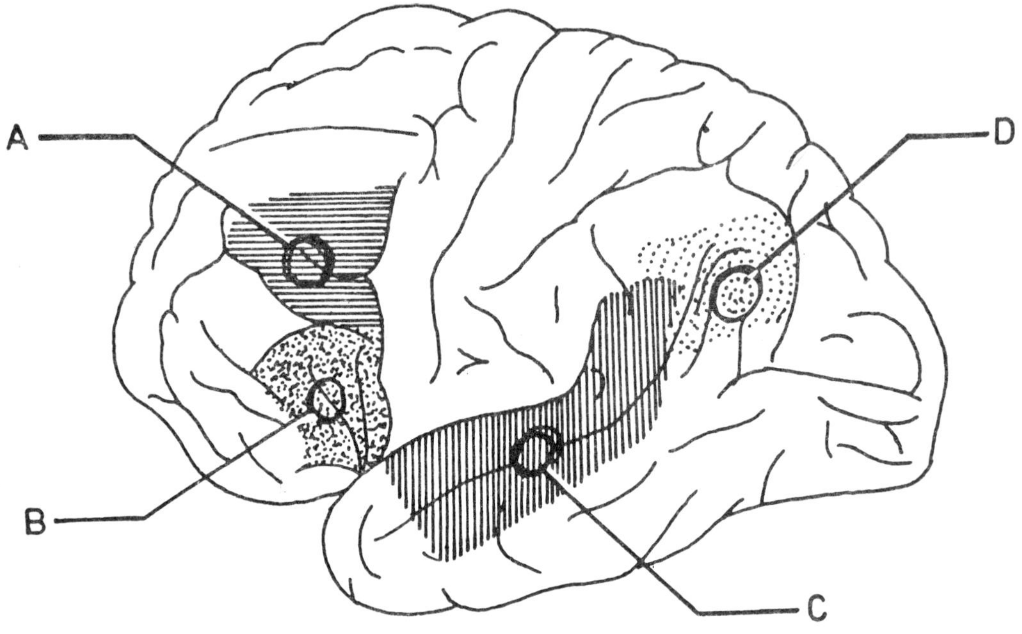

Fig. 15.1
Localisation of areas for power of expression.
A. Expression in writing - lesion leads to agraphia.
B. Expression in speech - lesion leads to aphasia.
C. Understanding spoken words - lesion leads to word deafness.
D. Understanding written words - lesion leads to word blindness.

The posterior part of the second frontal convolution governs the written speech.

The understanding of the spoken words i.e., auditory reception — is in the posterior part of the left superior temporosphenoidal convolution.

The visual reception area which governs the reception or understanding is in the posterior part of the first temporal convolution. (Fig. 15. 1)

Disorders of speech:

They can be classified in four main categories: 1. Aphonia, 2. Mutism, 3. Dysarthria, and 4. Aphasia or dysphasia (incomplete aphasia) : Dysphasia means difficulty in communication or expression of thoughts. Aphasia means absence in communication. (Aphonia and Mutism should be defined first as the cause of these conditions is usually not neurological).

1. **Aphonia:** Aphonia is failure of production of voice while speaking, which is due to local disease of the larynx and vocal cords. This can often be in a hysterical or debilitated patient.

2. **Mutism:** Mutism is usually due to psychological disorder and in this condition the patient makes no attempt to speak.

3. **Dysarthria:** In this condition the volume and content of speech is normal. However the pronunciation of words is defective due to difficulty in articulation of speech. The cause of this condition is an affection of the muscles of articulation. Thus, dysarthria is defined as a difficulty in articulation of speech due to involvement of muscles of articulation. The lesion may be central or peripheral.

Causes of dysarthria:

a. Due to pyramidal lesions.
b. Due to extra-pyramidal lesions.
c. Due to lower motor neuron lesions.
d. Due to cerebellar diseases.
c. Due to muscle diseases.

a. **Due to pyramidal lesions:** Spastic dysarthria is caused by bilateral damage to the pyramidal tracts. In this condition the tongue is spastic and so also the muscles of the pharynx. The jaw jerk is exaggerated. This condition is usually used by pseudobulbar palsy due to bilateral corticospinal tract damage, e.g. motor neurone disease and vertebro basilar insufficiency.

b. **Due to extra-pyramidal lesions:** Rigid dysarthria is due to rigidity of the muscles of the face, tongue and pharyngeal muscles, There is monotonous speech with words running into each other.

Palilalia: Repetition of a particular syllable is sometimes present.

Cause: Parkinson's disease and other extrapyramidal syndromes, dystonic cerebral palsy.

c. **Due to lower motor neuron lesions:** Here the muscles supplied by various cranial nerves are affected.

Paralysis of face - VIIth cranial nerve affection,

Paralysis of tongue - XIIth nerve affection,

Paralysis of palate - Xth, XIth cranial nerve affection.

The result is nasal twang in speech.

Cause: Motor neuron disease, infective polyneuritis, postdiphtheritic paralysis and bulbar polio encephalitis.

d. **Due to cerebellar lesions:** Inco-ordination of the muscles causes the speech to be slurred and irregular. The words may be spaced too far or too near and they may also be unnecessarily loud or soft (scanning, staccato, hot potato speech).

Causes: Cerebellar disease, hereditary ataxias, multiple sclerosis.

e. **Due to muscle disorders:** Myasthenia gravis causes a typical dysarthria. At the begin- ning of the speech, the voice is normal but at the end, practically at every sentence it trails off into hoarseness due to fatigue of the muscles. After a few seconds rest, again normal speech can be resumed.

4. **Aphasis or dysphasia:**

Examination for dysphasia starts at the time of history-taking. A completely aphasic or severely dysphasic patient will not be able to narrate his history at all. However, other abnormalities which will be discussed now may be suggested by listening to the construction of the sentence, words and their use, whether the words uttered have any meaning or whether they are of the patient's own construction and whether the patient goes on repeating the same words again and again.

Similarly, it should be noted whether the patient understands the question put to him. Sometimes he will not understand the order given to him verbally, but he may follow the same when it is demonstrated to him. (For instance, if the examiner orders "put up your left hand" the patient may not understand it and he may do nothing. However, if the order is accompanied by the examiner gesturing to lift the hand, the patient may immediately do so.)

The patient should be shown common objects and he should then be asked to name them. In more detailed neurological examination, where there is suspicion that speech areas are affected, the patient should be asked both to read and write.

Classification of aphasia:

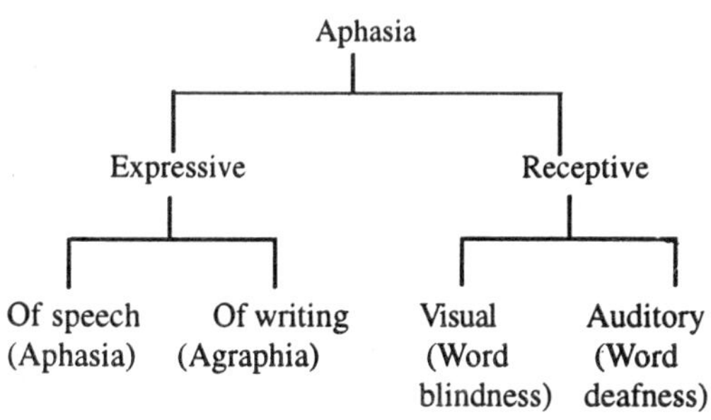

Aphasia can be classified roughly as shown above. However, in practice, though the main defect is of one type, there is always an overlapping of more than one type of defect.

Expressive aphasia of speech or motor aphasia:

In very severe degree of aphasia, there may be no speech at all or the patient may be able to utter only few words, that also incorrectly.

Lesion is in Broca's area and this is the most common defect encountered along with right sided hemiplegia in right handed patient (site of lesion is in the left hemisphere).

Nominal aphasia:

In this, the patient is unable to name the objects though he recognises them correctly. For instance if he is shown a pen he knows and answers that it is something with which one writes. If he is asked whether it is a comb, watch or any other object, he will answer negatively. Only when the examiner asks whether it is pen, he will answer in the affirmative.

Expressive aphasia of writing — Agraphia:

A pure agraphia is inability to write with other expressive and receptive faculties preserved. It is rare. Usually it is part of other aphasic states.

Receptive aphasia: The patient suffering from this condition will have a speech full of neologisms, paraphrasing and repetition of the same phrases. This is due to inability to understand words and sentences, either written or spoken. Hence, the patient is unable to recognise the mistake in his own speech.

Jargon speech: This presents as a severe defect of speech. The patient speaks words or sentences which are meaningless and have no place in the language.

This is produced by a severe defect in reception of both spoken and written speech.

Pure word deafness: The patient cannot understand the spoken word but his speech, reading and writing are normal.

Echolalia: In this the patient goes on repeating part of a phrase uttered by the examiner or someone else.

Alexia: It is the inability to understand written

speech. Pure alexia is rare. In this, the patient is unable to understand written orders but all the other components of speech are normal.

Alexia is commonly associated with agraphia (described above). The combination is also known as visual asymbolia and is much more common than pure alexia. The patient cannot read or write spontaneously in this defect.

Stammering and stuttering:

This defect is more commonly psychological. However, in developing children it can be associated with ambidexterity.

II. **Examination of Cranial Nerves:**

Ist cranial (olfactory) nerve:

Functions: This nerve carries the sensation of smell from the nasal mucosa to the olfactory bulb. From here the impulses pass through the olfactory nerve and tract to the periamygdoloid and prepyriform areas of cortex.

Test: Because of the frequent interference with the function of this nerve due to local causes like common cold the examination of its function is of limited value.

Small bottles containing substances of familiar odour are used. The patient is asked to smell them and identify the odours after closing one nostril by digital pressure and then the procedure is repeated on the opposite side. The use of ammonia or acetic acid should be avoided as they irritate the pain nerve endings of the trigeminal nerves.

The patient may identify the smell and name it correctly or sometimes the odour is smelt but he is unable to name it correctly. Both these may be considered as normal.

Anosmia means loss of sensation of smell. Causes are (in absence of common cold) :

1. Head injury with or without fracture of the base of skull in anterior fossa.
2. Tumours.
3. Distended cerebral ventricles in obstructive hydrocephalus.
4. Meningitis.
5. Tabes dorsalis.

Parosmia: It is a condition where any smell evokes a response. of unpleasant sensation. Causes are (in absence of common cold) :

1. Head injury.
2. In depression due to psychological causes.
3. Uncinate fits.

The IInd cranial (optic) nerve:

Function: This nerve carries the visual impulses from the retina. The fibres carrying visual sensations ascend through the optic nerves. Then at the level of optic chiasma, the fibres carrying impulses from the medial half the retina (which carry impulse from the temporal half of the visual field) cross to the opposite side. From here the impulses go through the optic tract to the lateral geniculate body, and superior colliculus. Here the optic radiation fibres originate and they end in the occipital cortex, where the visual reception centres are situated.

The function of the optic nerve is to be tested in three phases :

1. Acuity of vision,
2. Field of vision,
3. Colour vision.

1. **Acuity of vision:** By the bedside, the examiner relies on ordinary routine methods to test the acuity of vision.

The first precaution is to test each eye separately (by closing the other). The patient is asked to look at a distant object and identify it. Or he can be asked to look at a wall clock and tell the time. Near vision is tested by asking the patient to count the examiner's fingers held at a reasonable distance. If this is not possible, the procedure is repeated by bringing the hand progressively nearer the eye. If the patient cannot count them or is unable to see them at all he is tested for perception of light by directing a torch beam in the eye. Only when the perception of light (P.L.) is absent the eye can be considered as totally blind.

The visual charts (Snellen's chart for distant vision and Jaeger's type chart for near vision) are usually not used for routine physical examination of the nervous system.

Field of vision: Method: The field of vision is tested at the bedside by the confrontation method. The patient and the examiner face each other and the distance between the two should be roughly one metre. Each eye is tested separately and the examiner covers his own eye on the corresponding side. The patient's other eye is closed by the patient's hand. He is asked to keep on looking steadily in the examiner's eye without shifting his gaze from side to side. Then the examiner takes his finger as far out as possible in the four quadrants, in which the field of vision is to be tested, i.e., in the superior, inferior, lateral (temporal) and medial (nasal) quadrants. The finger is then gradually brought nearer and the patient is asked to say at what point he starts noticing it. This should be compared with the examiner's own field of vision (taking it for granted that it is normal).

After this, both eyes should be uncovered and the patient should be asked to look in the examiner's eyes. The examiner takes both his fingers in the lateral fields and the wriggling fingers are brought nearer. This will detect the visual inattention commonly seen in parietal lobe disorders, where though the visual fields are normal only the object on the unaffected side is appreciated. (Fig. 15.2(a) and 15.2(b)

Colour vision: At the bedside the colour vision can be tested roughly by showing the patient any red, green or yellow coloured object. Only gross defect can be made out in this fashion.

In more accurate testing, the patient is asked to match the shades of a particular colour. Holmgron's wools are usually used for this purpose. Colour vision is affected in cortical lesions or it may be congenital defect.

IIIrd (oculomotor), IVth (trochlear), VIth (abducens) nerves:

Functions: 1. Control of the external ocular movements. 2. Elevation of the upper eyelid. 3. Regulation of the pupillary reaction by the autonomic nerves, running in relation to these nerves.

Test : The following tests may be conducted :

1. to note the presence of ptosis,
2. to test the external ocular movements and any strabismus produced by their paralysis,
3. to inspect the pupils and test them for reactions of light and accommodation,
4. to detect and analyse nystagmus.

1. **Ptosis and squint :** This can easily be noted while looking at the patient without any special effort. Exophthalmos and enophthalmos also should be checked. Ptosis may be due to paralysis of the oculomotor nerve or due to sympathetic paralysis. Lid can be raised voluntarily in sympathetic paralysis while in the oculomotor paralysis, the frontal muscles contract to compensate for the drooping eyelid and hence the forehead appears wrinkled (may even lead to frontal headache).

Myasthenia gravis can also cause ptosis due to muscle weakness.

2. **External ocular movements and paralytic strabismus:**

The patient is asked to follow the examiner's finger which is then moved in all the four directions. The head of the patient is fixed with the examiner's other hand.

In ocular muscle paralysis the following information can be derived immediately.

(a) Failure of outward movement of the eyeball means weakness of the abducens nerve (VIth nerve).

(b) If there is inability of downward movement when the eyeball is deviated inwards, the weakness is of superior oblique muscle and hence it is due to weakness of the trochlear (IVth nerve).

(c) All other abnormalities will mean oculomotor (IIIrd nerve) lesion. Eye movements caused by different muscles are shown in Fig. 15.3. Paralytic squint occurs due to unopposed action of the normal muscles. Hence, in IIIrd nerve paralysis,

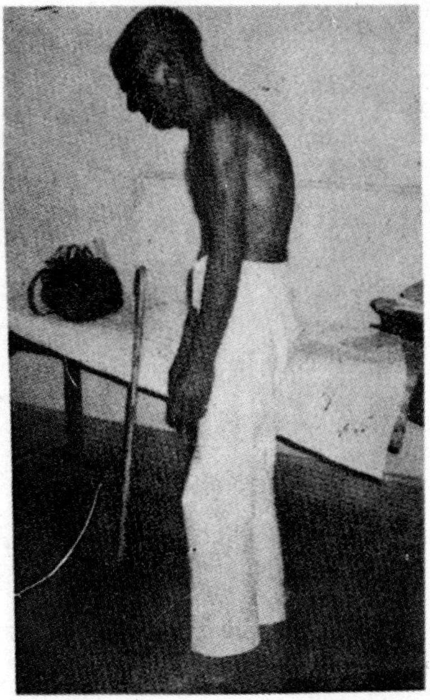

Pl. 15.1 Parkinsonian Posture

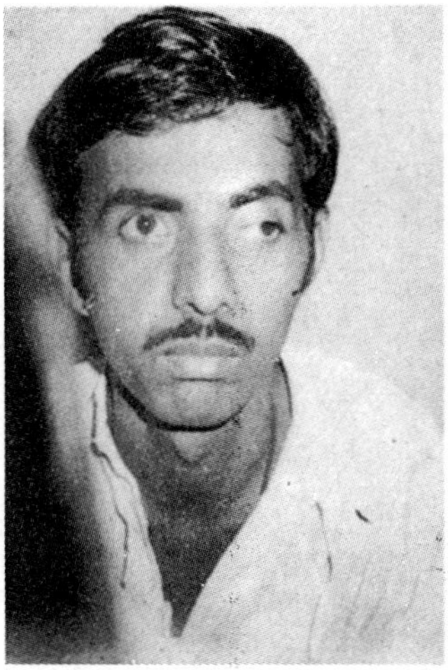

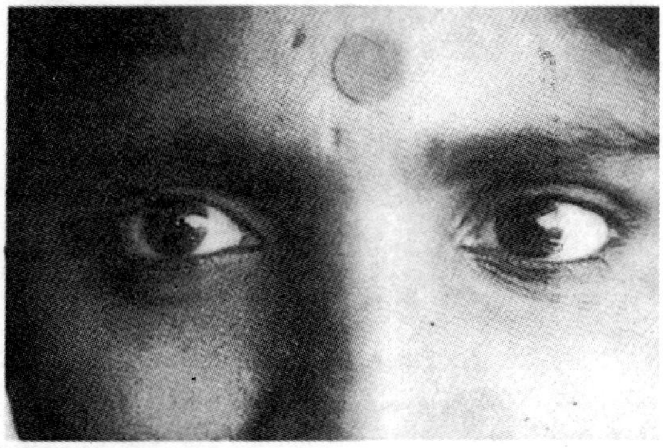

Pl. 15.2 a and b Ocular nerves

a) I I Ird nerve paralysis on (L) side resulting in ptosis, eyeball deviated to lateral aspect.
b) Lateral rectus palsy (L) eye - note that the eyeball is deviated to medial side. (Refer to text for details).

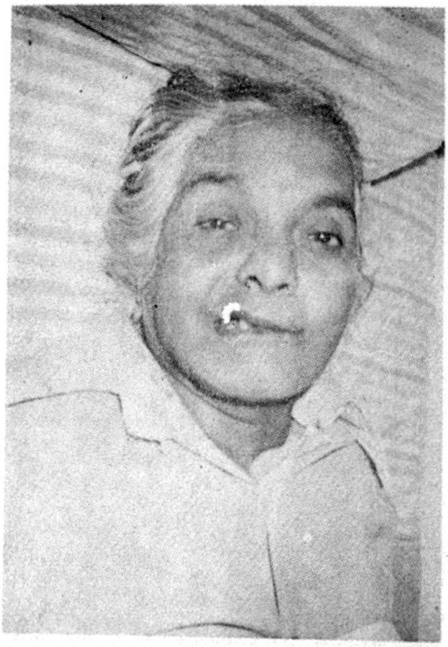

Pl. 15.3a Supranuclear facial palsy(L) side.
Note absence of naso labial fold.
Note presence of creases on forehead

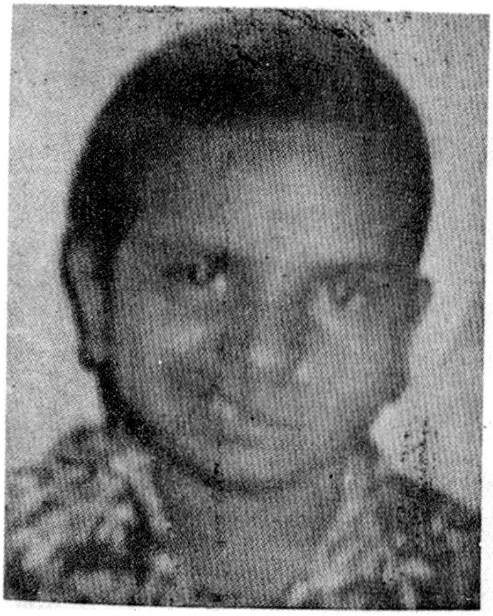

Pl. 15.3b Infranuclear facial palsy (L) side.
Note absence of labial fold.

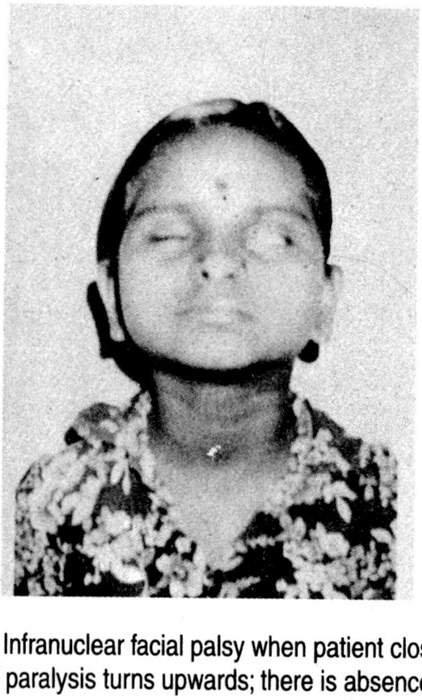

Pl. 15.3c Infranuclear facial palsy when patient closes eyes,
the eyeball on the side of paralysis turns upwards; there is absence of creases on forehead.

(Refer to text for details)

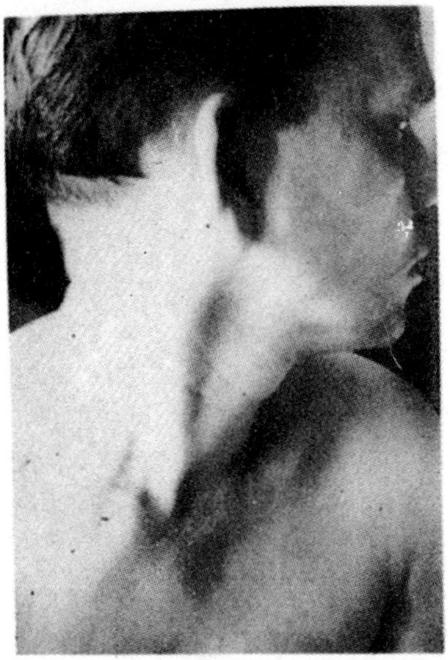

Pl.15.4a Sternomastoid - both the heads of sternomastoid are prominent when head is turned to opposite side.

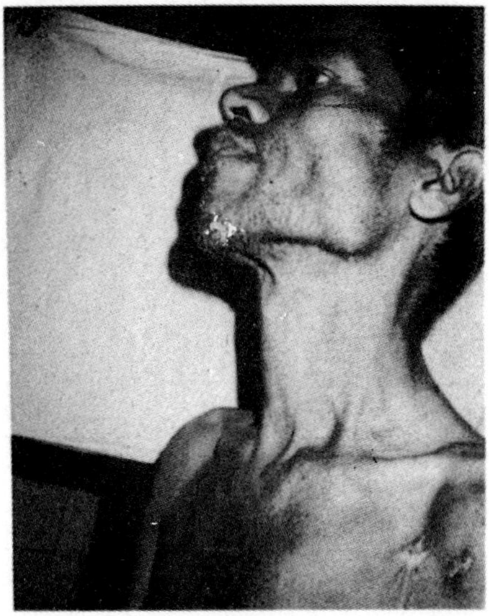

Pl.15.4b Wasting of sternomastoids.

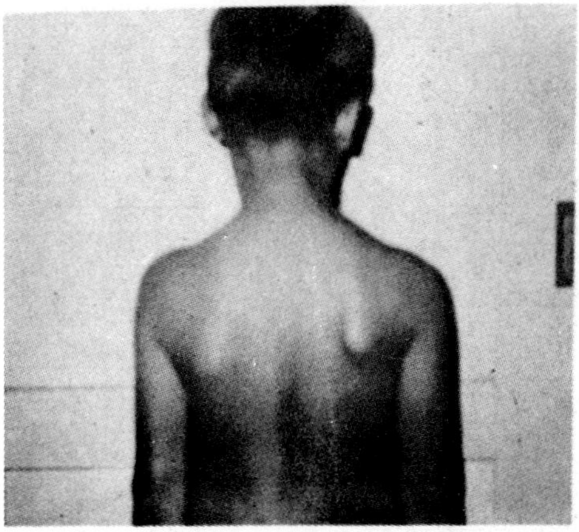

Pl.15.4c Trapezius - curvature of the neck is flattened on (L) side due to paralysis.

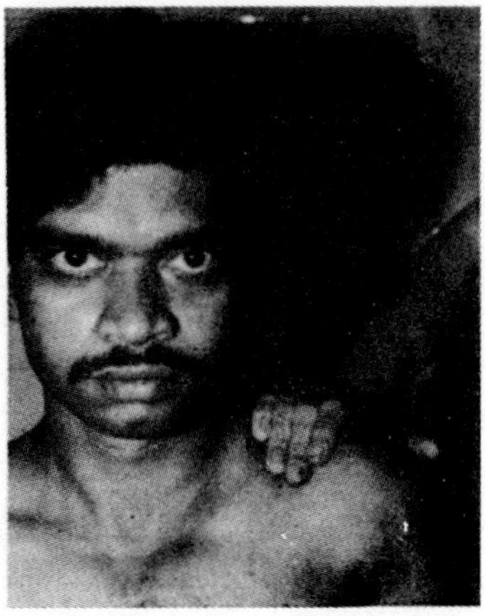

Pl. 15.4d Trapezius - Tested by asking patient to lift the shoulder against gravity and against resistance.

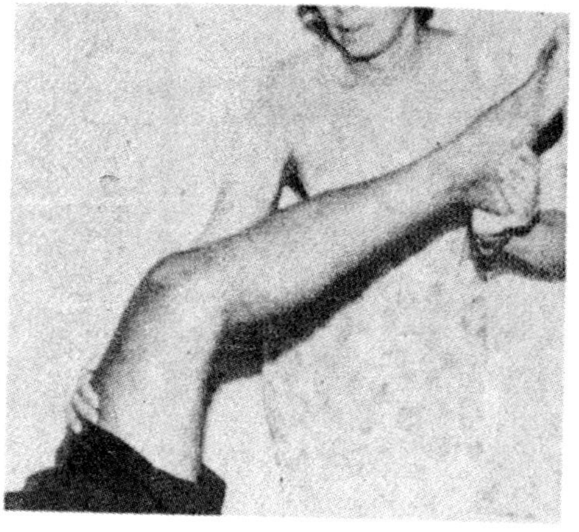

Pl. 15.5a Kernig's sign

Pl. 15.5b Brudzinski's neck sign
Note flexion of thighs and knees
on attempting flexion of neck
which is stiff.

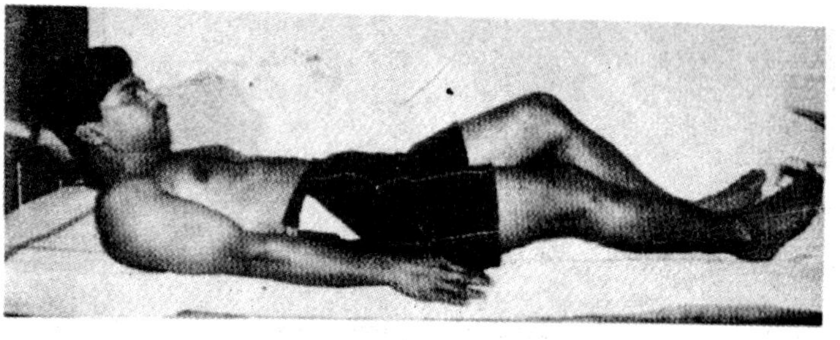

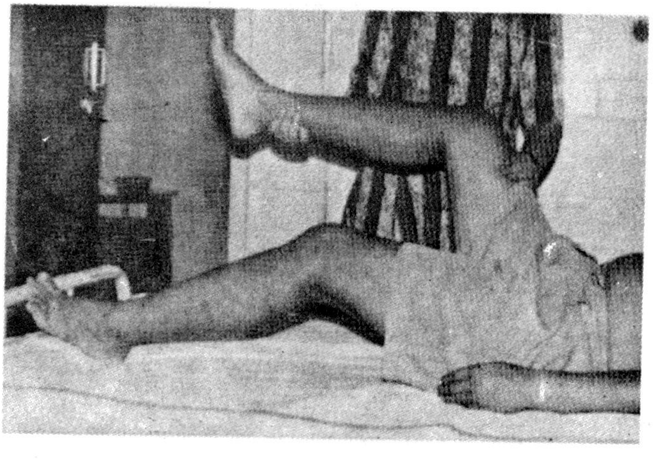

Pl. 15.5c Brudzinski's leg sign
Note the flexion of the other limb

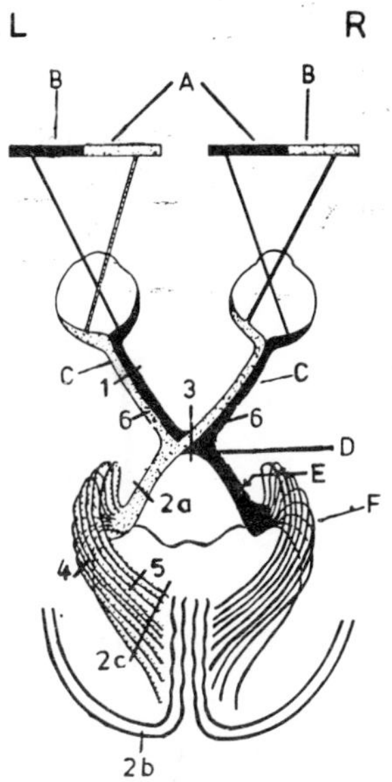

Fig. 15.2 (a)

Field of vision, the optic nerve and lesions at different sites leading to various abnormalities in field of vision.
A. Nasal field of vision. B. Temporal field of vision. C. Optic nerves. D. Optic chiasma. E. Optic tract. F. Optic radiation.
Note that fibres for temporal fields of vision cross while those for nasal fields of vision do not cross.

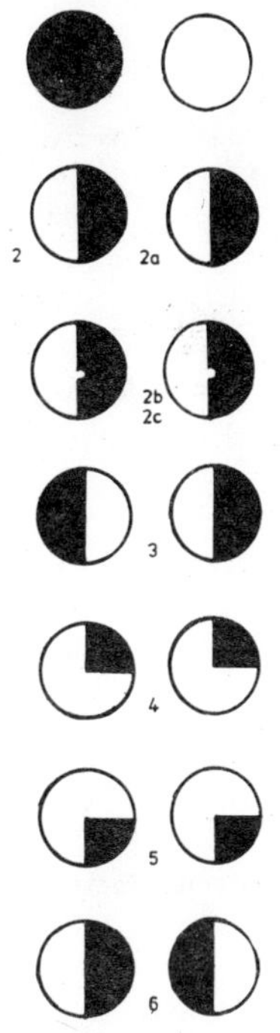

Fig. 15.2 (b)

Interpretation of defects of fields of vision.
Refer to Fig. 15.2 (a) for sites of lesion 1 to 6.

The common abnormalities of the field defects which are detected by this method of confrontation, due to neurological disorders are as follows:-

1. Complete blindness in one eye. Cause - Optic nerve lesion due to a. injury b. Retrobulbar neuritis c. Optic nerve compression.

2. Homonymous hemianopia (Commonest field defects). Cause - Lesions of optic tract, optic radiation fibres, or occipital cortex.
   a. If due to optic tract lesion - it is usually complete and incongruous without macular sparing.
   b. If due to lesion in optic radiation - it is usually incomplete and congruous with macular sparing.
   c. If the lesion is in the occipital cortex hemianopia is complete and congruous with macular sparing.
   WERNICKE's hemianopic pupillary reaction may be helpful to distinguish the site of the lesion as follows :
   If a light (slit lamp) is shone on the blind hall of the retina and the pupils react, the lesion must be either in optic radiation or occipital cortex.
   This is due to the fact that fibres for the light reflex travel in optic tract and not in optic radiation. Hence, when the lesion is in the optic tract there will be an absence of pupillary constriction after shining light on blind half of retina.
   Causes - Vascular accidents, cerebral tumours, vascular anomalies, injuries.

3. Bitemporal hemianopia due to lesions in optic chiasma - in its central portion (very common). Causes - Pituitary tumours. Craniopharyngioma. Supracellar meningioma. Hypothalamic neoplasms. Optic chiasma gliomas.

4. Superior quadrantic hemianopia - occurs in temporal lobe lesions, for inferior fibres of optic radiation which govern the superior field of vision and sweep around temporal horn of lateral ventricle.

5. Inferior quadrantic hemianopia occurs in parietal lobe lesion.

6. Binasal hemianopia - Very rare - Theoretically due to lateral portions of optic chiasma being involved - eg., i. Basal meningitis leading to local fibrosis. ii. More commonly due to local causes like glaucoma.

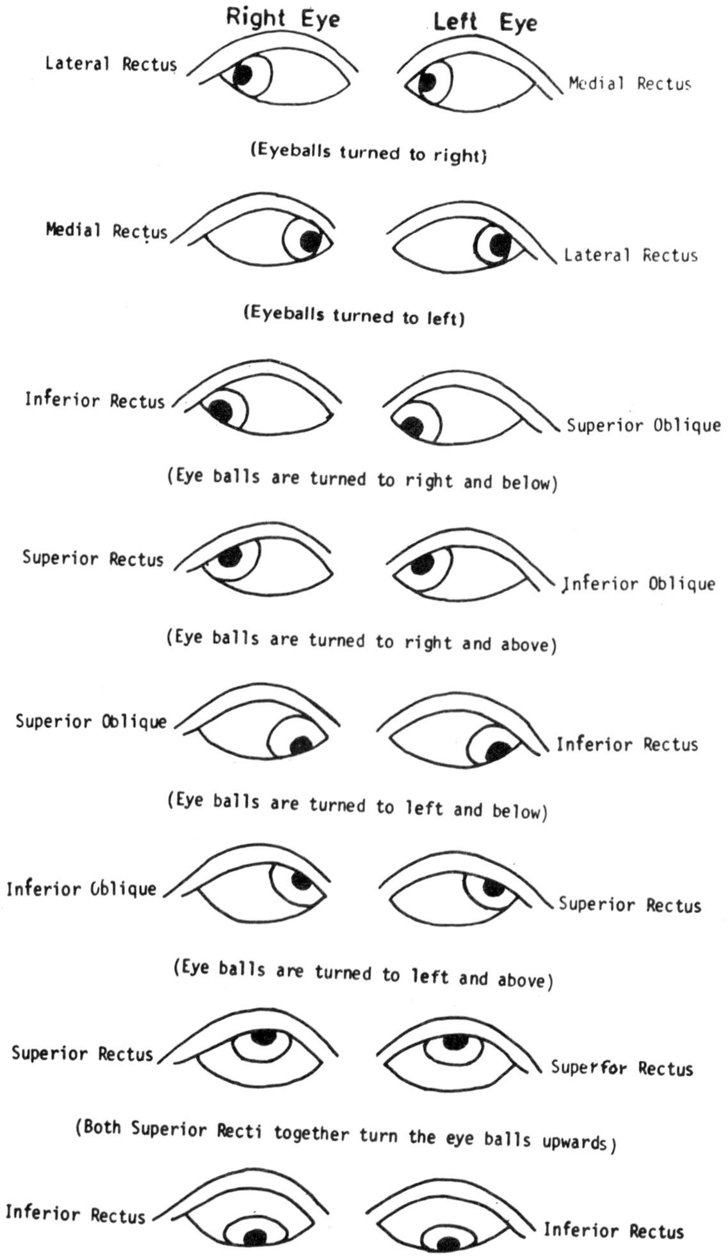

Fig. 15.3
Movements of eyeballs (Diagrammatic representation)

Lateral rectus is supplied by VI Cranial Nerve Abducens
Superior oblique is supplied by IV Cranial Nerve Trochlear
All other muscles are supplied by IIIrd Cranial Nerve Oculomotor

there will be a divergent squint due to the unopposed action of the lateral rectus muscle as shown in Fig. 15.4, the pupil also is dilated due to parasympathetic paralysis. (Pl. 15.2 (a) & (b))

In VIth nerve paralysis, there will be an internal squint. Squint is rare in IVth nerve paralysis.

In milder forms of cranial nerve palsies the squint will be evident only when the ocular movements are being tested. This is due to the weakness of the affected muscle causing lesser movement on one side.

Diplopia may be complained of by the patient during history-taking or it may be apparent when the external ocular movements are being tested. Two points should be remembered :

(a) The two images in diplopia will separate further if the eyeballs are moved in the direction of the paralysed muscle.

(b) The more peripheral image (false image) signifies the eye that is paralysed.

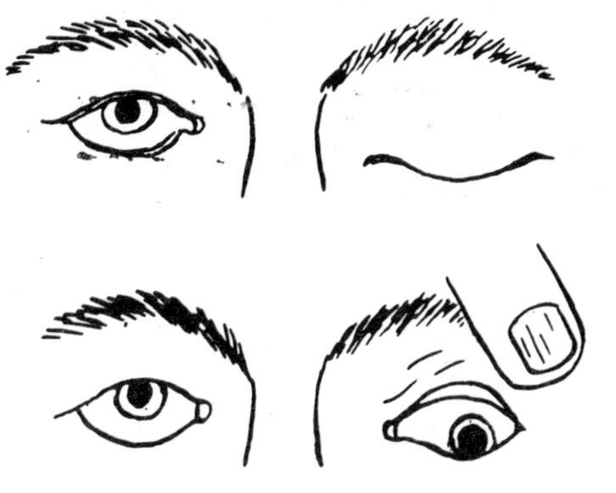

Fig. 15.4
IIIrd nerve paralysis of left eye
Note complete ptosis of left eye. On opening the upper eyelid passively, the pupil is deviated to lateral side due to pull of lateral rectus; it is dilated - because of paralysis of parasympathetic fibres and overaction of sympathetic fibres.

3. **Inspection and test of the pupils for reactions of light and accommodation :** In a normal person, the pupils are central, circular, equal and they react to light, accommodation and ciliospinal reflex.

(a) Pupil may be constricted (miosis) on one side pathologically due to sympathetic lesion as in Horner's syndrome. Horner's syndrome consists of miosis, ptosis, enothalmos, dryness and warmth on same half of the face. It is commonly due to lesions of the superior cervical ganglion (described in detail later).

(b) Mydriasis (dilated pupils) is due to paralysis of the parasympathetic fibres. These fibres arise in the Edinger-Westpal and the pretectal nuclei. They travel along with the IIIrd nerve and synapse at the ciliary ganglion in the orbit. Lesions of these fibres anywhere including their passage in the IIIrd nerve will cause a dilated pupil. Mydriasis is also commonly due to use of mydriatric, seen especially in nurses and medical students.

The light reflex (LR): In eliciting the LR the patient should be asked to look at a distant object in order to eliminate the contraction of pupil due to accommodation. The light reflex is elicited by directing a bright beam of light in one eye and noting the reaction of the pupil. (The other eye should be closed so that the pupil which is being tested does not contract due to consensual light reflex as a result of the effect of light on the other pupil.) The reaction of constriction should be brisk. Then, the examiner's hand should shield the light so that the rays shine only in one eye and the pupillary reaction in the other eye can be noted for the consensual reaction.

The accommodation reflex: This is conducted as follows :

The patient should be instructed to look at a distant object. Then, the examiner's finger should be suddenly placed very near the bridge of the nose (in mid line). This should result in constriction and convergence of the pupils.

Physiology of Light Refex and Accommodation Reflex

Pupillary Reactions:

(a) **Parasympathetic pathways:** to control irido-

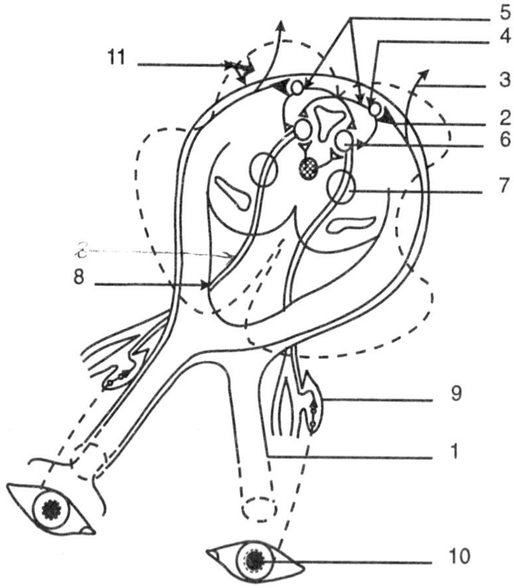

Fig 15.5
Showing parasympathetic pathways for pupillary constrictor muscles

1. Optic nerve,
2. Fibres for light reflex,
3. Fibres proceeding as optic radiation,
4. Edinger - Westpal nucleus (parasympathetic nucleus),
5. Fibres connecting both E-W nuclei (These account for consensual light-reflex),
6. Oculomotor nucleus,
7. Red nucleus,
8. Oculomotor nerve,
9. Ciliary ganglion,
10. Pupillary constrictor muscles.
11. Lateral geniculate body

constrictor fibres (ring like).

(b) **Sympathetic pathways:** to control radially arranged irido-dilator fibres.

(a) **Parasympathetic pathways:** (Fig. 15.5)

Impulses of light are conveyed by both optic nerves to both the lateral geniculate bodies. Few fibres after relay in lateral geniculate bodies end in both Elinger-Westpal nuclei (which are a part of oculomotor nucleus).

Edinger-Westpal nucleus is parasympathetic component of the IIIrd nerve. Fibres from this mucleus travel along with oculomotor nerve and relay in ciliary ganglion. Post-ganglionic fibres also travel with oculomotor nerve and supply the irido-constrictor muscles of iris.

Light reflex: When light is directed in one eye both pupils show constriction because fibres from lateral geniculate bodies end in both Edinger-Westpal nuclei. Damage to these fibres (from lateral geniculate bodies to Edinger-Westpal nucleus) leads to absence of light reflex.

Accommodation reflex: Edinger-Westpal nucleus is adjacent to IIIrd nerve mass which controls medial rectus muscle. So that when both these medial recti muscles are activated in an attempt to converge the eye, Edinger-Westpal nuclei become active and pupils constrict.

(b) **Sympathetic pathways:**

The sympathetic supply is ipsilateral. There are 3 neurons :

Ist - Hypothalamus to thoracic spinal cord.

2nd - From spinal cord to superior cervical ganglion.

3rd - From superior cervical ganglion to pupil.

Horner's Syndrome:

When the site of lesion is in the sympathetic pathway the result is Horner's syndrome.

i. Ptosis of eyelid of variable degree, but voluntary elevation of eyelid is preserved. Because smooth muscle fibres in upper eyelids are supplied by sympathetic nerves.

ii. Marked congestion of conjunctiva (because of loss of vasoconstrictor activity).

iii. Impaired or absent sweating over forehead because sympathetic fibres of blood vessels of face and sweat glands travel through superior cervical ganglion.

Abnormalities of pupils:

(a) **The Argyll Robertson pupils:** Classically these are small irregular pupils which do not react to light, but react to accommodation. They respond poorly to mydriatics and the size of the two pupils may differ.

Usual cause of this condition is syphilitic infection but it can occur in other mid-brain lesions like sclerosis or local tumours and also diabetes.

(b) **Holmes-Adie's syndrome:** Usually seen in young females as a dilated pupil on one side which does not react to light. However on testing for accommodation the pupil contracts slowly after initial delay and then it may become smaller than the normal pupil. The dilatation which brings it back to its original size is also very slow. It may be associated with absent knee and ankle reflexes. Usually it is asymptomatic, but the patient's complaint of sudden blurring of vision in one eye may draw attention to it.

(c) **Pupil reacting to light but not to accommodation reflex** (also called reversal of Argyll-Robertson pupil): This occurs in post-diphtheritic paralysis of accommodation and also occurs in brainstem lesions and in Parkinsonism.

(d) **Hippus :** Alternate contraction and dilatation of the pupil after light reflex is rarely seen. This is seen in patients suffering from chorea, meningitis or multiple sclerosis. It is quite common in normal healthy individuals.

4. To detect and analyse nystagmus:

Test: The patient is asked to look at a fixed point (the examiner's finger) which then should be gradually moved outwards, inwards and downwards. In outward movement, the eyelids should be raised to note the nystagmus properly.

Nystagmus will be seen as a to-and-fro movement of the eyeballs. It can be horizontal (most common) or vertical according to the direction of its movement. It can either be of the pendular variety in which case both the to-and- fro movements are equal or jerky with a slow and rapid component, and it can be rotatory, when a short to-and-fro rotation of the eyeball is seen.

Causes :

(a) **Pendular nystagmus:**

Due to visual defects from childhood, Albinism and miner's nystagmus(due to working in poor illumination).

(b) **Jerky nystagmus:**

i. Disturbances of vestibular system like Meniere's disease (usually accompanied by vertigo), acoustic neuroma, upper cervical cord lesions.

ii. **Vertical nystagmus (nystagmus in which the movements are up and down):**

Due to brainstem vascular lesions, multiple sclerosis, syringobulbia, Arnold chiari malformation and encephalitis.

iii. **Rotatory nystagmus:**

Labyrinthine diseases, brainstem lesions.

The Vth cranial nerve - (trigeminal):

Functions : Sensory: To carry all modalities of sensations from the anterior part of the scalp and the eye. To carry the general sensations like touch, pain, temperature but not taste, from the anterior two-thirds of the tongue.

Tests: Touch, pain and temperature should be tested over the areas supplied by the three divisions of this nerve.

The areas should be forehead and upper part of the side of nose (for the ophthalmic division). The upper lip and the malar region should be tested for the maxillary division. The anterior part of the tongue and the chin should be tested for the mandibular division. (Fig. 15.6)

The special points to be remembered about the distribution of this nerve (sensory) are that it supplies the anterior upper pinna. The areas supplied by it and the second cervical segment meet a little posterior to the vertex.

The skin over the angle of the jaw is not supplied by this nerve. It is supplied by the cervical nerves.

The abnormal findings and their causes:

(a) Total sensory loss of all the three divisions

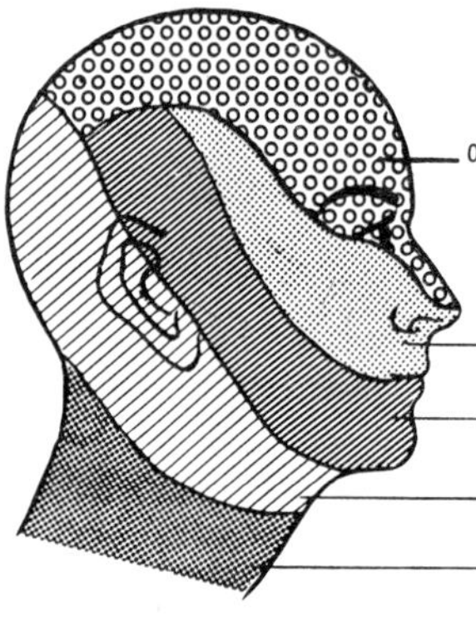

Fig. 15.6
Cutaneous supply of trigeminal nerve (V)
Note that CI has NO cutaneous distribution

of the nerve will indicate a lesion of the ganglion or sensory root.

Causes: Tumours eroding the base of the skull, chronic basal meningitis (tuberculosis, sarcoid) or injuries to the base of the skull. Partial lesions of the ganglion: herpes zoster, partial lesions of the root, acoustic neuroma causing compression.

(b) There may be a sensory loss of only one or two divisions of this nerve.

Ophthalmic division: 1. Compression by carotid aneurysm in the cavernous sinus or 2. By local tumours of facial bone in orbital fissure.

All the sensations may not be lost but there may be a loss of only pain and temperature sensations. This dissociated sensory loss is usually due to syringobulbia in foramen magnum anomalies. It is present on one side of the face and on the opposite side of the body in posterior inferior cerebellar artery thrombosis.

Loss of touch sensation along with the other sensations preserved is a feature of lesion in the pons affecting the principal sensory nucleus. Lesions are usually vascular but can be neoplastic. Rarely hyperaesthesia is the clinical abnormality and it is found in herpes zoster.

Corneal reflex: Described under superficial reflexes (also tested for Vth nerve).

Motor Functions: Muscles supplied by the Vth nerve are: masseters, pterygoids, temporalis, tensor tympani.

Masseters, pterygoids and the temporal muscles are tested as follows : The patient is asked to clench his jaw and the muscles, masseters and temporalis are palpated and compared. The medial pterygoids are tested by asking the patient to open his jaw. In case of weakness on one side, the jaw will be pushed toward the paralysed side.

The lateral pterygoids should be tested by asking the patient to move the jaw from side-to-side.

Causes: A lower motor neuron lesion as seen in motor neuron disease or myopathies leads to wasting of temporalis and masseter muscles.

VIIth Cranial Nerve: (Facial nerve)
Functions:

1. Motor innervation of the muscles of the face which control emotional and facial movements.
2. Supplies the platysma and stapedius.
3. Carries the sensation of taste from the anterior two-thirds of the tongue.

Method of examination: Even before specific examination, the patient's face should be observed and the following points should be noted :

1. The wrinkles on the forehead and the nasolabial folds.
2. The movements of the mouth on talking and smiling.
3. The presence of blinking should be noted and whether the eyeballs turn up with every blink.

Tests: The movements can be tested as follows by asking the patient

1. to raise the eyebrows,
2. to frown,
3. to shut his eyes tight and asking him to screw the eyeballs and to resist opening them,
4. to show his teeth,

5. to smile and open the jaw at the same time (which movement will make the platysma stand out).

A practical point which should be remembered is that instead of trying to explain verbally to the patient which action is desired, it is better to show him what is expected of him and then ask him to mimic it.

Taste on the anterior 2/3rds of the tongue should be examined by putting a drop of solution of the four primary tastes: sweet, salty, sour and bitter (sugar, salt, citric acid and quinine).

In between tests for taste the mouth should be cleaned by water.

Interpretation of facial paralysis:

1. Upper motor neuron (UMN) palsy
2. Lower motor neuron (LMN) palsy
3. Emotional facial palsy
4. Bilateral facial (UMN) or (LMN) palsy.

(1) In upper motor neuron (supranuclear) facial palsy, only the lower half of face is affected. The angle of the mouth is not raised and the nasolabial furrow does not deepen. The closure of eyes due to contraction of the orbicularis oculi, the creasing of the forehead and frowning are preserved. Emotional movements are preserved. Lesion is in cerebral cortex downwards up to the facial nucleus in the pons. (Fig. 15.7)

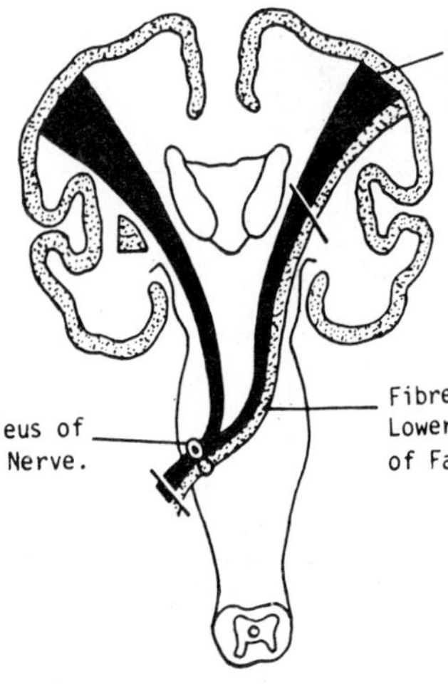

Fig. 15.7
Supranuclear connections of facial motor nucleus

Fibres to upper pan of the face - Note the bilateral innervation.

Fibres to lower part of the face - Note the unilateral innervation.

Nucleus of VII nerve. Any lesion at VII nerve nucleus or distal to it leads to lower motor neuron facial palsy.

(2) In lower motor neuron (infranuclear) facial palsy the wrinkling of the forehead and blinking of eyes is absent. The eyeball turns upwards on the affected side when the patient tries to close his eyes. The angle of the mouth cannot be raised and the nasolabial furrow remains obliterated. (Pl 15.3(a) & (c))

Lesion is in the course of facial nerve from the nucleus downwards. To localise the lesion in the course of facial nerve when the paralysis is affecting the whole face, a brief knowledge of the course of facial nerve is essential.

The nucleus of the VIIth nerve is situated in the pons and it is anterior and lateral to the VIth nucleus. The fibres of the facial nerve after their origin from the nucleus hook around the VIth nerve nucleus. Then they leave the pons and enter the internal auditory meatus with the auditory nerve. At the anterior boundary of the vestibule of the inner ear the nerve bends sharply forward and downwards. Geniculate ganglion lies at this angle. Then it enters the facial canal. Immediately distal to the geniculate ganglion it gives off the greater superficial petrosal nerve to the sphenopalatine ganglion and then the nerve to the stapedius. After this, it is joined by the nerve-chorda tympani. The nerve then emerges from the stylomastoid foramen. (Fig. 15.8)

Lesions at different levels (Fig. 15.9): For the sake of convenience the lesions are described from

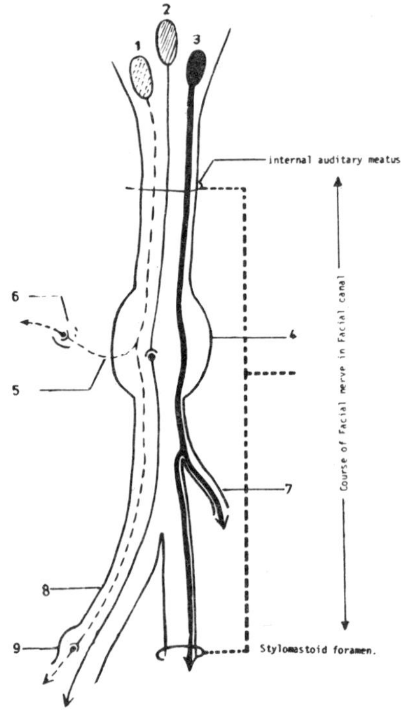

Fig. 15.8

Facial Nerve : Its various nuclei and diagrammatic representation of the course of (Facial nerve from the internal auditory meatus to stylomastoid foramen.)

1. **Superior salivary nucleus** (Parasympathetic nucleus).
2. **Sensory nucleus** — gustatory nucleus solitarius which receives sensations of taste from anterior 2/3rds of tongue
3. **Motor nucleus.**
4. **Geniculate ganglion** — Note that gustatory fibres synapse in this ganglion.
5. **Greater superficial petrosal nerve** carrying with it few parasympathetic fibres for lacrimal gland.
6. **Sphenopalatine ganglion** — Parasympathetic fibres relay here.
7. **Nerve to stapedius** — emerges soon after geniculate ganglion,
8. **Chorda tympani nerve** is given off soon after nerve to stapedius is given off. Parasympathetic fibres which supply salivary glands are carried by this nerve; so also afferent gustatory impulses from anterior 2/3rd of tongue travel via this nerve.
9. **Submandibular ganglion** - the parasympathetic fibres synapse here.

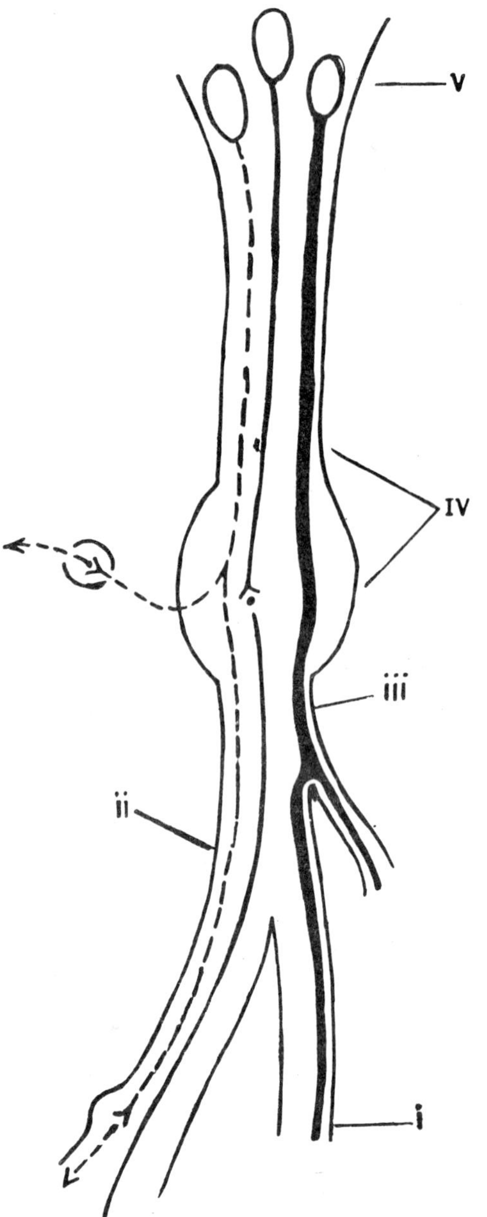

Fig. 15.9

Lesions of facial nerve at different sites.
Refer to text for i to v. Refer to Fig. 15.8 for various branches of facial nerve and their various levels.

distal to proximal part of the nerve. Refer to Fig. 15.9 for lesions I to V.

(i) Lesion at the stylomastoid foramen (Bell's palsy):

(a) Facial paralysis affecting all the facial-muscles on that side.

(b) Taste of anterior two-thirds of the tongue not impaired.

(ii) Lesion in the facial canal above the junction of the chords tympani but below the geniculate ganglion and nerve to stapedius:

(a) Complete facial paralysis.

(b) Loss of taste over anterior two-thirds of the tongue.

(iii) Lesion below the geniculate ganglion and above the nerve to stapedius:

(a) Complete facial paralysis.

(b) Loss of taste.

(c) Hyperacusis.

(iv) Lesion at the geniculate ganglion or proximal to it:

(a) Complete facial paralysis.

(b) Absent lacrimation.

(c) Salivation and taste also affected.

(d) May affect the auditory nerve.

(v) Lesion in the pons:

(a) Complete facial paralysis.

(b) Vlth nerve paralysis.

3. **Emotional facial palsy:** Weakness of the face (UMN) as manifested by deviation of the angle of the mouth is present only on smiling but is absent on voluntary movements (lesions in the thalamus).

4. **Bilateral facial palsy:** i. Pseudobulbar palsy is due to bilateral U.M. lesion. ii. Bilateral lower motor neuron palsy (Bulbar palsy) e.g., leprosy, 2. infective polyneuritis, 3. myasthenia gravis and muscular dystrophies.

The VIIIth Cranial (Auditory nerve):

Functions: It has two main divisions:

(a) The cochlear,

(b) The vestibular.

(a) The cochlear part carries the sound from the receptor end organs to the cochlear nuclei the medulla. The fibres are relayed to the superior temporal gyrus.

(b) The vestibular part: The labyrinthine impulses are carried first to the vestibular ganglia and then to the cerebellum and are connected to oculomotor nuclei, the temporal lobes, the nuclei of the upper cervical nerves and the spinal cord.

Method of examination of cochlear division:

Hearing is tested commonly by closing one ear and whispering in the patient's other ear. The whisper can be replaced by the ticking of wrist watch. Tuning fork with vibration of 256/sec can also be used. If the patient is unable to hear on one side, then the following two tests are employed to determine whether the lesion is in the nerve or in the middle ear (bone).

Rinne's test: A tuning fork is struck gently and the patient is asked to hear the sound. Then it is placed on the mastoid process and the patient is asked to state the precise moment when he stops feeling the vibrations. Then the fork is brought immediately near the meatus. Normally it should be heard.

In nerve deafness both air and bone conduction will be diminished as compared to the normal ear but the air conduction remains better than the bone conduction. In the middle ear disease, bone conduction will be better than air conduction.

Rinne's positive is the normal response and Rinne's negative means middle ear deafness.

Weber's test: A tuning fork is placed in the centre of the forehead. The patient should be asked whether the sound is better heard in one of the ears or in mid-line of the head. In bone (middle ear) deafness, it is better heard on the abnormal (affected) side, while in nerve deafness and in normal cases it is heard in the midline.

Audiometry is the test performed for quantitative measurement of the loss of hearing.

Method of examination of vestibular division:

The three tests commonly advised are usually beyond the routine of a neurological examination.

Symptoms of vertigo and the presence of nystagmus may be the only clues at the time of the usual interview.

The common tests used to test the vestibular function are:

1. The Rothmal tests.
2. The caloric tests.

Both will produce, nystagmus and giddiness by vestibular irritation and the presence and duration of these symptoms are taken into consideration in the interpretation of the results.

IXth Glossopharyngeal, Xth Vagus, XIth Cranial accessory nerves:

Functions: (i) To carry sensory impulses from the pharynx, tonsils, soft palate and posterior 1/3rd of the tongue. (ii) To carry the sensation of taste from the posterior 1/3rd of the tongue, (iii) Motor innervation of the palate and pharynx and the larynx.

Tests: 1. The patient's voice is noted. 2. A nasal twang suggests palatal paralysis and a hoarse voice suggests vocal cord involvement. 3. The palatal movements are tested as follows :

The patient is asked to open the mouth and say "Ah"; normally the uvula should remain in the midline with palate arching symmetrically.

If the uvula is deviated to one side there is a paralysis of the palate on the opposite side, because the uvula is pulled by the normal muscles to the normal side.

If there is no movement of palate and pharynx, it is due to bilateral nuclear medullary lesion or a bilateral upper motor neuron lesion (pseudobulbar palsy). In these cases the paralysis is accompanied by dysphagia, nasal regurgitation and nasal speech.

Unilateral or bilateral nuclear involvement can occur in bulbar polio — Gag reflex (given below) is absent in these cases.

Gag reflex:

It is tested by a throat swab being used to irritate one side of the back of the throat. This should result in contraction of the pharynx, elevation of the palate with retraction of the tongue.

IX-X nerve lesion is usually the cause of the loss of gag reflex.

Taste: Posterior 1/3rd of the tongue is examined for taste. It is a very difficult procedure as it is impossible to avoid anterior 2/3rd of the tongue.

Examination of vocal cords: Usually not carried out at bedside clinical neurological examination.

The spinal XI : Spinal accessory nerve:

Function : Motor supply to the sternomastoids and the trapezium. (PI 15.4 (a), (b), (c) & (d))

Test: Sternomastoids, i.e., head falling backwards or forwards shows severe bilateral weakness. Sternomastoid is tested as follows: The examiner's hand is kept on one side of the face and the patient is asked to turn his head towards it. The other sternomastoid normally becomes prominent. Both the sides should be tested one after the other, the size of muscles on both the sides is compared and the power assessed. Easier way of comparing the size is by keeping the hand on the forehead and by comparing both the sternomastoids.

Bilateral sternomastoid weakness which is not severe is easily noticed by asking the patient to sit up from supine position. The head will typically lag behind. The platysma may stand out during this procedure.

Trapezius (spinal accessory and $C_{3,4}$) is tested as follows :

The curve of the trapezium is checked from the back. Then the patient is asked to lift up his shoulders (as in shrugging) and this action should be opposed by the examiner for testing the power.

Bilateral trapezius and/or sternomastoid paralysis is seen in motor neuron disease and polyneurtis. It is also commonly seen in muscular dystrophy and in motor neuron disease.

Unilateral asymmetrical weakness is common in poliomyelitis.

The XIIth (hypoglossal) nerve:

Functions: Motor movements of the tongue.

Tests: 1. Surface, size and position of the tongue should be noted. 2. The patient is asked to protrude his tongue out. 3. The power of the muscles on each side of the tongue can be tested by asking the patient to press the cheek from inside and testing its thrust from outside.

In unilateral lower motor neuron lesion, there is wasting of the tongue on that side with exaggeration of the longitudinal folds. On protrusion the tongue deviates towards the paralysed side. Fasciculation may be observed on the affected side.

In bilateral lower motor neuron lesions, the tongue is atrophied and the protrusion is difficult. Speech is greatly impaired. In nuclear lesions, there is marked fasciculation (bulbar palsy as in motor neuron disease).

In upper motor neuron lesion (pseudo-bulbar palsy) the tongue will be small and protrusion will be difficult but there will be no atrophy or fasciculation. The jaw jerk may be exaggerated. Motor neuron disease is the only disease wherein the features of both upper and lower motor weakness are combined.

III. Motor System:

The examination of the motor system is indicated into:

1. Nutrition of the muscles,
2. Tone,
3. Power,
4. Co-ordination,
5. Involuntary movements.

This scheme should be strictly adhered to and the normal and abnormal findings should be carefully noted.

1. Nutrition of the muscles:

Before testing in detail, a general inspection of the musculature of the body should be carried out not only in lying down position, but if possible in both sitting as well as standing positions.

Any obvious deformity will easily be seen by this inspection and both congenital deformities and deformities caused by bone and joint diseases should be noted.

Then the patient should be examined in a systematic way to determine whether there is any wasting or hypertrophy.

The best method to follow will be inspection of the face, shoulder girdles, arms, hands, hip girdles, legs and feet. The muscles should be checked for atrophy, hypertrophy and fasciculations.

If there is any asymmetry the muscles should be measured on both sides by noting the circumference of the limb at an equal distance from a fixed bony symmetrical point on both sides (i.e., for calf muscles, 5 centimetres below the anterior tibial tubercle).

The muscles should be palpated for determining their consistency: either firmness or flabbiness.

Fasciculations, if present should be observed and the muscles in which they are present should be noted. Fasciculations indicate a chronic degeneration of the anterior horn cells or motor neuron supplying the muscles and is very helpful in localising the site of the lesion. It is a usual feature of motor neuron disease. It is also seen rarely in syringomyelia, cervical spondylosis, thyrotoxic myopathy, peroneal muscular atrophy.

If wasting is present it can be classified as follows:

A. Generalised muscular wasting:

(a) Seen in advanced motor neuron disease (with fasciculation and brisk deep reflexes).

(b) Myopathies (diminished reflexes and no fasciculation).

(c) Spinal muscular atrophy (with fasciculation and diminished reflexes).

B. Wasting mainly of proximal muscles:

(a) Facio-scapulo humeral dystrophy. The name of the disease itself suggests the muscles which are wasted. The wasting may be asymmetrical.

(b) Limb/girdle atrophy: Both the shoulder girdle and the hip girdle muscles are atrophied.

(c) Myotonia dystrophica: Facial muscles, sternomastoids and quadriceps are mainly involved.

(d) Pseudo-hypertrophic muscular dystrophy: Calves and hip girdles are predominantly affected. Pseudo-hypertrophy of calves is the most common feature. The arms are also involved showing either atrophy or hypertrophy. Mainly a disease of males and there may be pseudo-hypertrophy of deltoids also.

(e) Syringomyelia: Usually atrophy of the shoulder girdle with dissociated sensory loss over the face and the 'jacket area' on the thorax. (Fig. 15.10)

(f) Compression of the cervical cord: If the 4th and 5th cervical segments are compressed there will be a wasting of the muscles of shoulder girdle.

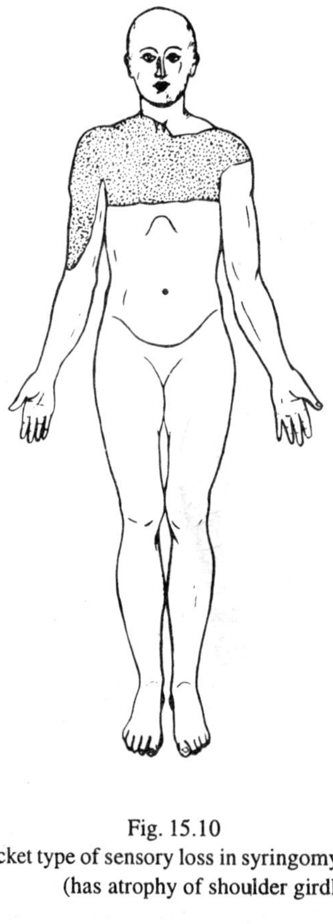

Fig. 15.10
Jacket type of sensory loss in syringomyelia (has atrophy of shoulder girdle).

Similarly, in cauda equina lesions, if the corresponding roots are compressed then the gluteal muscles will show atrophy.

C. Wasting of distal muscles in upper and/or lower extremities:

In the upper extremity the following are the causes of the wasting of small muscles of the hand and the forearm. The roots involved are C_7 T_1.

A. Anterior horn cells at this level may be affected :

(a) Motor neuron disease,
(b) Syringomyelia,
(c) Cervical cord compression,
(d) Poliomyelitis.

B. The motor root:
(a) Cervical spondylosis,
(b) Cervical cord tumours.

C. The brachial plexus:
(a) Due to injury,
(b) Cervical rib — compressing the brachial plexus.

D. Trauma or infection (leprosy) — affecting the peripheral nerves.

In the lower extremities the peripheral muscles are wasted due to

A. Cauda equina lesions (motor root)
B. Polyneuritis (peripheral nerves)
C. Peroneal muscular atrophy (muscle)

Peripheral wasting in both upper and lower extremities is seen mainly in chronic peripheral neuritis (alcoholic, diabetic or vitamin deficiency being the main causes) and in peroneal muscular atrophy.

2. **Tone:** Various definitions and descriptions of tone are available, but the simplest clinical description would be 'the slight resistance that a normal healthy muscle offers to passive movement'.

Tone depends on: The local reflex arc, and its higher control.

The local reflex arc comprises of the muscle

spindles, the afferent fibres arising from them and ending in posterior horn cells. (Fig. 15. 11)

From posterior horn cells, the impulses are carried by internuncial neuronal fibres to anterior horn cells. The neurons (in anterior horn cells) concerned are gamma neurons (small) and alpha neurons (big). Gamma neurons are under the control of MRS (medial reticulo spinal tracts) and LRS (lateral reticulo spinal tracts). These tracts have facilitatory influence on gamma neurons. Alpha neurons are under the control of pyramidal tracts; these tracts have inhibitory influence on alpha neurons.

Normal tone is a state of resistance which the examiner can learn only by experience.

The abnormalities of tone are either increase of tone or decrease or loss of tone.

Increase of tone: The two main varieties are: A. Spasticity. B. Rigidity.

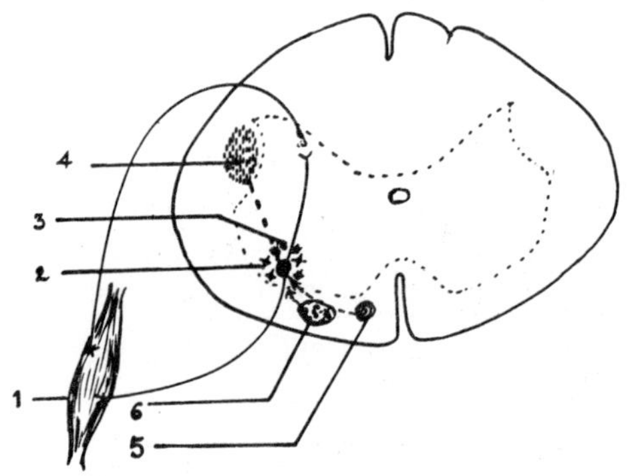

Fig. 15.11

Reflex Arc to maintain tone of muscles and connection with various tracts

1. Muscle spindle
2. (Big) Alpha neurons
3. (Small) Gamma neurons
4. Lateral cortico spinal tract
5. Medial reticulo spinal tract (MRS)
6. Lateral reticulo spinal tract (LRS)

Note that cortico spinal tracts control alpha neurons while lateral and medial reticulo spinal tracts control gamma neurons. These alpha and gamma neurons are connected with internuncial neurons in posterior horn cells.

A. **Spasticity:** When the examiner tries to move the limb in a particular way initially there is resistance and then there is a sudden overcoming of this resistance. This is described as clasp knife spasticity. This is usually more marked in the flexors of the upper limb and the extensors of the lower limbs. It is believed to be because of extra pyramidal overaction.

B. **Rigidity:** The resistance offered to passive movement is uniform in both the opposing group of muscles and is present throughout the range of movement.

It is also known as lead pipe rigidity. The other variant of the disorder is cog wheel rigidity. It is present when there are tremors in the limb which is being tested.

The cause of both the lead pipe and cog wheel rigidity is lesion in extra-pyramidal system.

Loss of tone: There is no resistance or very marked diminution in the resistance offered to passive movements and hence movements beyond the normal range are possible.

Common causes of this condition are : (A) A lesion of the local reflex arc. (B) Cerebellar disease, as cerebellum controls tone through proprioceptive impulses. (C) Neural shock.

(A) **A lesion of local Reflex Arc:** can be of

(a) Motor component.

i. Anterior horn cells: poliomyelitis, motorneuron disease.

ii. Motor nerves : peripheral neuropathy, nerve injury, nerve infection as in leprosy and polyneuritis.

(b) **Muscles:** myopathies, myasthenia gravis.

(c) **Sensory component:** tabes dorsalis, herpes zoster, sensory neuropathy.

In disease like syringomyelia or cord compression both the motor and sensory components will be affected.

B. **In cerebellar diseases:** There is a hypotonia on the same side associated with incoordination and pendular reflexes.

C. **In neural shock:** There is a temporary hypotonia which is later on replaced by the signs of pyramidal damage.

In meningitis there is an increased tone or rigidity which is of diagnostic value. This rigidity is protective by nature in the sense that the irritation of the meninges is minimised by preventing movements which may stretch the nerve roots coming out of the meninges.

Following signs which are diagnostic of meningeal irritation are based on the above principles.

Neck rigidity: This is evident when the examiner tries to flex the head passively. There is a spasm of extensors of the neck which prevents the flexion of the neck. The chin cannot be approximated to the chest and the patient's upper body may be lifted as a rigid single piece.

Kernig's sign: The thigh of the patient is flexed over abdomen and knee also is flexed. The knee joint is then extended slowly by holding the leg. When this sign is positive, extension of the knee is limited by spasm of the hamstring muscles and is accompanied by pain. (Pl 15.5 a,b and c)

Brudzinski's neck sign: When the neck is flexed while testing for neck rigidity, there is flexion of the hip and the knee.

Brudzinski's leg sign: The thigh is flexed over the abdomen with knee already flexed. When the knee is extended passively as in Kernig's sign, the other lower limb shows flexion at hip and knee.

Straight leg raising sign (Laseque's sign): When the patient's leg is raised passively by flexing the hip, normally it (extended leg) can be raised easily, practically and vertically. In meningeal irritation, there is pain and limitation of this movement.

3. **Examination of power:** This should be carried out in a systematic manner by testing the movements of muscles at every joint. Individual muscles or the groups of muscles should be tested depending on the need.

The muscles can be tested in either of the two ways:

(A) By asking the patient to perform a movement and then the examiner should resist the same throughout its performance. It is usually necessary to demonstrate to the patient what exactly he is supposed to do, i.e., if the flexors of the elbow are being tested then the examiner should demonstrate to him the same action passively at first or show it to him by putting his own limb through the same action.

(B) The patient is asked to complete the movement and retain the same position against the resistance applied by the examiner.

The power tested accordingly is then graded as follows :

Grade 0: No movement of the muscle at all and no flicker also.

Grade 1: Slight flicker of movement but no movement of the limb.

Grade 2: The patient can move the limb with gravity eliminated but not against it (i.e., in horizontal plane).

Grade 3: The patient is able to move the limb against gravity but not against resistance.

Grade 4: The patient is able to move the limb against gravity and against resistance, but not to the fullest extent.

Grade 5: Normal power.

Types of muscular weakness: (Fig. 15.12)

(A) due to upper motor neuron lesion,

(B) due to lower motor neuron lesion.

(A) **Due to upper motor neuron lesion:** Lesions of the upper motor neuron usually produce weakness of movements rather than that of individual muscles. In the upper extremity the abductors and the extensors are the most affected. The finer movements of the fingers and the movements of the thumb suffer the most in upper motor neuron lesions and recover the last if at all.

Similarly the dorsiflexors are the worst affected

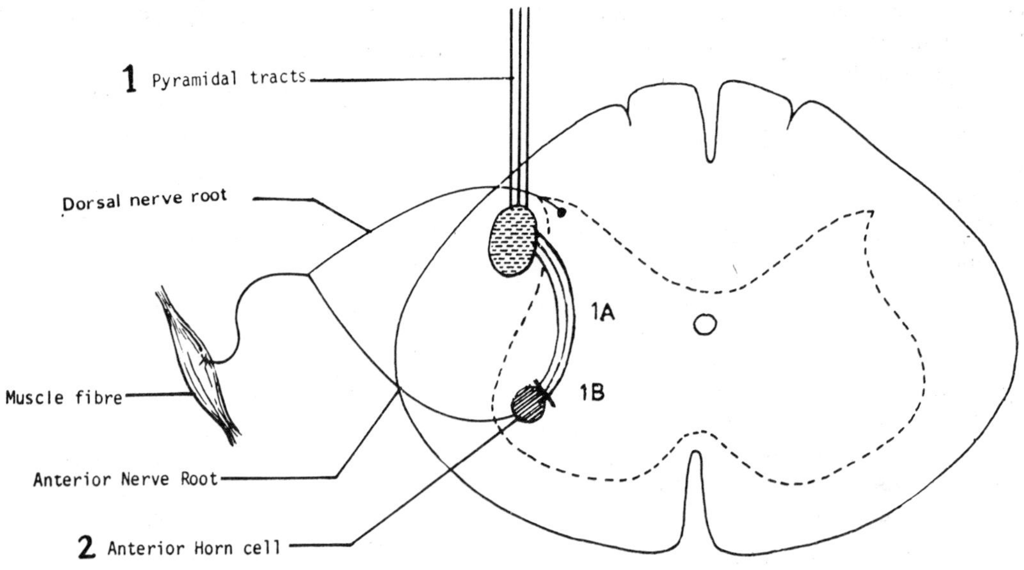

Fig. 15.12
Demarcation of upper motor neuron - lower motor neuron
1A. Part of pyramidal fibres which end in anterior horn cells
1 B. Exact site where the fibres end in anterior horn cells
Lesions anywhere up to 1B is upper motor neuron
Lesions anywhere from 2 onwards is lower motor neuron.

in the lower extremities and they are also the last to recover. The lesion may be anywhere from motor cortex in cortico-spinal tracts up to anterior horn cells (anterior horn cell not included).

(B) **Due to lower motor neuron lesion:** This produces severe individual muscle weakness with wasting. The paralysis is localised to the segments which are affected in cord or motor root lesions and may be bilaterally symmetrical in peripheral neuropathy. The lesion can be anywhere from anterior horn cells up to the muscles which are innervated.

The main differences in these two types of weakness are as follows:

Upper motor neuron paralysis	Lower motor neuron paralysis
i. Paralysis of movements	i. Paralysis of individual muscle.

Muscles groups affected.	
ii. No atrophy (only slight disuse atrophy may be seen).	ii. Marked atrophy of the muscles.
iii. Spasticity.	iii. Hypotonia.
iv. Exaggerated deep reflexes.	iv. Loss of deep reflexes.
v. Extensor plantar reflex.	v. Absent or normal plantar reflex.
vi. Fasciculations absent.	vi. Fasciculations may be present.

C. **Myastbenic weakness:** Myasthenic weakness is typically seen in myasthenia gravis. Here the severity of weakness may vary from time to time but always increases with repeated use of the muscle and may progress to total paralysis. A period of rest, even short, will restore it to its normal state.

Tests for individual muscles and groups of muscles:

The important muscles and groups of muscles whose weakness is encountered in routine neurological practice are described here.

While testing the action it is necessary to palpate the muscles to feel for their contraction. (Pl 15.6 to 15.13)

1. Supraspinatus (Suprascapular C_5):

Action abduction of the arm from the side up to 30^0. Tested by applying resistance to abduction when arm lies near body.

2. Deltoid (Circumflex $C_{5,6}$) forms round curvature of the shoulder :

i. Action tested by applying resistance after initial abduction.

ii. When the elbow is flexed, the hand rests on iliac crest and

(a) the arm is brought forwards against resistance. Muscles acting are deltoid (anterior fibres) and pectoralis major; the action is medial rotation and flexion at shoulder,

(b) when the arm is brought backwards against resistance, muscles acting are deltoid (posterior fibres), latissimus dorsi and teres major. The action is lateral rotation and extension at shoulder.

Wasting of deltoid causes flattening of shoulder (squaring of shoulder).

3. Pectoralis major: Lateral and medial pectoral nerves. ($C_{5,6,7,8}T_1$)

i. forms anterior axillary fold,

ii. Medial rotation and flexion as above.

iii. Abduction: Raise arm at horizontal level and flex elbow. Try to bring down the arm against resistance.

4. Teres major ($C_{6,7}$): Forms posterior axillary fold (alongwith latissimus dorsi). Action is alongwith posterior fibres of deltoid as above.

5. Latissimus dorsi ($C_{6,7,8}$): Its actions are extension, abduction medial rotation at shoulder, seen prominently as posterior axillary fold and can be felt, if patient coughs. The muscle also pulls the trunk upwards and forwards when the arm is raised for holding railing while climbing.

6. Serratus anterior (nerve to serratus anterior $C_{5,6,7}$): Lateral and forward movement of the scapula which is tested by pushing the arm against resistance (or wall). In weakness of this muscle the scapula will stand out prominently (winging of the scapula).

7. Rhomboids (Rhomboidal nerve C_5): Causes retraction of the scapula which is tested by taking the elbows backwards with hands on the hips.

8. Infraspinatus (Suprascapular $C_{5,6}$) : Lateral rotation of forearm backwards. Forearm flexed at the elbow and held by the side of body (lateral rotation is tested).

9. Biceps (Musculo-cutaneous $C_{5,6}$) : Flexion and supination of the elbow. Tested by flexion of extended forearm against resistance.

10. Triceps (Radial $C_{6,7,8}$): Extension of flexed forearm. Tested against resistance.

11. Brachioradialis (Radial $C_{5,6}$): Flexion of forearm at the elbow which is tested by flexing the extended elbow. It stands out when supine or semiprone elbow is flexed against resistance.

12. Supinator teres (Median $C_{6,7}$): Supination of forearm (Note that biceps is also supinator of forearm).

13. Pronator teres (Median $C_{6,7}$): Pronation of forearm.

Pl. 15.6 a,b,c,d,e,f,g,h, and i, Testing actions of different groups of muscles at shoulder girdle and certain important features. (Refer to text for details).

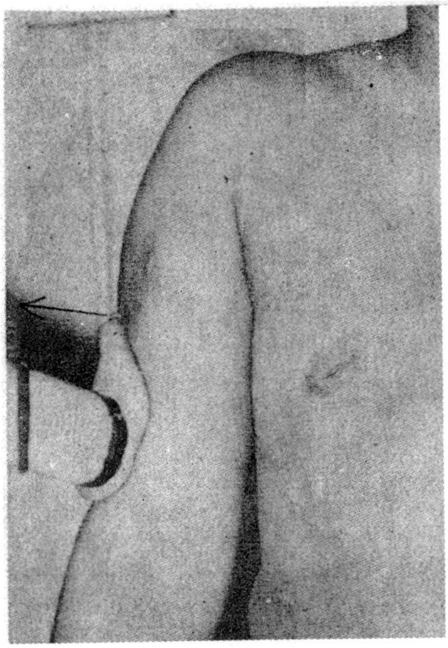

Pl. 15.6a Supraspinatus - Initial 30 degrees abduction. Tested by applying resistance to arm when it lies near body. Note rounded curvature of shoulder due to deltoid.

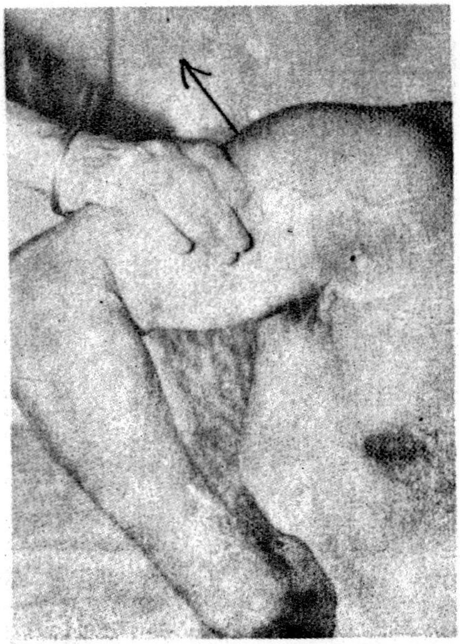

Pl. 15.6b Deltoid - Abduction beyond 1st 30 degrees Tested by appling resistance to arm.

(Refer to text for details)

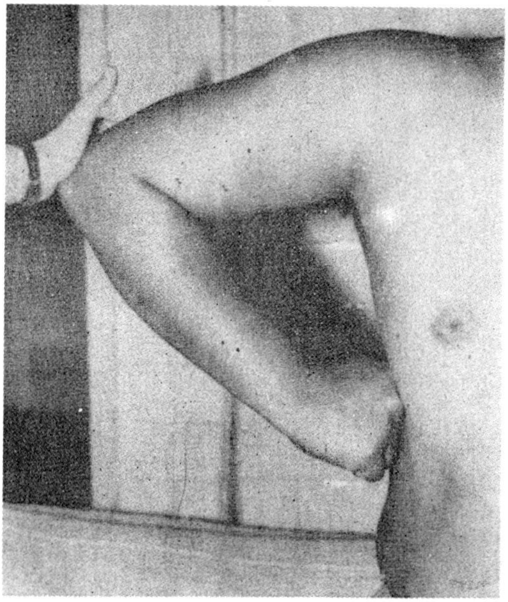

Pl. 15.6c Deltoid - Abduction beyond 90 degrees. After fixation of scpula by serrtus anterior.

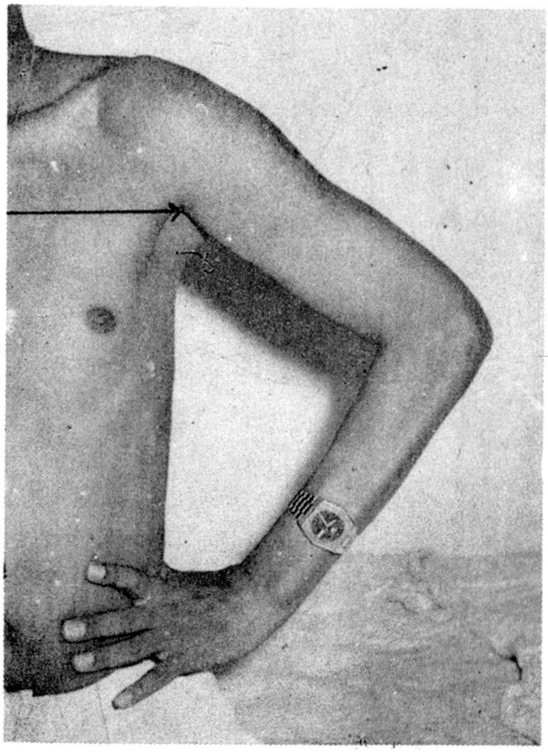

Pl. 15. 6b Anterior axillary fold formed by pectoralis major.

(Refer to text for detalis)

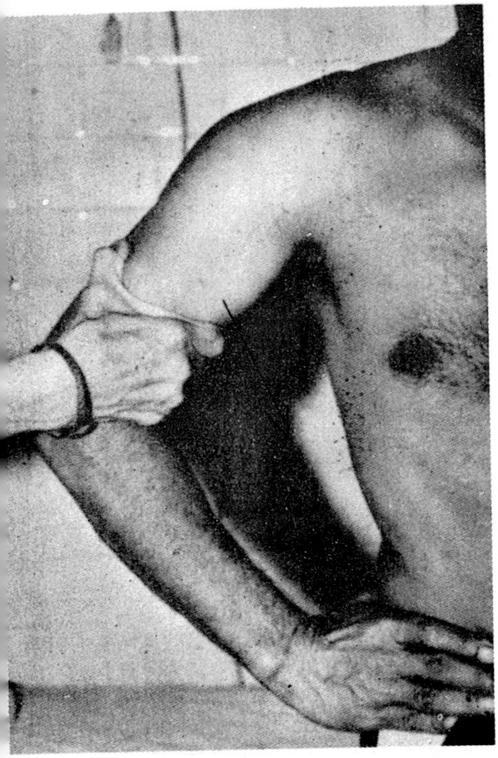

Pl. 15.6e Pectoralis major and latissimus dorsi-Adduction at shoulder tested by adducting abducted arm against resistance.

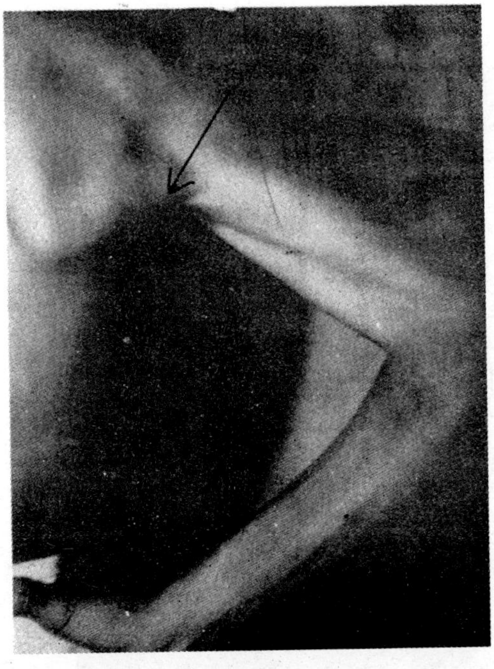

Pl. 15.6f Posterior axillary fold - Formed by latissimus dorsi and teres major.

(Refer to text for details)

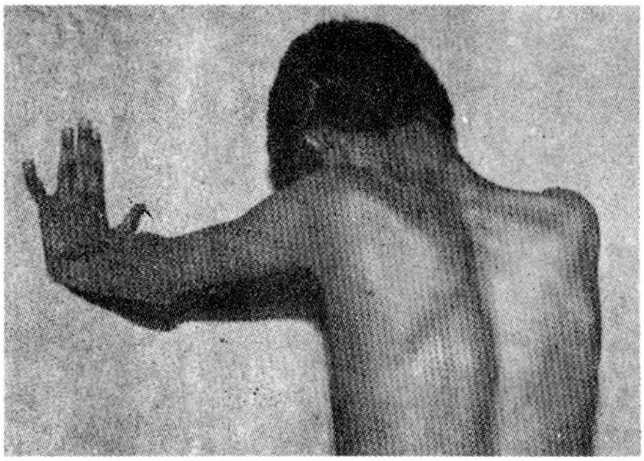

Pl. 15.6g Serratus anterior - Lateral and forward movement of scapula against resistance

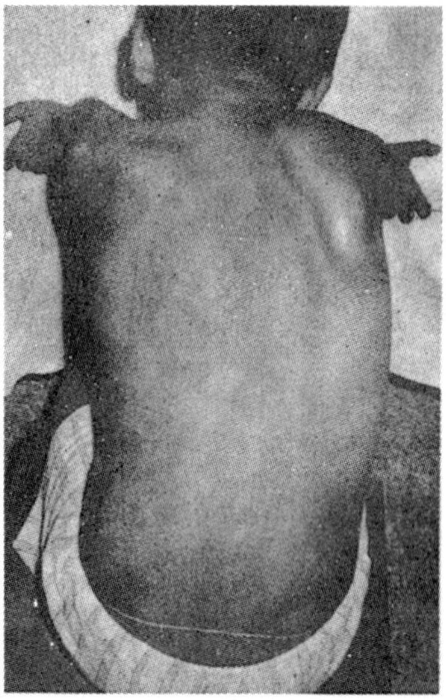

Pl. 15.6h Winging of scapula (R) - Paralysis of serratus anterior on (R) side.

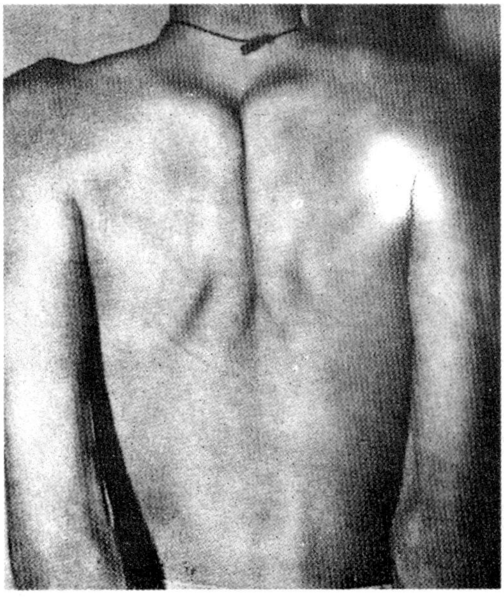

Pl.15.6i Rhomboids - Retraction of scapulae

(Refer to text for details)

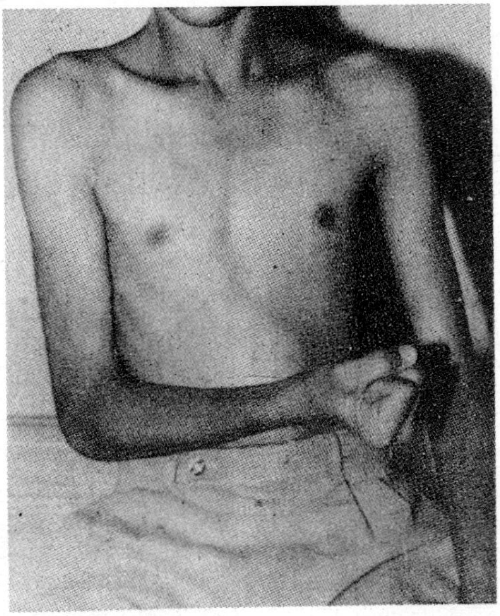

Pl. 15.8a Medial rotators of shoulder - Anterior fibres of deltoid pectoralis major

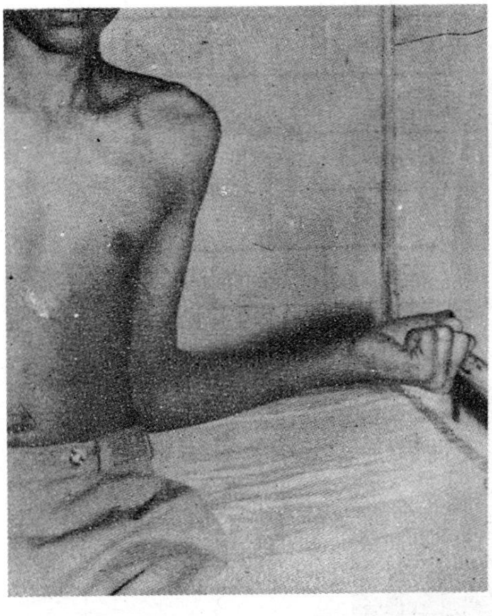

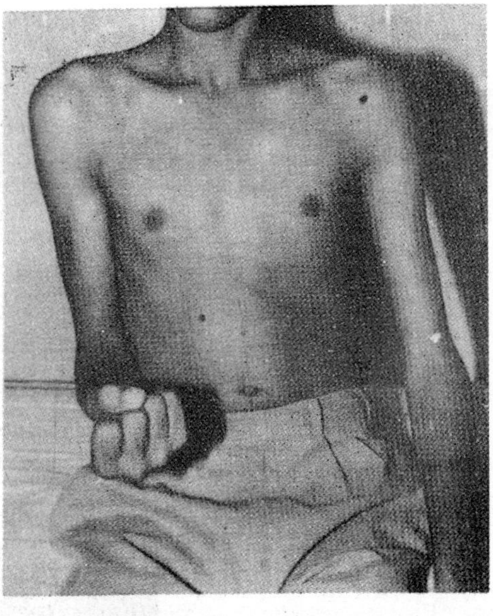

Pl.15.8 b and c Lateral rotators of shoulder - Posterior fibres of deltoid and infraspinatus. Medial and lateral rotation at shoulder are tested by flexing the elbow and holding it by side of body as in 8c.

(Refer to text for details)

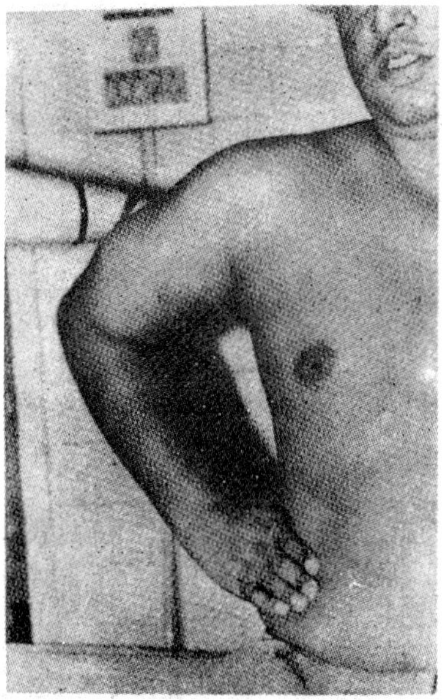

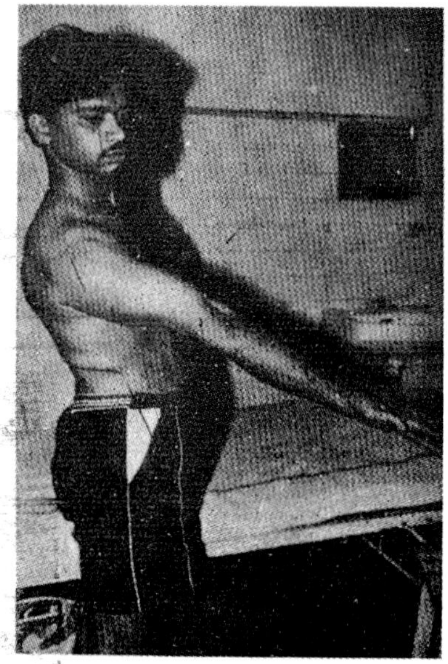

Pl. 15.7a Flexors of shoulders - Anterior fibres of deltoid
Pectoralis

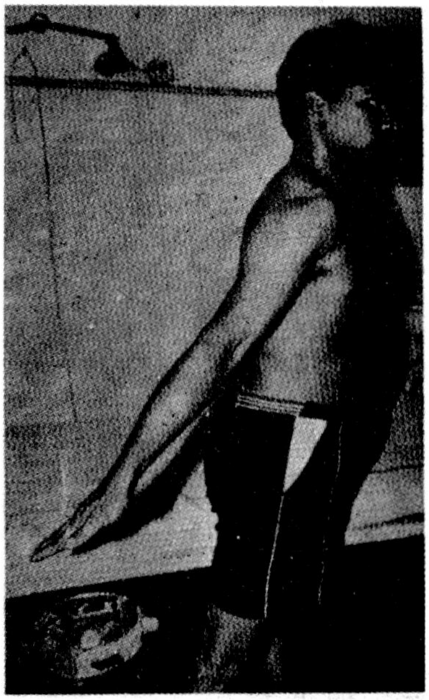

Pl. 15.7b Extensors of shoulder - Posterior fibres of deltoid
Teres major

Pl. 15.9a, b, c, d, and e Groups of muscles of forearm. (Refer to text for details)

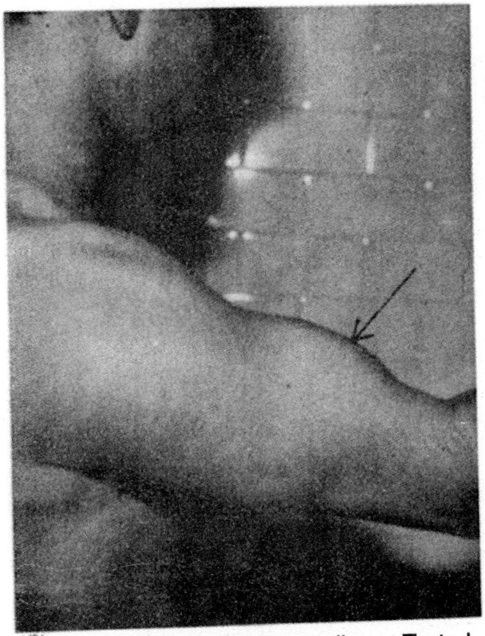

Pl. 15.9a Biceps - Flexion at elbow - Tested by applying resistance.

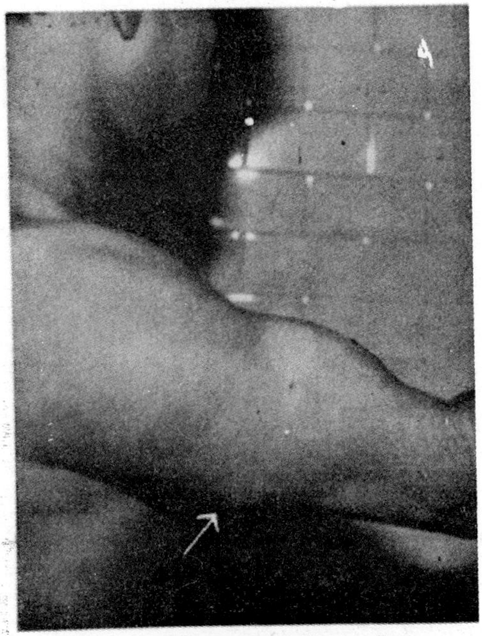

Pl. 15. 9b Triceps - Extension at elbow - Tested by applying resistance. Note prominence of biceps and triceps.

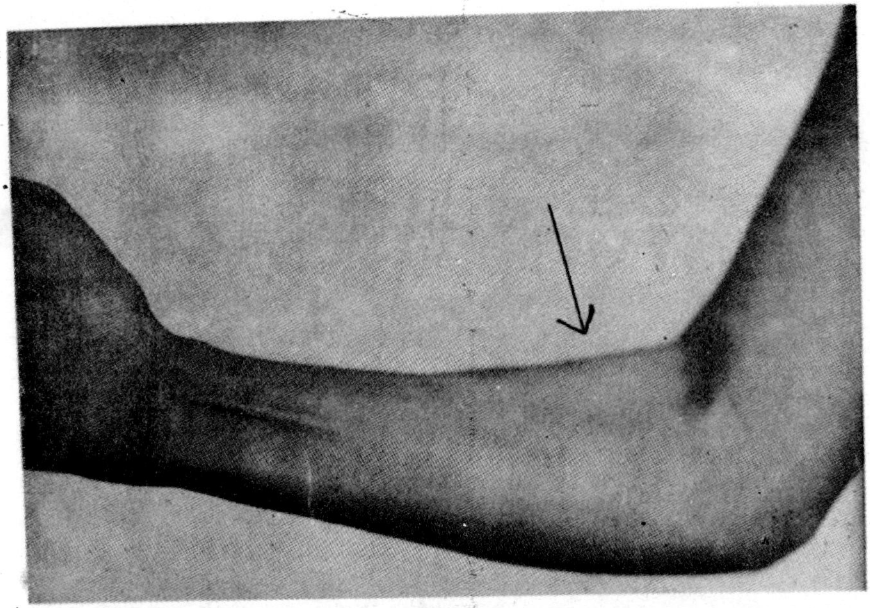

Pl. 15. 9c Brachioradialis - flexion at elbow
Note the tendon of brachioradialis

(Refer to text for details)

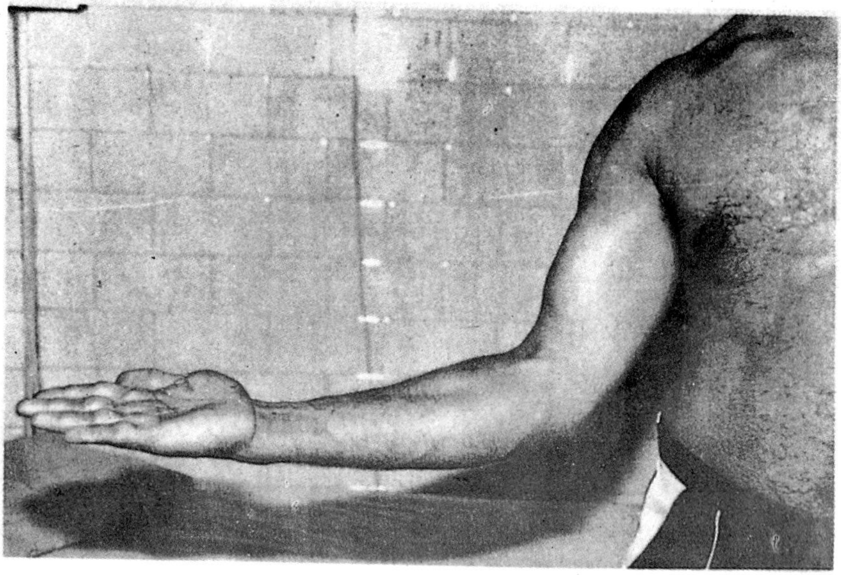

Pl. 15.9d Supinator - Supination of forearm

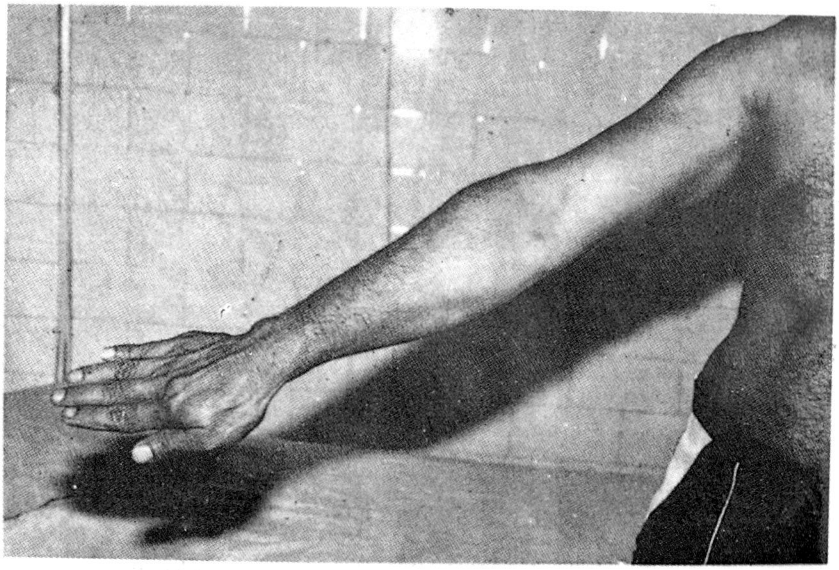

Pl. 15.9e Pronator teres - Pronation of forearm

14. Extensors of wrist: Extension at wrist is brought about by
   i. Extensor digitorum (Radial $C_{7,8}$)
   ii. Extensor carpi radialis (Radial $C_{6,7,8}$)
   iii. Extensor carpi ulnaris (Ulnar $C_{7,8}$)

Extension at wrist tested by extending flexed hand at wrist in prone position against resistance and gravity.

15. Ulnar deviation of wrist:
   Extensor carpi ulnaris } (Ulnar $C_{7,8}$)
   Flexor carpi ulnaris
16. Radial deviation of wrist:
   Extensor carpi radialis - (Radial $C_{6,7,8}$)
   Flexor carpi radialis (Median $C_{6,7}$)
17. Flexors of wrist:
   Flexor carpi ulnaris (Ulnar $C_{7,8}$)
   Flexor carpi radialis (Median $C_{6,7}$)
   Flexor digitorum superficialis (sublimis) - (Median $C_{7,8}$ T_1)
   Flexor digitorum profundus - (Median and Ulnar C_8 T_1)
   Tested by flexing extended hand against resistance.
18. Flexor digitorum superficialis : (sublimis) (C_8 T_1)
   Flexion of middle and proximal phalanges.
19. Flexor digitorum profundus (C_8 T_1)
   Flexion of distal phalanges.
   Flexion of mainly distal, middle phalanges is tested together by feeling grip the hand.
20. Extensor digitorum (Radial $C_{7,8}$) Extension at metacarpophalangeal joints.
21. Muscles of hand:
   Extensor pollicis longus, Extensor pollicis brevis, Abductor pollicis longus } (Radial $C_{7,8}$)
   Opponens pollicis, Abductor pollicis brevis, Flexor pollicis longus, Flexor pollicis brevis } Median nerve

Lumbricals: (lateral) Ist two : Median; (medial) 3rd and 4th: Ulnar

Interossei, Abductor digiti - minimi, Abductor pollicis } Ulnar nerve

All these are supplied by C_8 T_1 (median and ulnar)

a. Extension of thumb - Extension at metacarpophalangeal joint by extensor pollicis brevis. Extensor pollicis longus causes extension at interphalangeal joint. Extension takes thumb away from fingers in the same plane.

b. Flexion of thumb - Flexion at metacarpophalangeal joint by flexor pollicis brevis. Flexor pollicis longus causes flexion at inter- phalangeal joint. Flexion brings the thumb across the palm.

c. Adduction of thumb - Aductor pollicis longus and brevis. The thumb is brought at right angles to the palm.

d. Adduction of thumb: Adductor pollicis. (Thumb lies in the line with the other fingers. Tested by holding paper between thumb and index finger). (Supplied by ulnar Nerve C_8 T_1).

e. Opposition (Pinching movement) : Flexion of the proximal joint of the thumb tested by asking the patient to touch the little finger with the thumb.

Lumbricals: Flexion at the metacarpophalangeal joints tested by trying to flex the extended fingers at the metacarpophalangeal joints (for lumbricals).

Lumbricals and Interossei: form common aponeurosis - cause extension at inter-phalangeal joints.

Dorsal interossei are tested by asking the patient to separate the fingers and maintain this abduction against resistance.

Palmer interossei are tested by adducting the extended fingers. The power can be tested by inserting a piece of paper between the fingers, and the examiner trying to pull it out.

The first palmer interosseus tested by the patient trying to bring the abducted index finger to an imaginary line passing through longitudinal axis of the middle finger.

22. Abdominal muscles T_8 L_1 : Abdominal muscles are tested by palpating them when the patient lying on his back attempts to raise his head. Umbilicus will move upwards if weakness of the lower abdominal muscle is present (there may be a local bulge of the weakened muscle).

23. Intercostal muscles (intercostal nerves T_1 to T_{12} : Movements of these muscles are observed

during inspiration and expiration.

24. Extensors of the spine (posterior rami of the spinal nerves) : Patient lies prone and attempts to lift the head and shoulders above the bed level).

25. Flexors of thigh: (Pl 15.14 to 15.16)

i. Iliopsoas : (Femoral $L_{1,23}$). causes flexion of thigh over abdomen. Also raises trunk and pelvis forwards against resistance from recumbent to sitting posture.

ii. Sartorius (Femoral $L_{2,3}$): flexes leg on thigh, therefore called 'tailor's muscle'. The flexors are tested by applying resistance to leg while flexing thigh.

26. Adductors of thigh: Longus, brevis and magnus (Obturator $L_{2,3,4}$) adduction tested by applying resistance to abducted thigh (with knee flexed when patient attempts to adduct.

27. Extensor of thigh-Gluteus maximus (in-ferior gluteal L_5 $S_{1,2}$) : Extension of thigh and lateral rotation at hip. Maintains erect posture by maintaining position of pelvis. It is tested as follows: Patient lies in prone position and flexes knee. Pelvis is fixed by examiner and patient is asked to raise the knee on his own and against resistance. It is also lateral rotator.

28. Abductors and medial rotators of thigh-Gluteus medius and minimus (superior gluteal L_5 S_1): Most important in maintaining upright posture. Weakness leads to sinking of pelvis on affected side. Tested as follows: patient lies in lateral position and knee is flexed. Then the knee is raised against resistance and gravity (lateral movement of the thigh).

29. Medial rotators of thigh: Gluteus medius and minimus.

30. Lateral rotators of thigh : Gluteus maxi- mus, Obturator muscles.

31. Extensor of knee-quadriceps (Femoral $L_{2,3,4}$): Powerful muscle in maintaining upright position of lower limbs. It gets wasted quickly in case of paralysis whenever knee joint is affected and also by disuse. Tested by extension of flexed knee against resistance.

32. Hamstrings (Sciatic L_5 $S_{1,2}$): It is main flexor of knee. Patient lies in prone position and leg is flexed over thigh against resistance and the tendons of'biceps and semitendinosus stand out prominently.

33. Gastrocnemius and soleus - Medial popliteal $S_{1,2}$: Plantar flexor of foot. Flexor of knee first examine the belly of muscle for wasting or pseudo-hypertrophy.

Can be tested in two ways, patient lies in prone position and plantar flexion, is attempted against resistance.Tendo-achillis becomes prominent.

Another way of testing gastrocnemius is by asking patient to walk on toes or to raise heel off ground in upright posture.

34. Dorsiflexors of foot : All supplied by deep peroneal nerve.

Tabialis anterior ($L_{4,5}$)
Extensor hallucis longus } (L_5 S_1)
Extensor digitorum longus

Dorsiflexion tested by applying resistance to plantar flexed foot, during dorsiflexion. Also tested by asking patient to walk on his heels.

35. Extensor hallucis longus (L_5,S_1): Extends phalanges of big toe, also dorsiflexor of foot.

36. Extensor digitorum longus (L_5,S_1): Extends phalanges of other toes and dorsiflexor of foot.

37. Invertors of foot: Inversion is tested by inverting plantar flexed foot.

Tibialis posterior ($L_{4,5}$)
Tibialis anterior ($L_{4,5}$)

38. Evertors of foot: Eversion is tested by everting plantar flexed foot. Peroneus longus and brevis (L_5 $S_{1,2}$)

39. Flexor digitorum longus ($S_{2,3}$): Flexion of phalanges of toes, also plantar flexor of the foot.

40. Flexor hallucis longus - (Tibial nerve $S_{2,3}$) Flexion of phalanges of big toe, also plantar flexor of the foot.

41. Perineal muscles should be tested in cauda equina lesions by stroking gently skin around anus. The external sphinctar shows brisk contraction, i.e., anal reflex (see also page 235).

The above list was a review of individual and groups of muscles, their root innervation and the method to test them for power. The following list will give an idea of the muscles supplied by the root segments. It must be remembered that the muscles mentioned are supplied by more than one root and the root mentioned is one of the two or three roots supplying the muscles.

C_3 spinal accessory trapezius
C_4 diaphragm
C_5 deltoid,
C_6 biceps, brachioradialis, pronator teres,
C_7 triceps,
C_8 interossei and long flexors of the fingers,
T_1 thenar and hypothenar muscles, lumbricals,
T_2 - T_{12} intercostal muscles,
$L_{1,2}$ iliospoas,
L_3 quadriceps femoris,
L_4 adductors of thigh,
L_5 S_1 abductors of thigh
L_5 Peronei,
$L_{4,5}$ tibialis anterior and posterior,
S_1 gastrocnemius, hamstrings,
$S_{1,2}$ glutei,
$S_{3,5}$ perineal muscles.

These should be tested particularly in the patient who complains of a spinal lesion, i.e., if the examiner suspects a root lesion say at the level of $C_{8,}$ interossei should be tested carefully for the signs of wasting weakness and fasciculation and for adduction and abduction of fingers.

4. Co-ordination:

Co-ordination can be defined as harmonious movement of muscle groups with correct sequence of appropriate muscles. It is normally controlled by sensory tracts, cerebellum, vestibular apparatus and power of muscles.

Tests:

The points to be remembered when testing co-ordination are as follows :

1. The patient may not be able to perform the necessary action due to loss of power causing swaying of the limb.

2. The test should be explained carefully to the patient, if necessary by mimicking the action required.

Co-ordination tests in the upper extremities:

1. The patient should be asked to extend both arms symmetrically and the fingers stretched. These are then displaced by tapping on the arms gently. Normally there is a very minimal displacement and the patient regains the posture immediately.

In cerebellar disorders the arm overshoots initially the position held by him and on tapping, there is a wide displacement. In parietal lobe lesions if the patient is asked to close his eyes, the arm may gradually change its position without patient being aware of it.

2. **Finger-nose test:**

The patient is asked to touch the tip of his nose by index finger. The arm should be kept by the side when starting this movement. At first the patient is asked to perform the movement by keeping the eyes open and his ability to perform the action correctly is noted. Then the test is repeated by closing the eyes.

In cerebellar disease there is a jerky movement of the finger but the patient can touch the tip of his nose properly (intention tremors). In posterior column lesions the movement is possible with eyes open, but with eyes closed there is a marked inco-ordination.

In lower extremities:

1. **Heel-knee test:**

The patient is asked to approximate at first the heel of the right foot to the left knee. Care should be taken to explain that this action is performed by lifting the leg clear off the bed without touching the other leg or the patient does this by sliding the foot upwards along the other leg. Then he is asked to slide the heel up and down over the shin. In cerebellar disease, the lifted heel overshoots the knee and there is marked incoordination with tremors in performing the action of sliding the heel up and down the shin.

In posterior column lesion, the inco-ordination is marked when the eyes are closed which can be compensated when the patient keeps his eyes open and does the same action.

2. Toe-finger test:

The patient in lying down position is asked to

lift his toe and touch it to the examiner's finger. The same overshooting with inco-ordination as described above will be present in cerebellar lesions and the test will be practically impossible with the eyes closed in posterior column lesion.

3. **Romberg's test:**

If a patient is able to stand, inco-ordination can also be tested as follows : He is asked to stand with feet close together and toes touching each other. If he is able to do this then he is asked to close his eyes and stand in the same fashion. In sensory ataxia (posterior column lesion) if he closes his eyes, he sways and may even fall down (Romberg's test +ve). Romberg's test is +ve in sensory ataxia but has no relation with cerebellar ataxia. (In cerebellar ataxia the patient may lose his balance whether eyes are open or closed.)

Special tests for inco-ordination : Due to cerebellar involvement:

1. **Dysdiadokokinesis or adiadokokinesis:**

Adiadokokinesis is the inability to perform repetitive alternate movements quickly. This can be tested by asking the patient (a) to pronate and supinate the forearms rapidly, and (b) to clap rhythmically. In cerebellar involvement, he cannot do so on the affected side.

2. **Rebound phenomenon:**

The patient is asked to flex his forearm at the elbow against resistance and then the forearm is released suddenly. The patient is unable to stop the flexion and may hit his own face.

3. **Dysmetria:**

Ability to stop a particular movement as described is lost in cerebellar affection - patient is unable to judge the range of movements.

In finger-nose test, it is evident by the finger past the tip of the nose or stopping only when it hits the nose with greater force than intended.

The patient should be asked to close eyes and hold his one upper or lower limb in particular position. Then he should put the other limb in same position. He is unable to do so because of the inability to judge the range of movements.

4. **Pointing and past-pointing:**

This test is performed by, at first asking the patient to touch the examiner's finger by his finger. The action is repeated once or twice and then the patient is asked to do it with eyes closed. The examiner's finger is held in the same fixed position.

In cerebellar disease, the finger past points the examiner's finger on the affected side.

5. **Barany's pointing test:**

Patient is asked to outstretch both upper limbs, straight and parallel to each other. In cerebellar disease the ipsilateral limb will deviate outwards. If he closes his eyes and is asked to move the limb and bring it back to the same previous position he cannot do so on the affected side.

6. **Walking tests:**

If the patient suffering from a unilateral cerebellar disease is asked to walk on a straight line he will sway and deviate towards the affected side.

In bilateral or midline cerebellar disease, the gait will be drunken and the patient will sway on either side.

In unilateral cerebellar disease, if the patient is to go round a chair or a stool, he will come nearer and nearer the chair if the affected side is pointing towards it (centripetal). He will move in wider and wider circles if the side affected is opposite to the central object (centrifugal).

5. **Involuntary movements:**

Analysis of involuntary movements will require very careful observation of the patient and also a detailed knowledge of involuntary movements of various types.

I. The points to be noted in observation should include :

1. Which parts of the body are affected?

2. Whether the movements occur constantly, episodically or periodically.

3. Whether they are present at rest or during movements or at both times.

4. Effect of voluntary movements on the involuntary movements.

5. Alteration due to eye closure, if any.

6. Whether they disappear during sleep.

7. Whether there is awareness of these movements.

These points are noted by examining the patient as a whole when he is lying down. If possible then he should be asked to stand up and walk. Then he should be asked to stretch the hands straight which will make tremors evident. Then his grip should be tested to find out whether voluntary movement increases the involuntary movement. Lastly, the finger movements are tested by asking him to perform acts like buttoning his shirt, handwriting, etc.

II. Common abnormal movements observed generally are enumerated below :

1. Due to involvement of extrapyramidal system
   - i. Chorea,
   - ii. Athetosis,
   - iii. Dystonia,
   - iv. Hemiballismus,
   - v. Myoclonus,
   - vi. Tremor,

2. Due to other causes
   - i. Hysterical tremor,
   - ii. Intention tremor,
   - iii. Spasmodic torticollis,
   - iv. Craniocervical spasm,
   - v. Tics and habit spasm,
   - vi. Writer's cramp.

3. Miscellaneous involuntary movements
   - i. Fasciculation,
   - ii. Myokymia,
   - iii. Myoedema (myotatic irritability),
   - iv. Spasm.

The description of involuntary movements due to extrapyramidal system are discussed elsewhere. The description of other involuntary movements is given below.

Involuntary movements due to other causes :

(i) **Hysterical tremors:**

a. Bizarre picture.

b. Do not correspond to any known types of organic tremors.

(ii) **Intention tremors:**

a. Precipitated due to a willed movement.

b. Absent when the limb is relaxed and during the early part of the voluntary movement.

c. Jerky, rhythmic oscillation with attempt at precise movement.

d. May persist for a short time after the action is over.

e. Rarely head involved (titubation).

f. Cause : cerebellar disease.

(iii) **Spasmodic torticollis —**

a. Forced turning of head on one side with elevation of the chin and lowering of the occiput.

b. Spasms of the sternomastoid.

c. Causes could be extrapyramidal lesion (drug induced or otherwise) or of psychogenic origin.

(iv) **Cranio-cervical spasm:**

a. Muscles of the face and neck involved.

b. Spasm starts suddenly and stops suddenly.

c. May be abolished in sleep.

(v) **Ties and habit spasms:**

a. Irregular facial movements.

b. Not due to organic disease.

c. Repetitive movements such as blinking, contraction of the platysma, etc.

d. Most common in the face and shoulder girdles.

(vi) **Writer's cramps:**

a. Usually seen in people who have to write or perform continuous stereotyped work.

b. Initial words while writing are clear, then the hand goes into spasms and the patient is unable to continue.

c. Cause : psychological.

3. **Miscellaneous involuntary movements:**

(i) **Fasciculation:**

a. Irregular twitching of the muscle bundles.

b. Easily seen in large muscles.

c. Increased by irritating or slapping the muscles.

d. indicates chronic or slow degeneration of motor neuron, e.g., motor neuron disease.

e. Fibrillation is a misnomer applied to the same movement. It denotes contraction of single muscle fibres and seen on EMG and in the tongue muscles.

f. Present during sleep.

(ii) **Myokymia:**

a. Rapid repeated fine contractions in the fibres of the same group of muscles.

b. May persist for minutes at a time.

c. Commonly seen in orbicularis oculi and eyelid muscles.

d. Sometimes coarse contraction of bundles of muscle fibres usually in a large muscle near the joint due to fatigue and neurasthenia.

(iii) **Myoedema (Myotatic irritability):**

a. Slow contraction and relaxation of muscle fibres on tapping.

b. May be seen on change in posture in a patient with hypothyroidism.

(iv) **Spasms:**

a. Tonic spasms seen in prolonged contractions in tetany, tetanus or in epilepsy for a brief duration.

b. Clonic spasms are repetitive contractions of opposing muscle groups.

IV. **Sensory System:**

The examination of this system constitutes the most difficult part of the neurological examination as the results of testing are subjective and are dependent upon the patient's interpretation of the stimuli administered.

The patient has to understand and to pay a great deal of attention when the tests are carried out and he should be told to interpret the findings as accurately as possible. This will mean that the patient has to be explained properly what is expected of him.

Methods of examination:

Sensory system is examined as follows:

1. Examination for touch, pain and temperature (superficial sensations).

2. Examination of joint sense, vibration sense, sense of position (deep sensations).

3. Examination of stereognosis and two-point discrimination, etc.

Examination of superficial sensations:

Touch : Touch is tested by using a piece of cotton wool rolled to point and touching it lightly to the skin (hairy parts sometimes offer difficulty, while touching the skin, hair may modify or exaggerate the impulse).

The first choice of the area to be tested will vary, but that part, which from the history can be said to be normal, is tested first. The patient is asked whether he feels the impulse and if so he is asked to describe the sensation. This will make the patient realise as to what type of test is going to be conducted and what sort of stimulus he should expect and interpret.

Then the patient is asked to close his eyes and the same stimulus is applied. He is asked to indicate verbally where he feels the sensation and whether he can localise it.

Then the sensory areas from face to foot should be examined systematically. Of course, special attention will have to be given to the parts which are likely to be abnormal.

Pain: A sharp pin with a blunt head is used for testing this sensation.

Just as in case of the examination of touch, the patient is first explained the test and then it is demonstrated to the patient in an apparently normal area. Then again a systematic examination for this sensation is carried out according to the dermatomes.

Another point to be remembered is that whenever possible, the examination should be conducted from an area of impaired sensation to the area of normal sensation. The patient is asked to indicate at what level he starts feeling the pain sensation normally and that level is carefully noted.

At this level there may be hyperalgesia, i.e., an exaggerated sense of pain before the area of normal sensation is encountered.

Temperature: Hot and cold sensations are examined by using test tubes or small glass bottles containing warm and cold water. Very hot and very cold temperatures should be avoided as they will stimulate the pain endings rather than thermal nerve endings.

The same principles as those used in touch and pain are followed.

The patient is asked to close the eyes and localise the temperature sensation as hot or cold.

Deep sensations (proprioceptive):

Joint sensations (sense of passive movement). This is tested as follows: The great toe in the lower extremity and either the thumb or the finger in upper extremity are selected for testing the joint sense (Fig 15.13).

Before testing, it is very carefully explained to the patient what he is supposed to say when the toe is put in either upward or downward direction. Usually 'up' and 'down' are the only expected answers and the corresponding positions of the toe are shown to the patient.

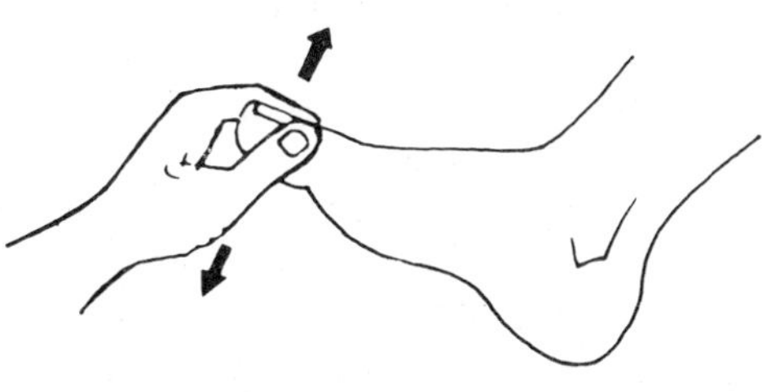

Fig. 15.13
Method of testing joint sensations. Note that the great toe is held in between two fingers from sides.

Then the finger or the toe is held in the examiner's finger sidewise. Otherwise the touch sensation and the pressure exerted by the finger will be registered and hence this will not be a test of joint sensations.

The patient is then asked to close the eyes and the test is carried on. A precise upward and downward movement should be done. So also an alternation between up and down positions should be avoided by the examiner as it is a very common experience that the patient who really cannot make out the joint position will give answers alternately, i.e., up-down-up-down which accidentally might coincide with the position of the finger being tested.

Vibration sense: A tuning fork (usually with a vibration of 128/cps) is chosen and after striking it is kept on the forehead or the clavicle of the patient. This enables him to understand what he is going to feel. The patient is then asked to close his eyes and the vibrating fork is kept on bony parts.

In the lower extremity, the medial malleoli, the patella, and the anterior superior iliac spines are tested successively if the patient cannot feel it on the lower level.

In the upper extremity the end of the radius and the olecranon are the common points chosen; over the trunk, costochondral junctions.

The two sides of the body are compared. As some patients might be confused and answer positively to the sensation of touch alone, it is necessary to try and cross check the patient's answers by applying a tuning fork which is not vibrating on to the bony part. A patient who has understood and has appreciated vibrations will answer in the negative.

Sense of position: The examination is conducted with the patient's eyes closed throughout.

1. Patient is asked to replace his arm in a particular position after the examiner has first put it in a particular position and then moved it away.

2. He is asked to mimic the position by the

other arm.

3. Legs are similarly tested.

Certain points about the sensory.system must be considered for correct interpretations of lesions in the sensory system.

Sensory pathways: Peripheral nerve carries at first all forms of sensations from where they reach the spinal cord or the brain-stem (in case of cranial nerves) via the sensory root.

The afferent fibres carrying touch, pain and temperature enter the spinal cord through dorsal sensory root, and relay in dorsal horn cells. After relaying, they ascend on the same side for 2-3 segments and then cross to the opposite side. While crossing, they lie very close to the spinal canal and the arrangement is as follows. The fibres carrying temperature lie closest to the spinal canal, those carrying pain are placed intermediate and those carrying touch are away from the spinal canal. This is important in dissociated sensory loss in syringomyelia. After crossing, the fibres carrying light touch form anterior spinothalamic tracts. Those carrying pain, temperature and also touch form the lateral spinothalamic tracts. In the lateral spinothalamic tracts, fibres carrying sensations from lower limbs lie outermost (hence are affected first whenever there is any spinal cord compression).

Proprioceptive impulses, joint sense, vibrations, light touch and tactile discrimination travel in the posterior columns of the spinal cord on the same side and they end in the nuclei Gracilis and Cuneatus. From there the fibres cross to the opposite side (sensory decussation) to ascend in the brain-stem as the medial emniscus. Spinothalamic tracts and sensory fibres carrying sensation from opposite side of face which travel through trigeminal nerve also join the medial lemniscus at the level of pons. From here they pass to the thalamus and then to the sensory cortex.

Thus sensations of touch are carried partly by posterior columns and partly by spinothalamic tracts.

The peripheral sensations of touch, pain and temperature are tested segmentwise or according to the root value of the skin area.

A complete diagram of dermatome distribution is seen in Figure 15.14 & 15.15. Fig 15. 15a shows dematomes and nerves of head and neck. Figs. 15.15b_1, c_1, d_1, e_1 & f_1 show dematomes of different parts of the body while Figs 15.15b_2, c_2, d_2, e_2 & f_2 show corresponding nerves of corresponding parts of the body.

However, for remembering the dermatomes when examining a patient clinically, the examiner should remember the important facts :

1. C_2 supplies the occiput (C_1 has no cutaneous supply).
2. C_5 supplies the lateral aspect of the tip of the shoulder.
3. C_7 supplies the middle finger.
4. Inner border of the forearm is supplied by T_1 and T_2.
5. Thorax is supplied anteriorly by T_3 to T_8 roots.
6. T_{10} supplies the level of the umbilicus (T_8 to T_{10} upper abdomen and T_{10} to T_{12} lower abdomen).
7. L_1 supplies the area from where the cremasteric reflex is elicited.
8. L_3,supplies the knee (anterior aspect),
9. L_5 runs diagonally across from the outer aspect of the tibia to the inner aspect of the foot.
10. S_1 supplies the lateral aspect of the foot including the little toe.
11. $S_{3,4,5,}$ supplies the saddle area, around the anus.

Sensory level (Relation between the root value and the vertebral level) : A student is quite likely to be confused with the usual description of the relation between these two.

However, it should be remembered that the spinal cord is shorter than the vertebral column and ends at the level of L_1 vertebra. Hence, the spinal segments do not correspond to the vertebrae in thoracic and lumber region (except in the highest cervical segments).

In the highest cervical region the spinal segments and the vertebral level correspond. In the

Pl. 15.10a, b, c and d. Groups of muscles acting at wrist.

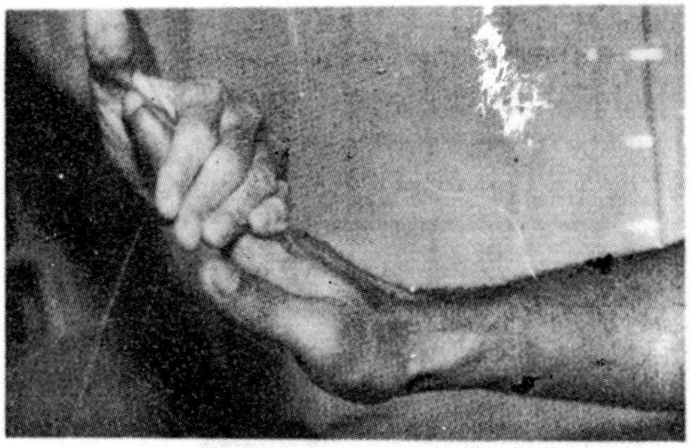

Pl. 15.10a Extenxors fo wrist
Extensor digitorum
Extensor carpi radialis
Extensor carpi ulnaris
Tested by extending flexed hand against resistance.

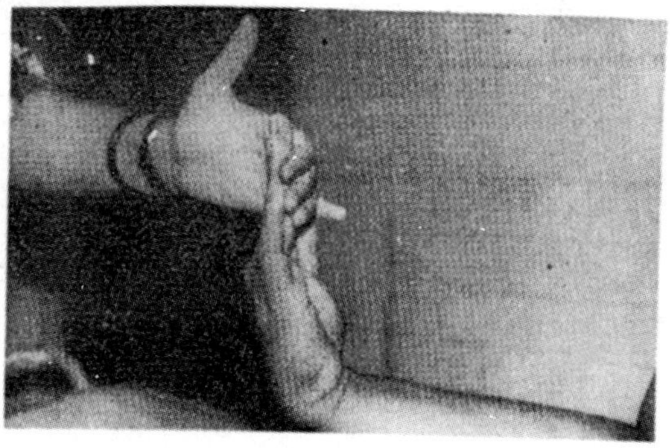

Pl. 15.10b Flexors of wrist
Flexor digitorum superficialis
Flexor digitorum profundus
Flexor carpi ulnaris
Flexor carpi radialis
Tested by flexing extended hand against resistance.

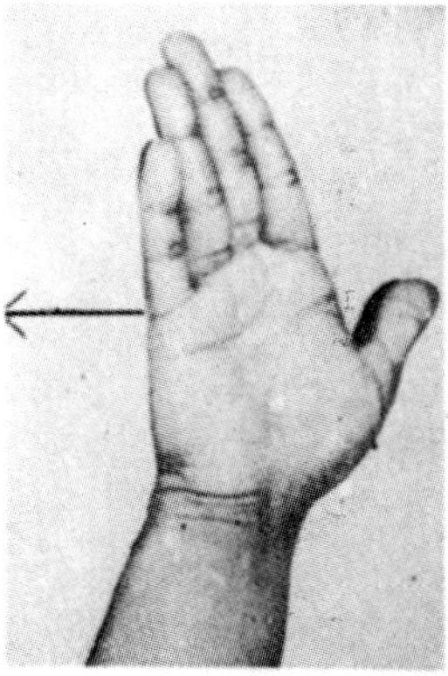

Pl. 15.10c Ulnar deviation - Flexor and extensor carpi ulnaris

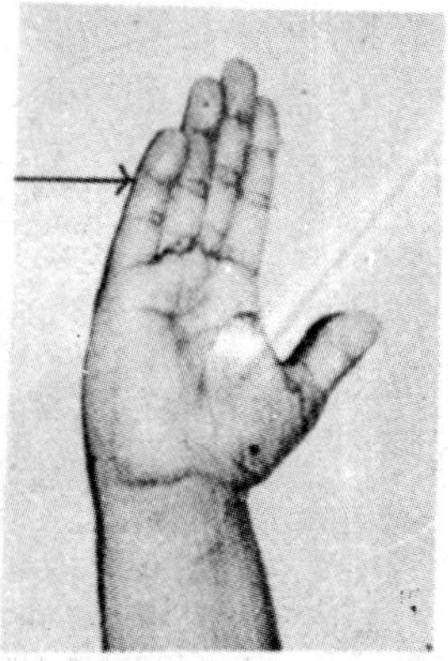

Pl. 15.10d Radial deviation - Flexor and extensor carpi radialis

(Refer to text for details)

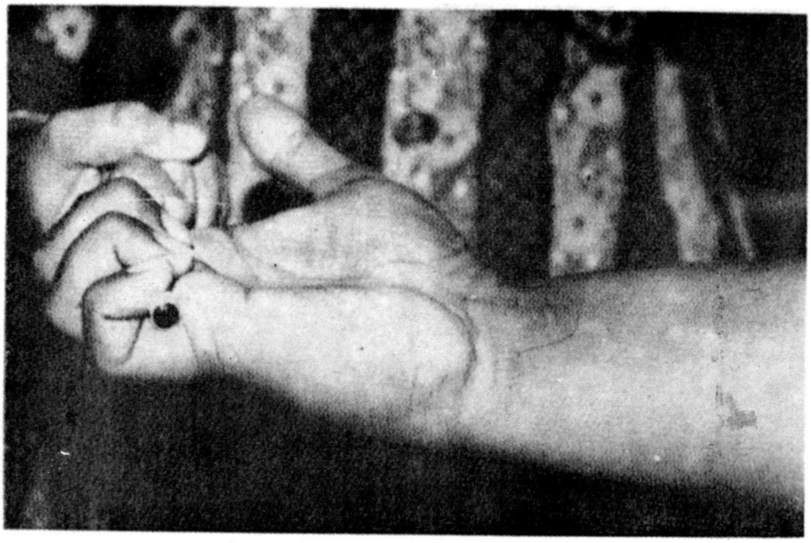

Pl. 15.11 Flexor digitorum superficialis and flexor profundus - flexion at proximal interphalangeal joints and distal interphalangeal joints respectively.

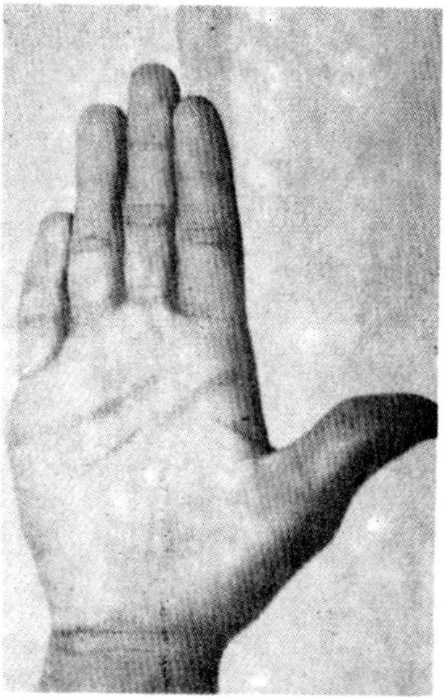

Pl. 15.12a Extension of thumb - thumb is away from finger in same plane.
Extensor pollicis brevis.

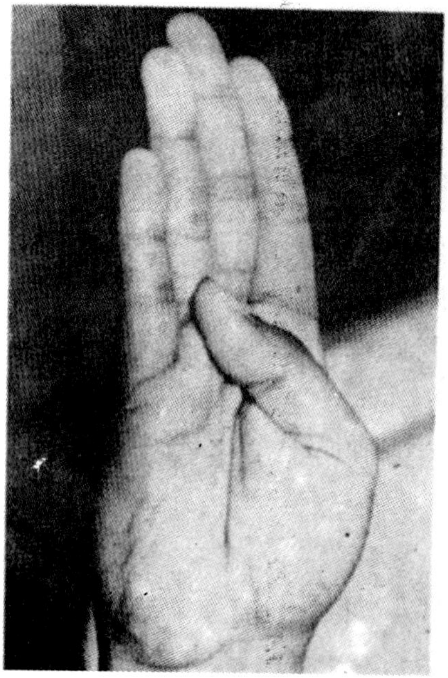

Pl. 15.12b Flexion of thumb - thumb in across the palm.
Flexor pollicis brevis

(Refer to text for details)

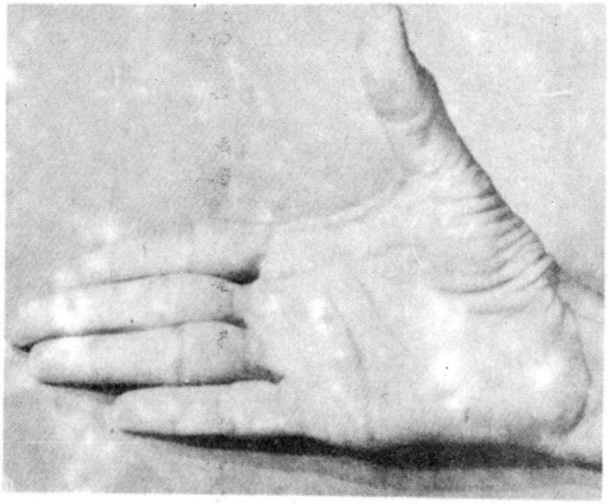

Pl. 15.12c Abduction of thumb
-thumb is at right angles to palm.
-Abductor pollicis longus and brevis.

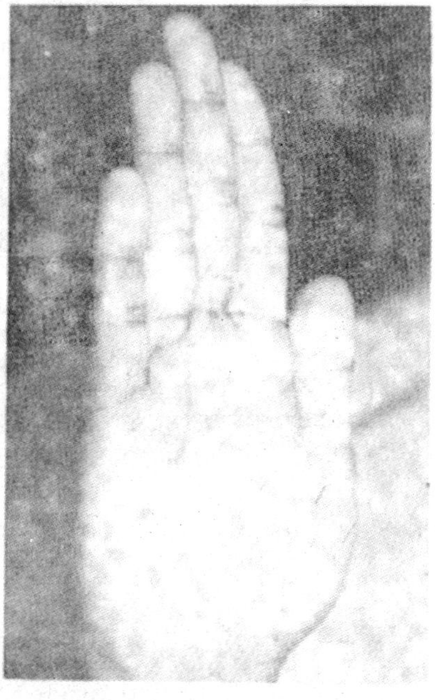

Pl. 15.12d Adduction of thumb - thumb is in line with fingers
-Adductor pollicis

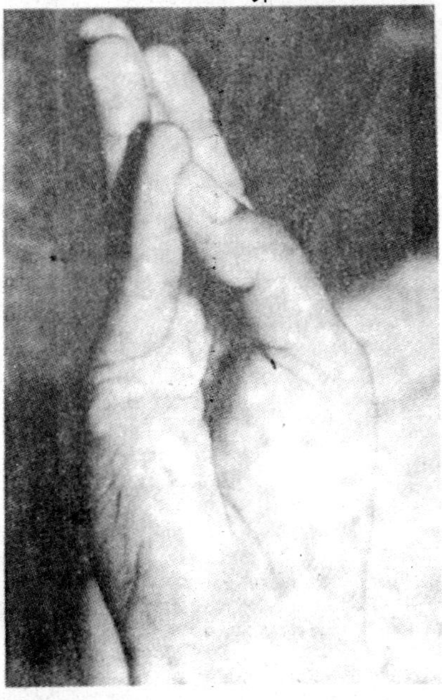

Pl. 15.12e Opposition of thumb - counting fungers
- Opponens pollicis

(Refer to text for details)

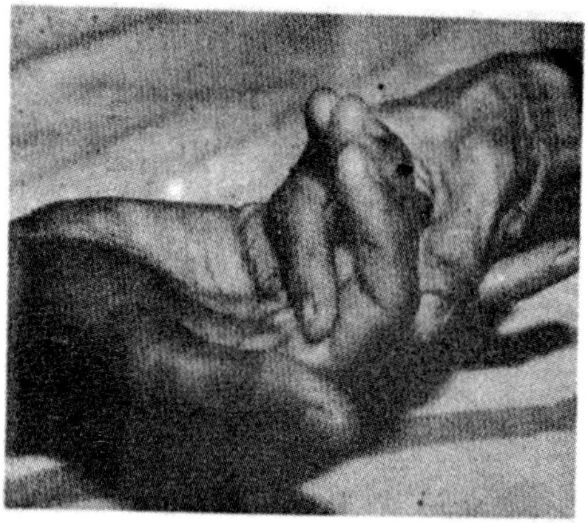

Pl. 15.12f Flexion at metacarpophalangeal joints. Lumbricals

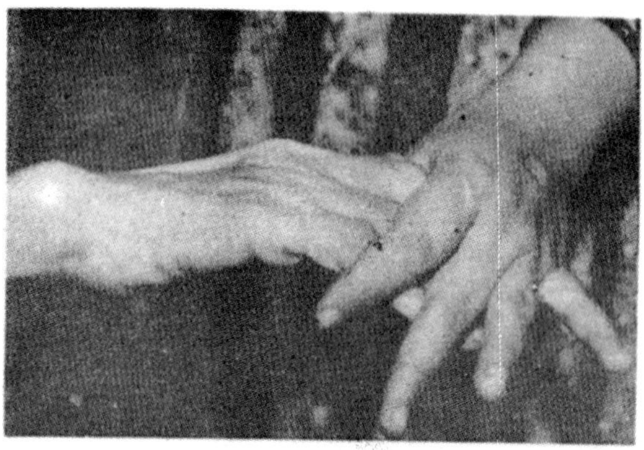

Pl.15. 12g Extension at interphalangeal joints. Lumbricals - interossei muscles

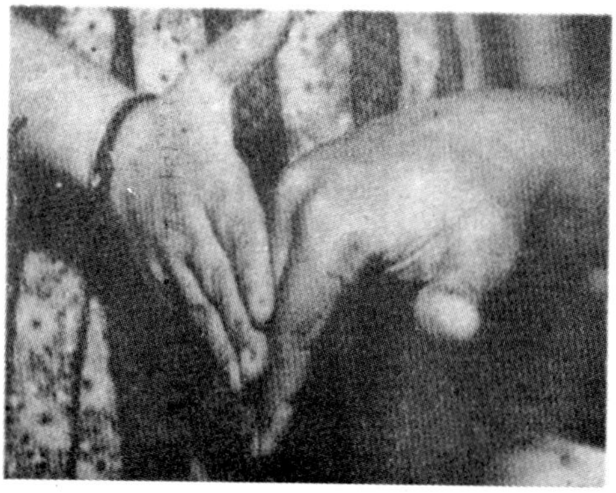

Pl. 15.12h Extension at metacarpophalangeal joints. Extensor digitorum

Pl. 15.13a, b Adduction and abduction of fingers (Refer to text for details)

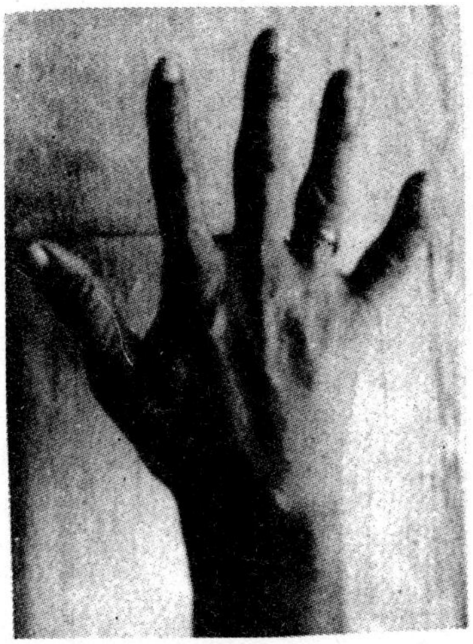

Pl. 15.13a Dorsal interossei
abductors of fingers

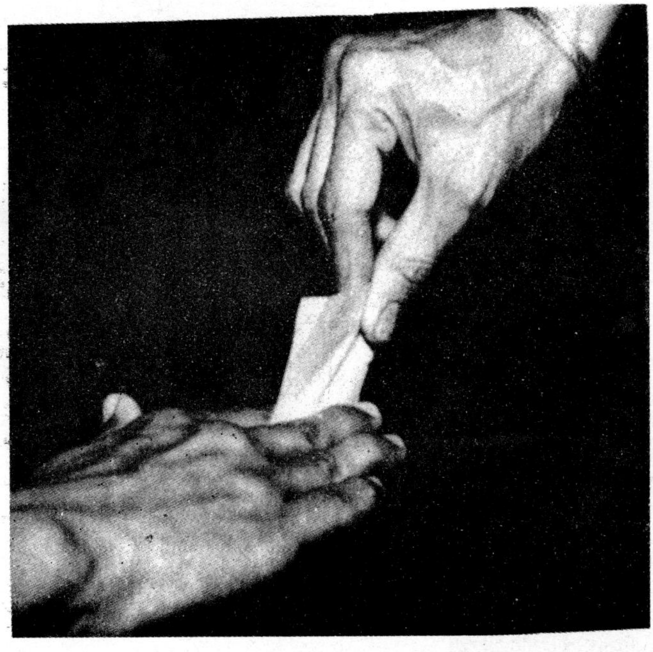

Pl. 15.13b Palmar interossei
adductors of fingers - Tested by inserting a paper in between two adjoining fingers. (53)

Pl. 15.14a, b, c, d and e Groups of muscles of thigh (Refer to text for details)

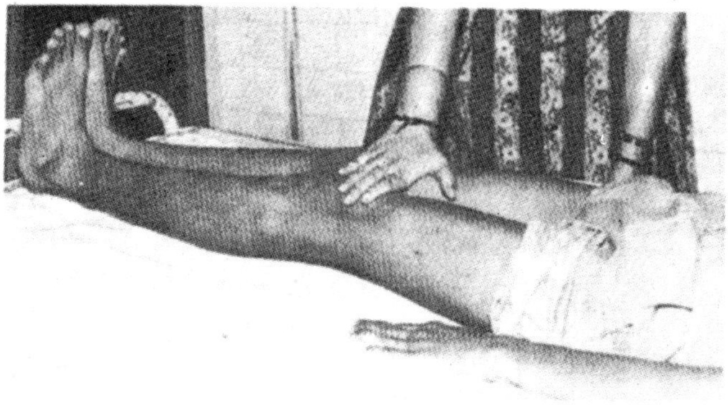

Pl. 15.14a Flexors - Ilio psoas
-Sartorius

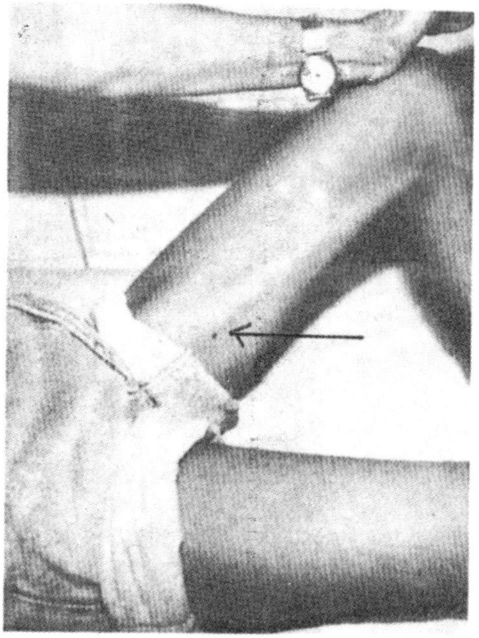

Pl. 15.14b Adductors - Longus brevis and magnus.
Note that adductor magnus becomes prominent

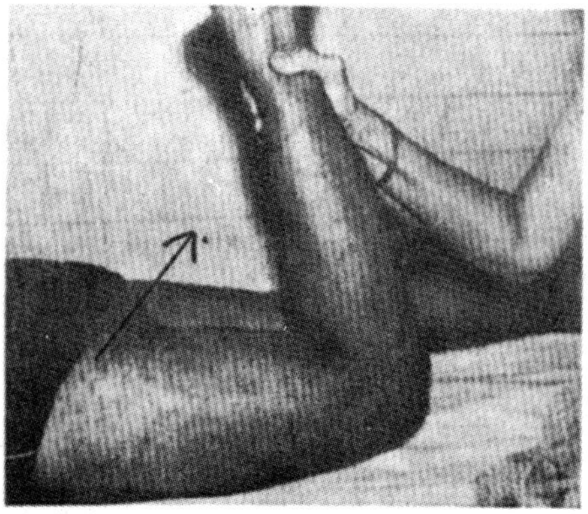

Pl. 15.14c Extensors - gluteus
maximus

(Refer to text for details)

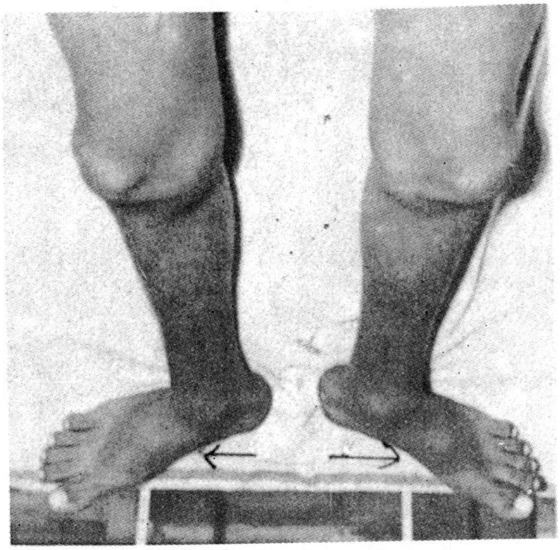

Pi: 15.14d Lateral rotator - gluteus maximus, obturator

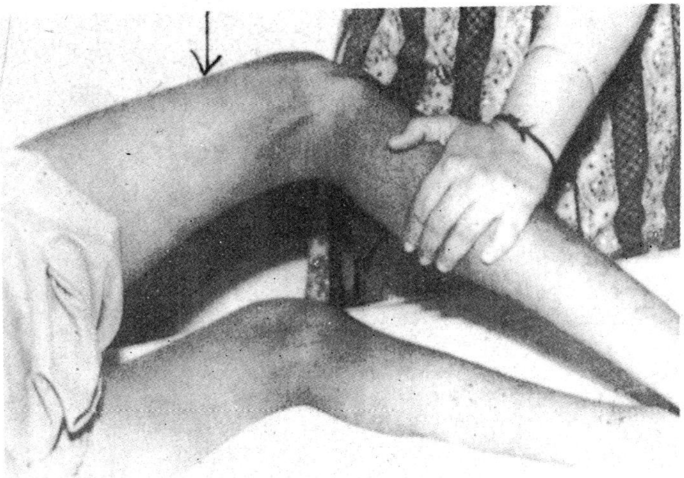

Pl. 15.14e Abductors - gluteus medius and minimus. Ideally tested in lateral position.

Pl. 15.15a and b Groups of mucles acting at knee. (Refer to text for details)

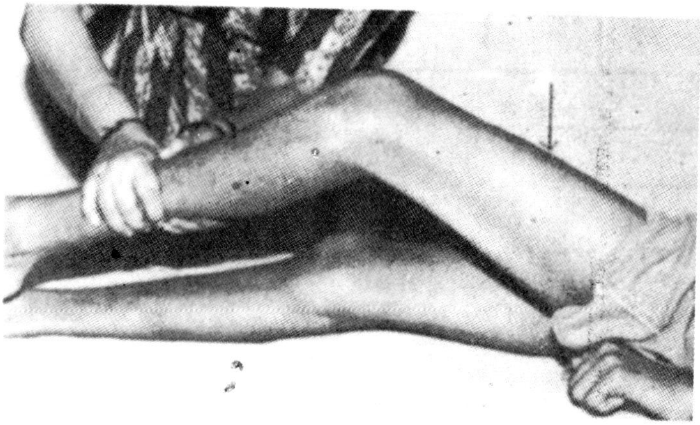

Pl. 15.15a Extensor of knee - Quadriceps
Note bulk of quadriceps when extension is attempted against resistance.

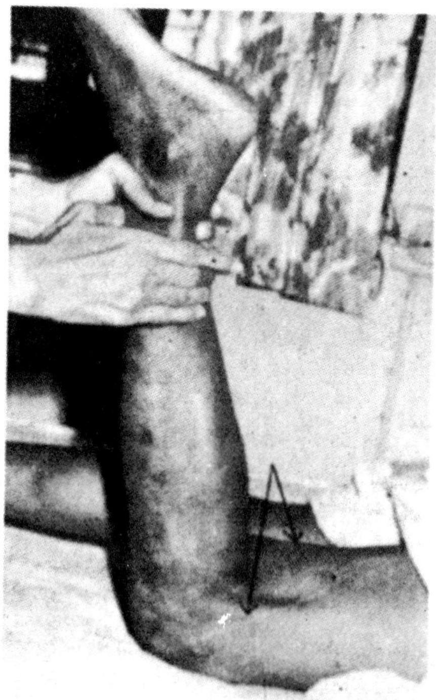

Pl.15.15b Flexors of knee - Hamstrings
Note prominent tendons of biceps femoris and semitendinosus - when flexion is attempted against resistance.

lower cervical segments there is a difference of *one* segment, i.e., C_8 spinal segment is opposite to C_7 vertebra. In upper thoracic area the difference is of *two* segments (i.e., T_3 will correspond to T_5 spinal segment); in mid-thoracic spine the difference is of *three* segments and the lumbar and sacral segments are all opposite $T_{11,}$ to L_1 vertebrae.

Cortical type of sensory loss:

The following tests are commonly carried out to determine the integrity of the sensory cortex.

1. **Stereognosis** is the ability to recognise a familiar object from the feel of its shape and size. It is the first sensation to be tested.

The examiner chooses a familiar object like a coin. It is placed in the patient's palm and he is asked to close his eyes and identify the object.

Stereognosis or a test of cortical function cannot be carried out when there is sensory lesion affecting touch and position sense. Hence, when there is anaesthesia or hyperaesthesia in the limb this test should not be necessarily interpreted as cortical type of sensory loss.

2. **Two point discrimination test:** A normal person can identify two separate points of stimulation when they are simultaneously applied (for instance two points of a divider). The ability to do so varies in different parts of the body.

The fingers are the most sensitive (5 mm separation) but the back and the dorsum of the foot, are the least sensitive (may be up to 5 cm).

The test is first explained and demonstrated by touching the two points on the hand by widely separating them. The two points are brought nearer and the patient is asked to differentiate them (with his eyes closed). The gap is gradually narrowed until the patient no longer recognises them as two separate points. This is compared then with the other side.

The point of the compass divider must be blunt or otherwise instead of testing for tactile discrimination, pain sensations will be stimulated.

The test is carried out as follows. The forearm is touched lightly on one side and the patient (with his eyes closed) is asked to say the side which he feels the stimulus, i.e., he should say, right when the right hand is stimulated. Then the other forearm (corresponding point) is touched alone when the patient will say 'left'. After repeating this once or twice, the examiner should touch both the extremities simultaneously.

In cortical type of sensory loss, the patient can feel the discrimination on unaffected side, he feels the touch only on the normal side and he forgets the touch on the affected side.

3. **Cutaneous localisation and number writing:** This is the ability of recognising letters written with a blunt point on the skin. After closing the eyes of the patient, the examiner draws letters or numbers on his palm. The patient is unable to recognise them in cortical type of sensory loss.

Some common forms of sensory loss: (Figs. 15.16 a to h shaded portion shows loss of sensations.)

1. Total unilateral loss of all sensations. This can occur due to severe lesion of the thalamus or due to hysterical reaction.

2. Unilateral hyperalgesia and hyperaesthesia. Partial lesions of the thalamus are the usual causes of this complaint.

The pains have a peculiar unpleasant character.

3. Unilateral loss of cortial sensations, and loss of position sense. A parietal lobe lesion between the thalamus and the cortex is the cause of this disturbance.

4. Loss of pain and temperature on one side of the face with similar loss on the opposite side of the body due to lesion of the medulla.

5. Bilateral loss of all forms of sensation below the level of lesion. This occurs in a severe and complete lesion of the spinal cord. A zone of hyperaesthesia may be present above the level of the sensory loss and denotes the level of spinal segment (transection of spinal cord).

If the upper level is not well defined and if there is no accompanying zone of hyperaesthesia the level of the lesion may be much higher than this level.

6. Contralateral loss of pain and temperature

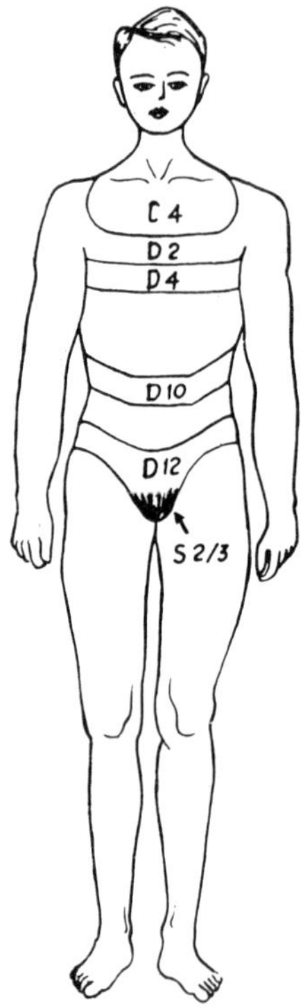

Fig. 15.14
Diagram showing dermatomes of trunk and genitals. Note that the dermatomes between C_5 to D_1 are utilised for upper limbs.

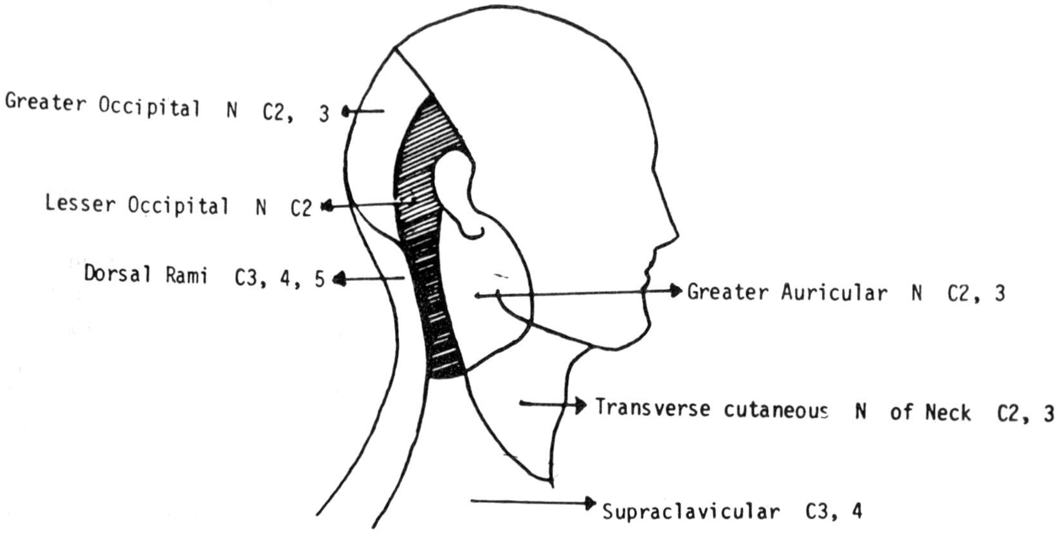

Figures 15.15 (a) to (f_2) show dermatomes and cutaneous supply of various parts of the body.

Fig. 15.15 (a)
Dermatomes and cutaneous supply of scalp and neck. Note that C_1 has no cutaneous distribution.

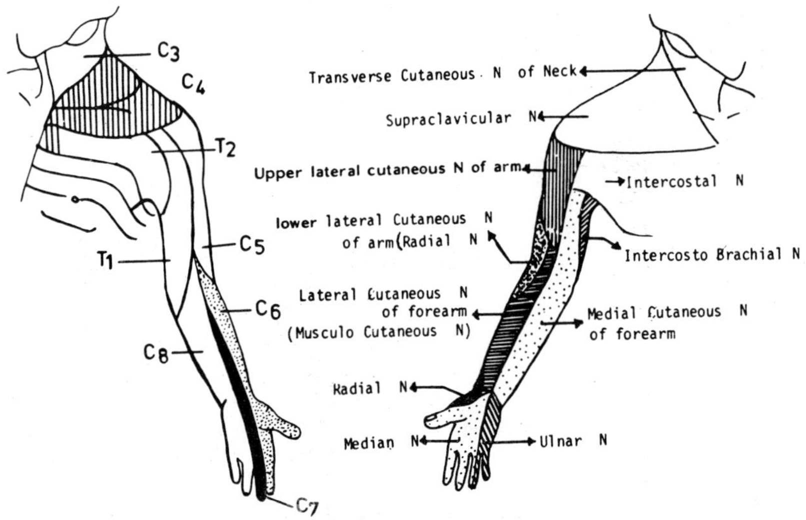

Fig. 15.15 (b_1) Dermatomes of front upper limb. Fig. 15.15 (b_2) Cutaneous supply of front of upper limb.

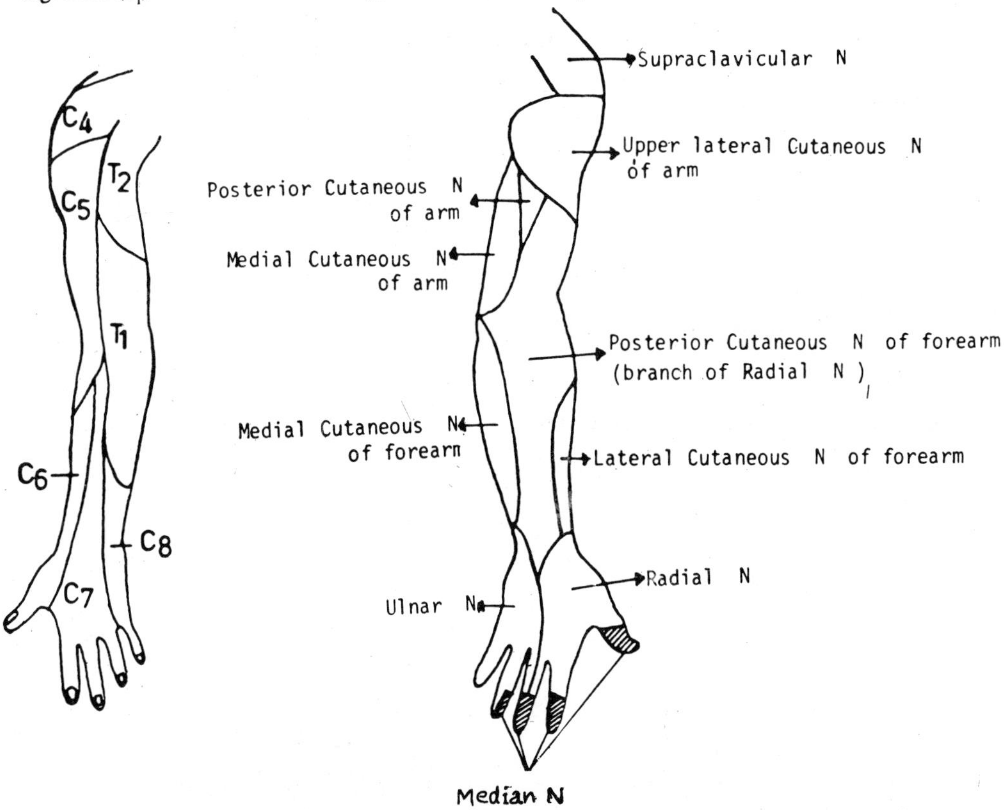

Fig. 15.15 (c_1) Dermatomes of back of upper limb. Fig. 15.15(c_2) Cutaneous supply of back of upper limb.

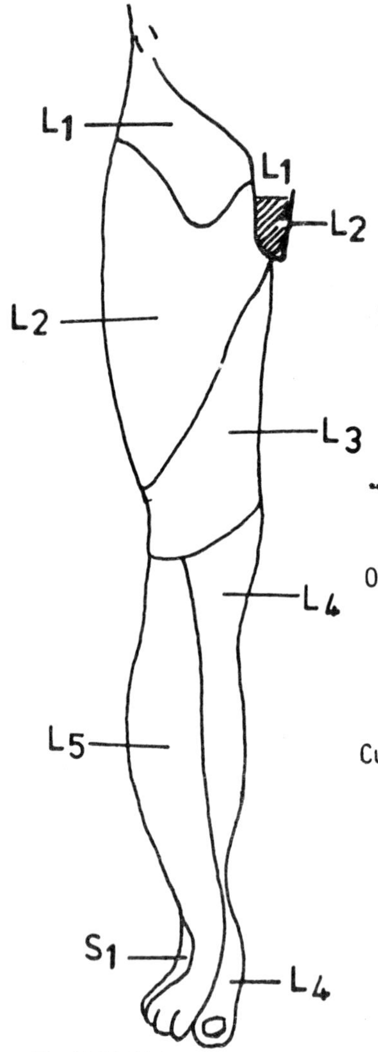

Fig. 15.15 (d_1) Dermatomes of front of lower limb.

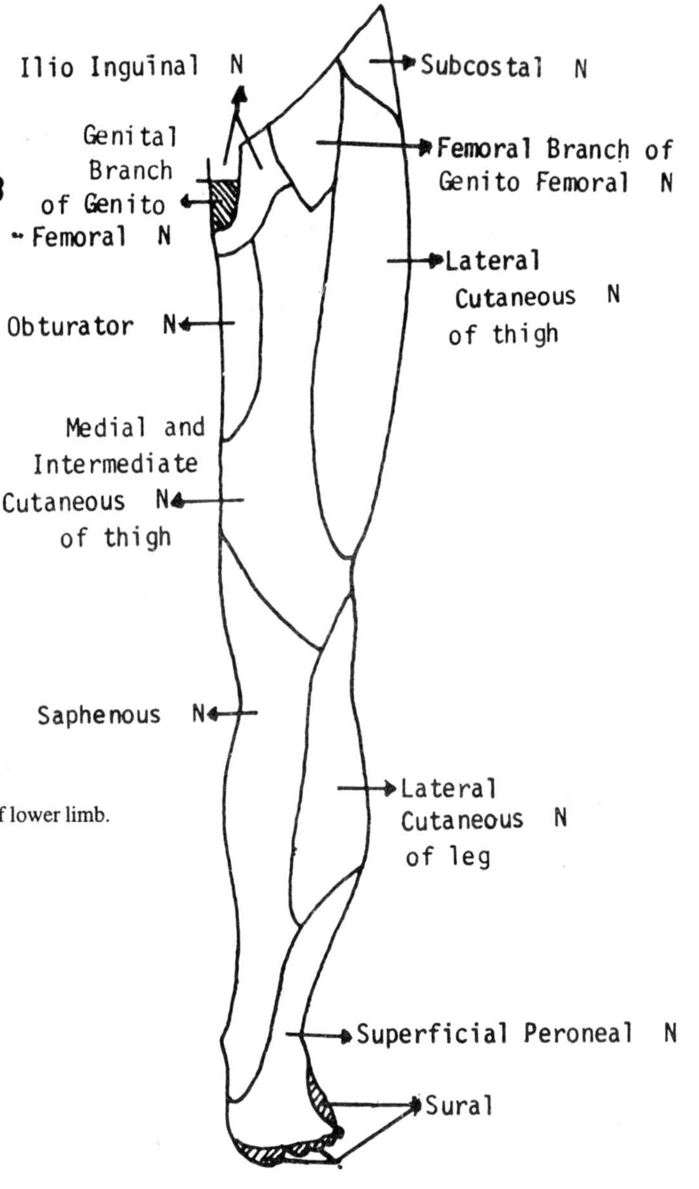

Fig. 15.15 (d_2) Cutaneous supply of front of lower limb.

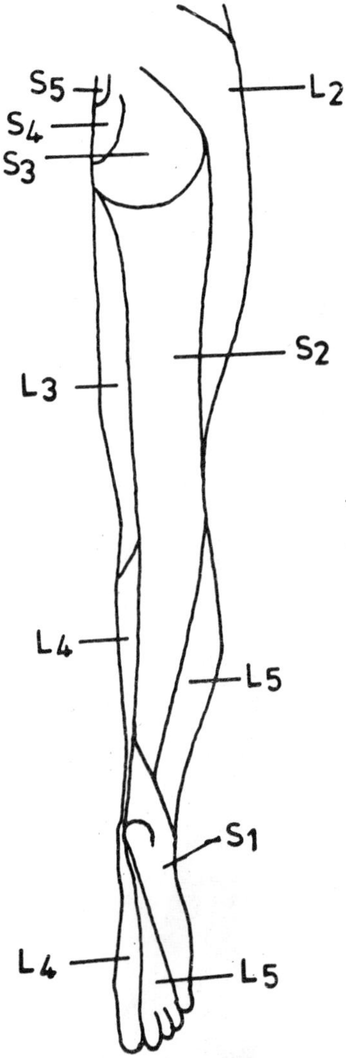

Fig. 15.15 (e_1) Dermatomes of back of lower limb.

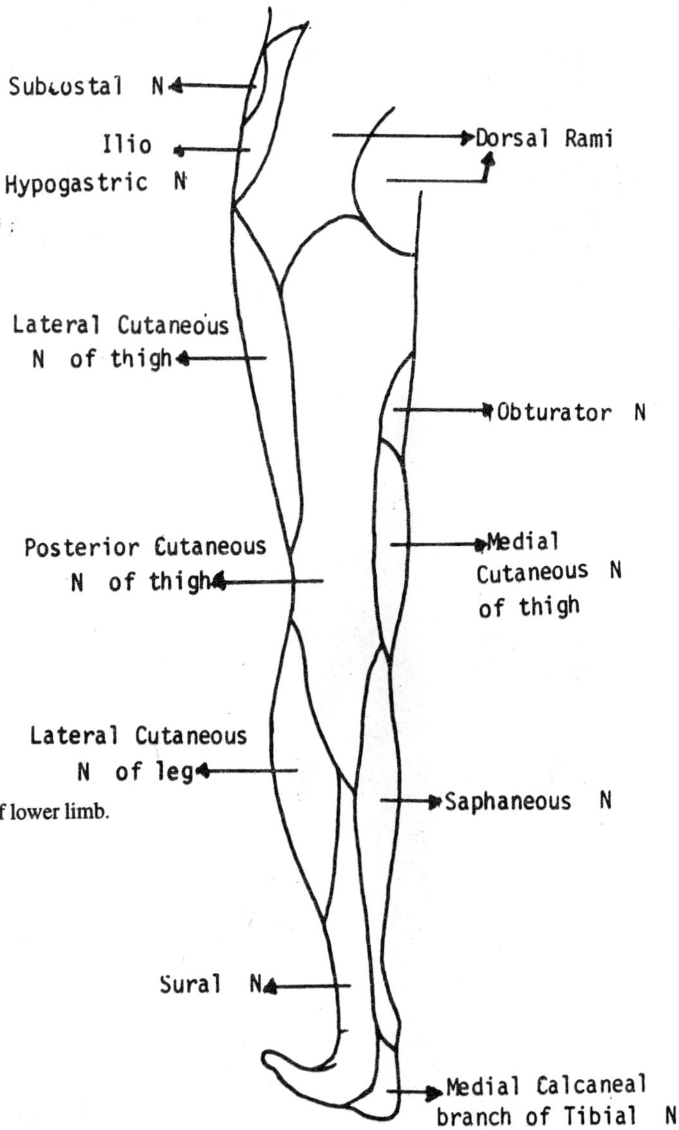

Fig. 15.15 (e_2) Cutaneous supply of back of lower limb.

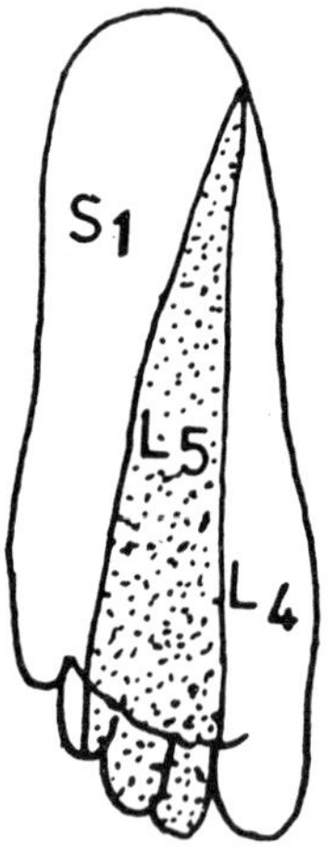

Fig. 15.15 (f_1) Dermatomes of foot.

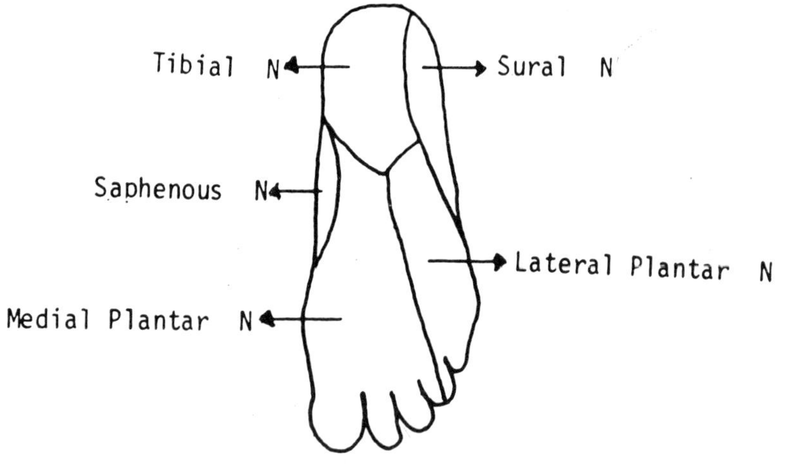

Fig. 15.15 (f_2) Cutaneous supply of foot.

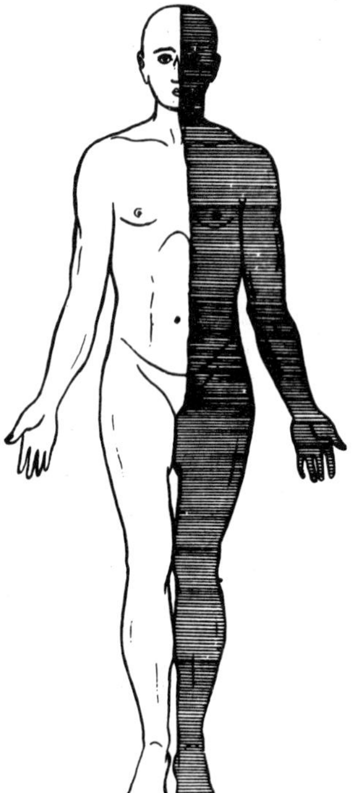

Fig. 15.16
Common forms of sensory loss
Fig. 15.16 (a) Hemianaesthesia is on contralateral side — lesion at thalamus.

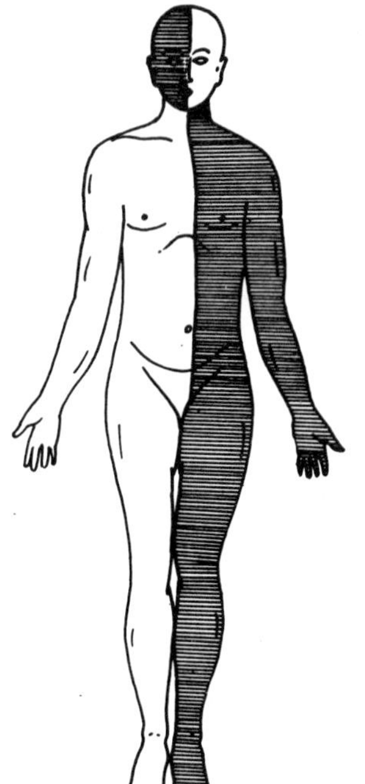

Fig. 15.16 (b)
Hemianaesthesia of body on ipsilateral side with anaesthesia of contralateral side of face-lesion at the level of medulla involving spinal tract of trigeminal (sensory nucleus) and sensory tracts due to involvement of vertebral artery.

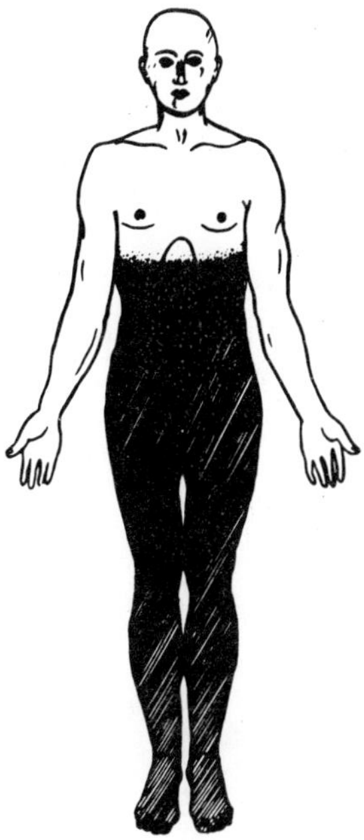

Fig. 15.16 (c)
Complete transection of spinal cord — Loss of all sensations and power below the level of lesion.

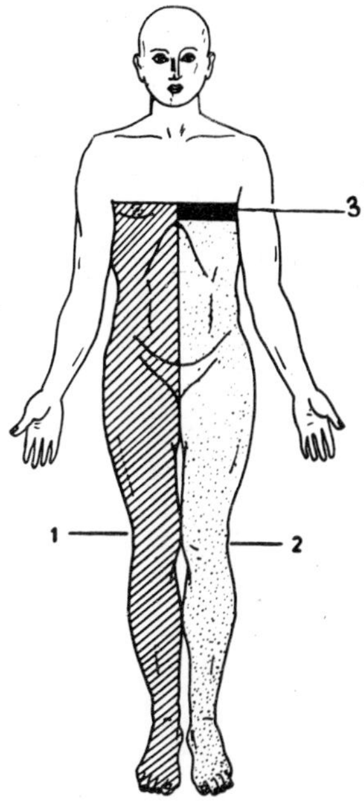

Fig. 15.16 (d)
Brown Sequard syndrome (hemisection (L)) side of spinal cord

1. Loss of pain temperature and touch to some extent on opposite side - as the fibres cross after entering spinal cord.
2. Loss of proprioceptive sensation on ipsilateral side as fibres do not cross till they reach medulla oblongata. Loss of power on ipsilateral side.
3. Band of hyperaesthesia on ipsilateral side above the level of loss of proprioceptive impulses.

sensations below definite level associated with ipsilateral loss of position, joint and vibrations. There is hyperalgesia on the ipsilateral side due to dorsal root lesion just below the level of transection. This occurs in hemisection of the spinal cord which is described as the Brown-Sequard syndrome. In Brown-Sequard syndrome, there is motor paralysis of the U.M.N. variety on the side of the lesion below its level. At the level of lesion, the anterior horn cells of the particular segment may be involved and there may be LMN paralysis of the muscles innervated by that segment.

Sensory involvement is as follows :

(a) Below the level of the lesion, the sensations carried by the posterior columns are lost up to the level of the lesion on the same side.

(b) On the same side, below the level of lesion, there may be a band of anaesthesia and loss of temperature sensation as the fibres crossing from these segments are affected before they cross to the opposite side.

(c) At the level of the lesion on the affected side, there will be a band of hyperalgesia due to the irritation of spinal segment.

(d) On the opposite side, there will be a loss of pain and temperature sensation from about 2 to 3 segments below the level of the lesion.

(e) Touch is less affected because it is carried by crossed and uncrossed fibres.

7. **Dissociated sensory loss:** Indicates a lesion of the intra-medullary variety, i.e., commonly syringomyelia which involves the fibres of pain and temperature sensation which are crossing to the opposite side.

The resultant loss is only of these sensations with touch and deep sensations being preserved (Jacket type sensory loss).

8. **Saddle anaesthesia:** Is the loss of sensa-

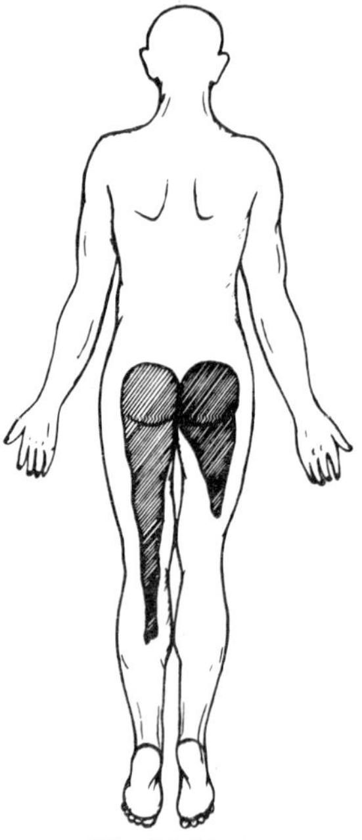

Fig. 15.16 (e)
Saddle shaped anaesthesia - lesion at cauda equina and conus medullaris.

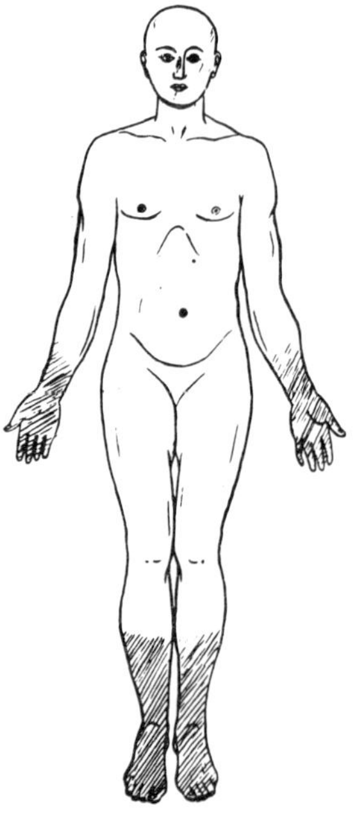

Fig. 15.16 (f)
Glove and stocking type of anaesthesia — polyneuritis.

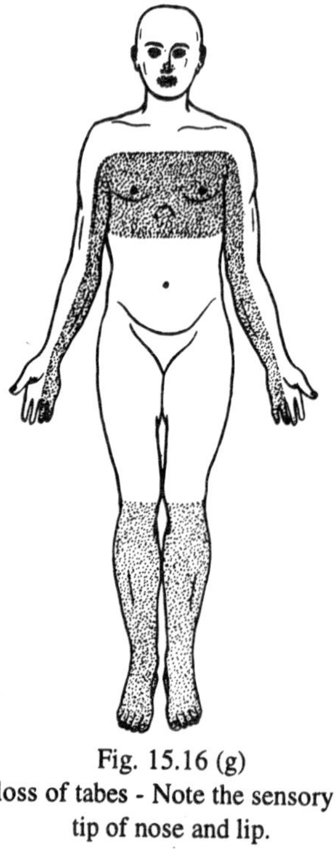

Fig. 15.16 (g)
Sensory loss of tabes - Note the sensory loss at the tip of nose and lip.

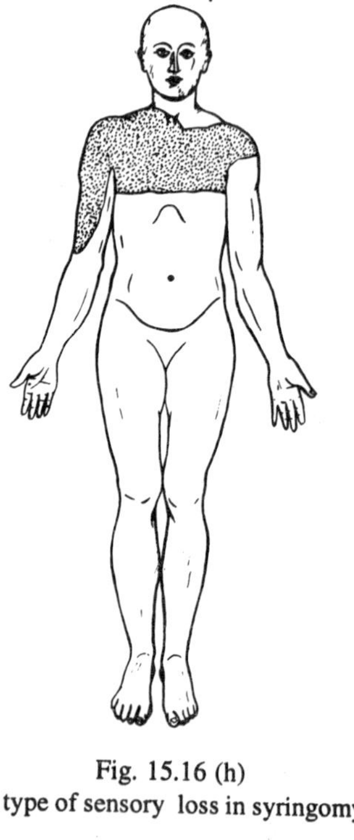

Fig. 15.16 (h)
Jacket type of sensory loss in syringomyelia.

Pl. 15.16a, b, c, d, e, f, g and h Groups of muscles acting at ankle joint and muscles of foot

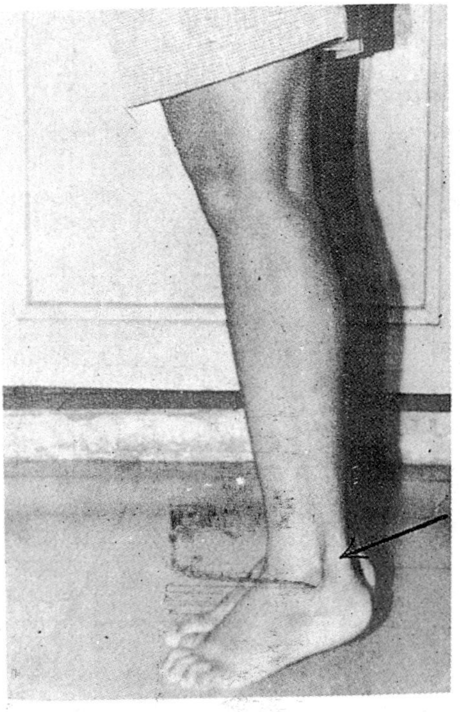

Pl. 15.16a Plantar flexor of ankle - Gastrocnemius tested by asking patient to walk on toes. Note the prominent tendon - tendo achillis.

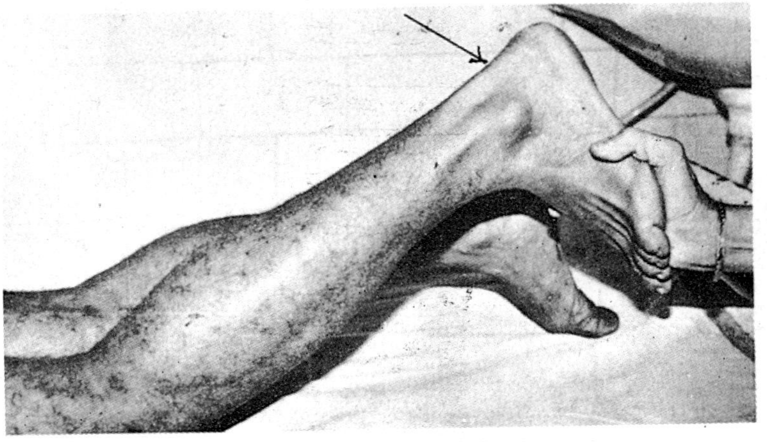

Pl. 15.16b Plantar flexors of ankle also tested by plantar flexion ((in prone position) against resistance.

(Refer to text for details)

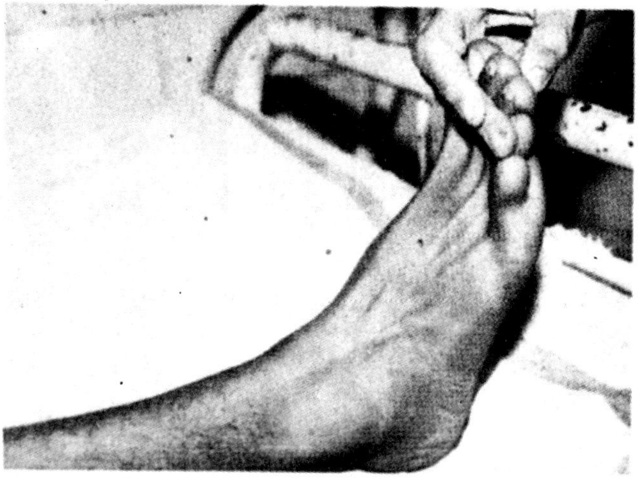

Pl. 15.16c Dorsiflexors of ankle - Tibialis anterior Extensor digitorum longus Extensor hallucis longus, Tested by applying resistance. Note that tendon of tibialis anterior stands out.

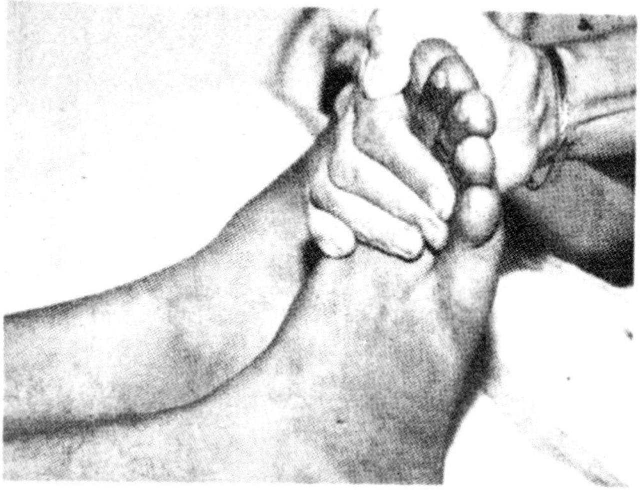

Pl. 15.16d Dorsiflexors of great toe and other toes.-Extensor hallucis longus brevis and Extensor digitorum longus

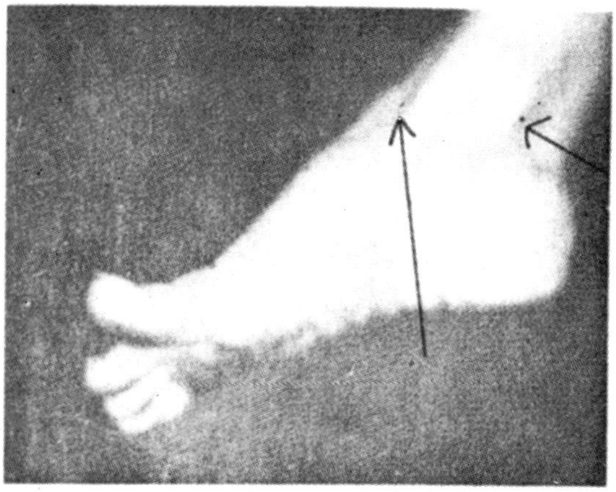

Pl. 15.16e Investors of foot - Tibialis anterior Tibialis posterior. Note the prominent tendons of tibialis anterior and posterior.

(Refer to text for details)

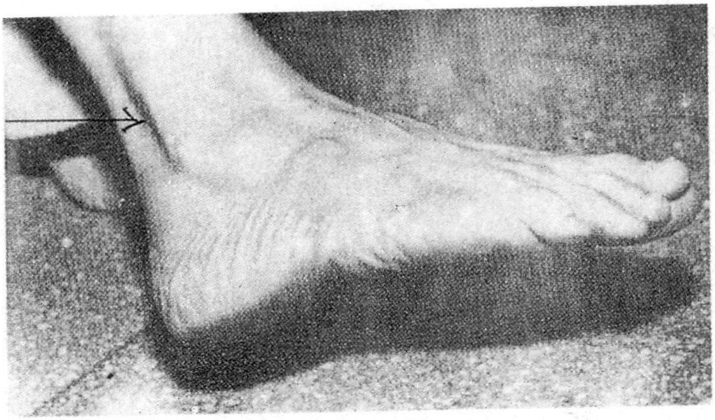

Pl. 15.16f Evertors of foot-Peronei.

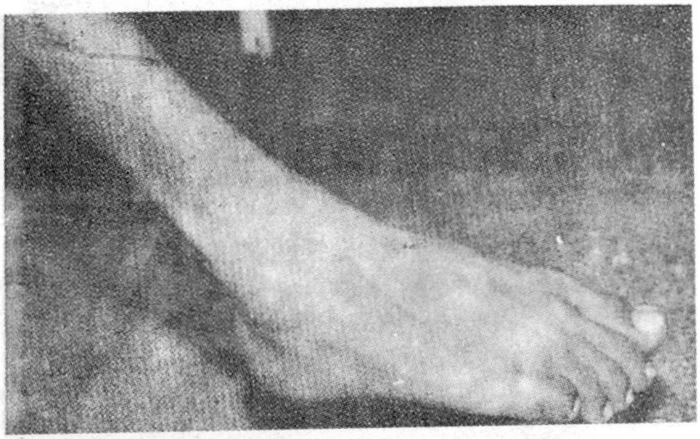

Pl. 15.16g Plantar flexor of toes - Flexor digitorum longus. Flexion at interphalangeal joints.

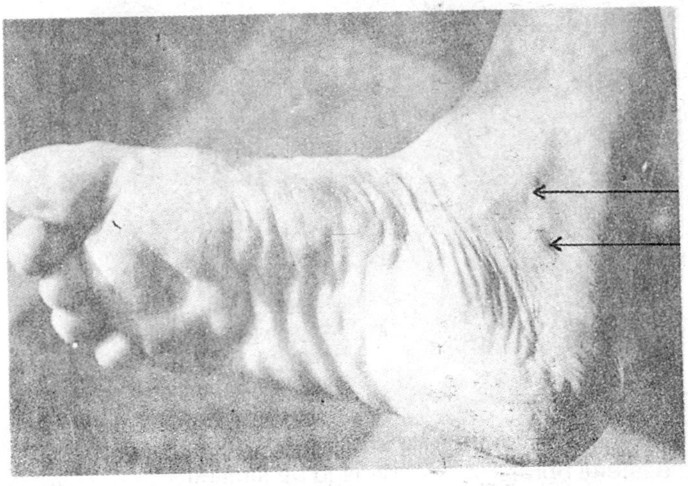

Pl. 15.16h Note the tendon of tibialis posterior at the posterior aspect of medial malleolus. The pulsating posterior tibial artery is well seen. (tendon and artery are shown by arrows.)

Pl. 151.17a, b Superficial reflexes (Refer to text for details)

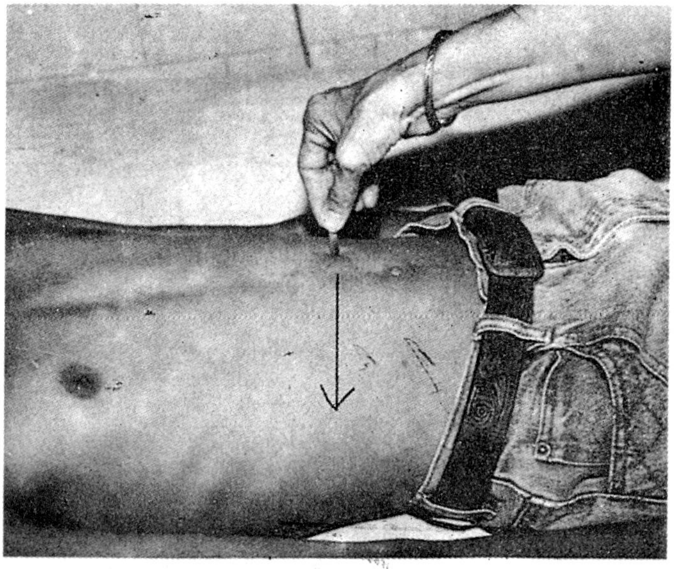

Pl. 15.17a Abdominal reflexes.
Note the direction in which the object is drawn across the abdominal wall.
Frm medial to lateral aspect.

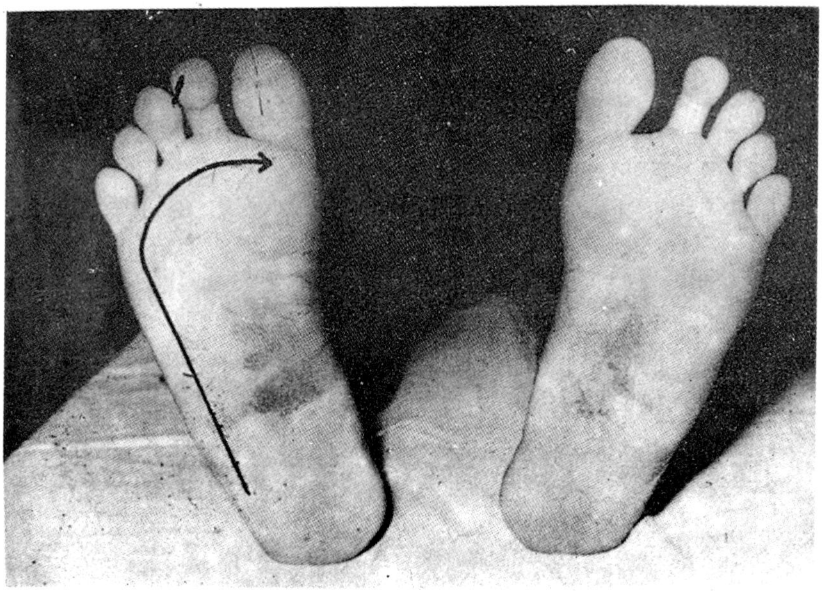

Pl. 15.17b Plantar reflex.
Note that extreme lateral border of the sole is to be stroked.

Pl. 15.18a, b, c, d, and e Deep Reflexes (Refer to text for details)

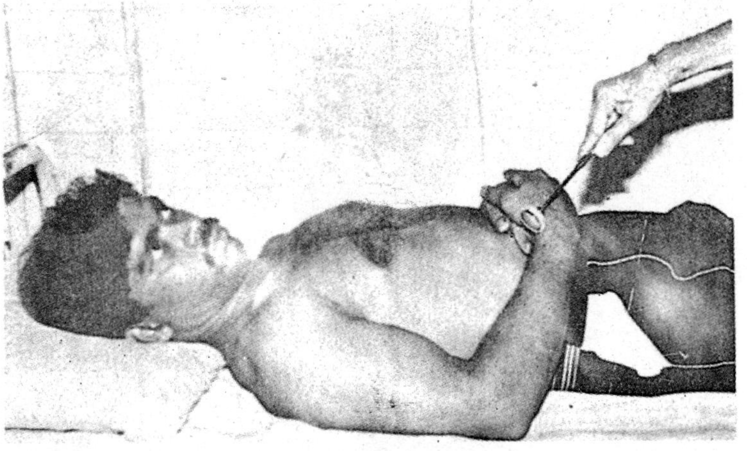

Pl. 15.18a Supinator reflex

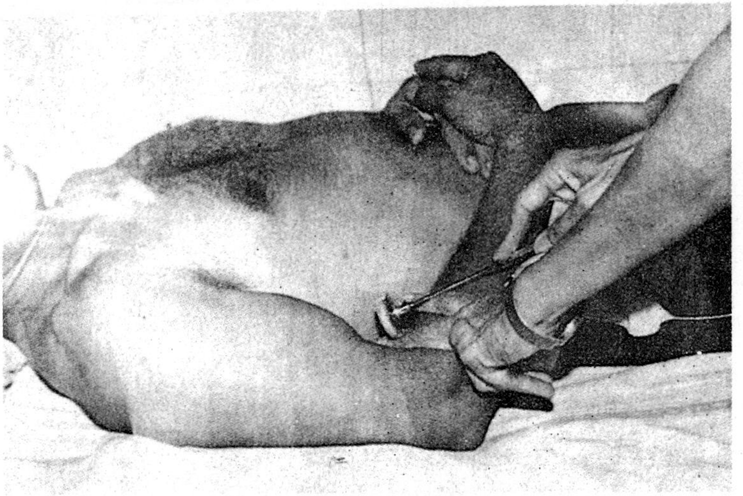

Pl. 15.18b Biceps reflex

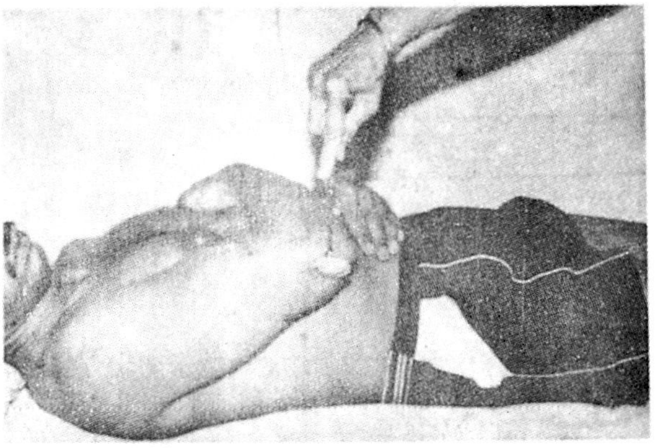

Pl. 15.18c Triceps reflex

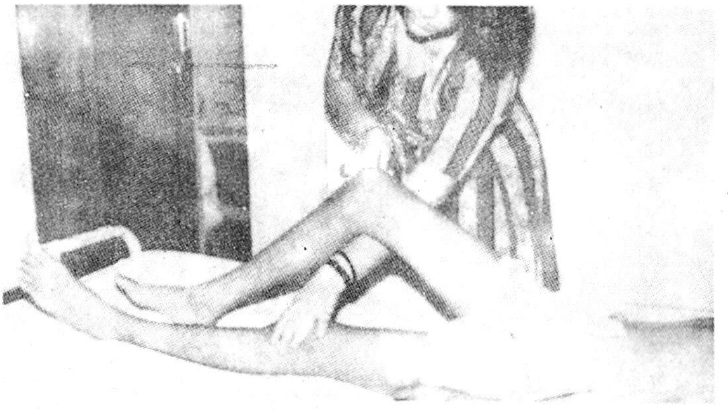

Pl. 15.18d Knee reflex

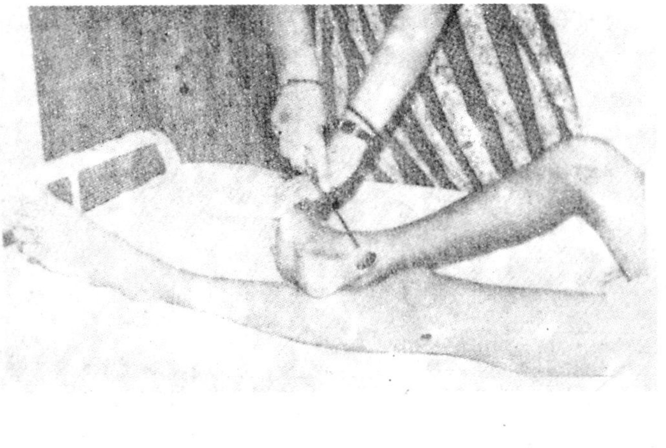

Pl. 15.18e Ankle reflex

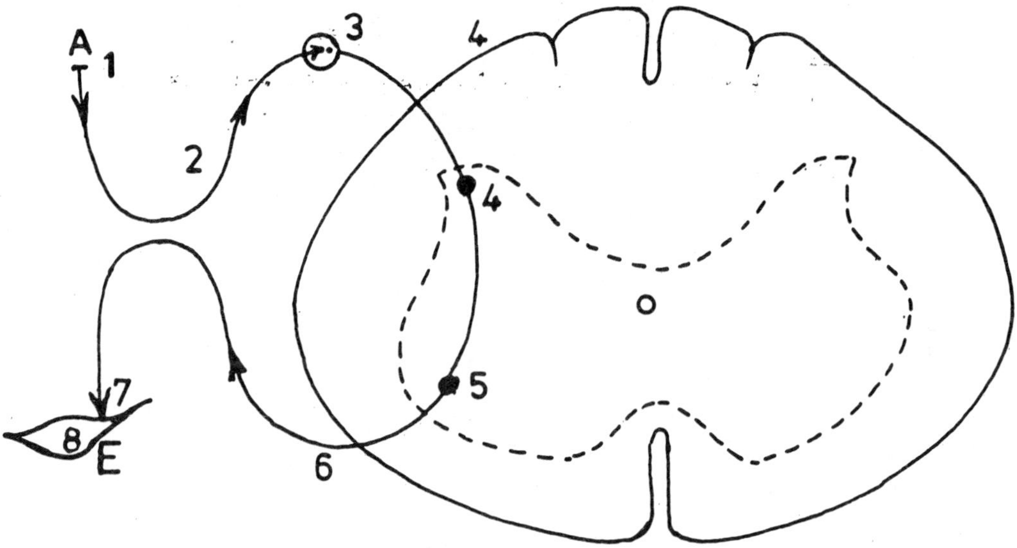

Fig. 15.17
Reflex arc and its components
A — Afferent E — Efferent
1. Receptor organ at the periphery, 2. Sensory nerve, 3. Sensory ganglion, 4. Spinal cord and posterior horn cell 5. Anterior horn cell, 6. Motor nerve, 7. Myoneural junction, 8. Muscle spindle

tions in the area supplied by $S_{3,4,5}$ nerve roots, due to lesion of cauda equina or conus medullaris.

9. **'Glove' and 'stocking' anaesthesia:** The name is given to the peripheral loss of sensations occurring in the distal parts of hands and feet due to peripheral neuropathy.

10. **Loss of joint and vibration sensations:** Occurs due to lesions of the posterior columns. Common causes are subacute combined degeneration, tabes dorsalis, Freidreich's ataxia, carcinomatous neuropathy and heavy metal (mercury) intoxications. Rarely seen in compression of the cord as an early or isolated symptom.

11. **Tabetic sensory loss:** There is a loss of sensation around the tip of the nose and lips and also over the chest and ulnar borders of both arms. This is accompanied by the loss of proprioceptive sensations (due to involvement of posterior columns) as described above.

V. **Reflexes :** Reflex action is tested clinically as:

1. Superficial reflexes,
2. Deep reflexes,
3. Visceral reflexes, which though included in the reflex action examination, are not usually examined clinically.

Important points in reflex activity: Every reflex depends upon the integrity of the following: (Fig.15.17)

1. A receptor organ on the periphery, 2. sen-

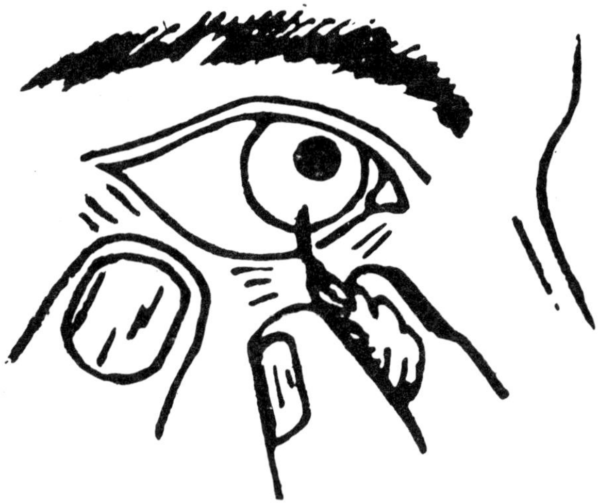

Fig. 15.18 : Method of elicitation of corneal reflex.

sory nerve which carries the impulse through, 3. the sensory ganglion to, 4. the spinal cord. In the spinal cord the impulse goes to, 5. the anterior horn cells or the motor cells from where the impulse is conducted, via, 6. the motor nerve to, 7. the myoneural junction to, 8. the muscle whose contraction (reaction) is judged as reflex activity.

In general, when considering deep reflexes, it can be stated that :

i. Reflexes above the level of the lesion in the spinal cord are normal.

ii. Those at the level of the lesion are absent.

iii. Those below the level of the lesion are brisk or exaggerated. In certain cases clonus can be elicited.

Superficial reflexes are abolished due to lesions at the local segment in the reflex arc. However, they are usually abolished by lesions of the pyramidal tracts. However, this does not hold true, at all times. Hence, the significance of the changes in these superficial reflexes for localising the lesion is limited.

The only important point of the greatest clinical importance is the plantar reflex. The very classical change in the plantar reflex from flexor to extensor response has the time-honoured clinical significance.

Superficial reflexes:

They are elicited by applying an irritating stimulus to either the skin or the mucous mem-brane. The contraction of muscles is the result of this reflex activity.

1. **Corneal reflex :** (Fig. 15.18) This should be tested by touching the cornea with a piece of cotton wool. The cotton wool should not touch the eye-lids or the conjunctiva. This is facilitated by asking the patient to look up as much as possible.

The normal response is bilateral blinking. No response will be present from either lid when the abnormal side is stimulated in the Vth lesions and a bilateral response is present when the normal side is stimulated.

In VIIth nerve lesions there is no response from the paralysed side, but there is blink reflex from the normal side.

Reflex arc : Afferent : trigeminal nerve
Efferent : facial nerve

2. **Conjunctival reflex:** Same procedure as above is repeated by touching the conjunctiva.

Reflex arc : Afferent : trigeminal nerve
Efferent : facial nerve

3. **Pharyngeal reflex** (gag reflex): Elicited by touching the back of the pharnyx by a swab (cot-

ton wool on a stick).

The result is the contraction of the pharyngeal muscles.

Reflex arc : Afferent : IXth nerve
Efferent : X-XIth (cranial) nerves.

4. **Palatal reflex:** When the soft palate is touched there is an elevation of the arch of the soft palate.

Reflex arc : Afferent: IXth nerve,
Efferent : X-XIth (cranial) nerves.

5. **Abdominal reflexes:** The patient should lie down relaxed and flat on his back. He should be explained what is to be done to him.

The abdominal muscles are stroked gently by a blunt object and not the sharp nail file which is the commonly used object. A pencil or key is slightly drawn across the abdominal wall from lateral to medial aspect and the contraction of the abdominal muscles in that particular quadrant is tested. The umbilicus is drawn in the same direction. (Fig.15.19) (Pl 15.17(a))

To avoid fallacies the pencil or the key should not be drawn in the direction in which the umbilicus will contract. In patients with absent abdominal reflexes, it will be possible to mechanically pull the umbilicus towards that quadrant giving a false positive result.

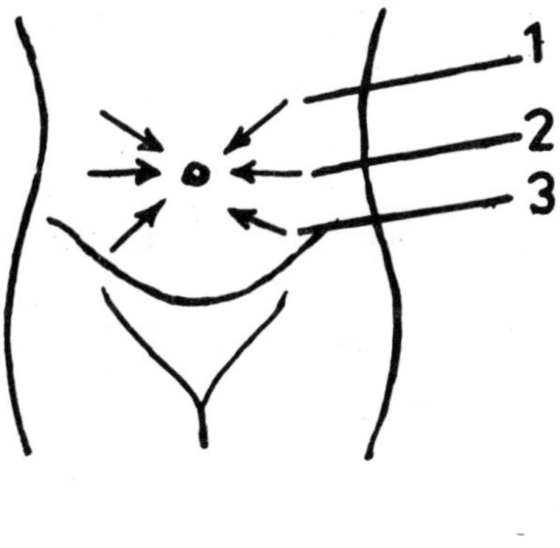

Fig. 15.19
Elicitation of superficial abdominal reflexes
Direction of elicitation is from lateral to medial
1. Upper segment - T_8
2. Middle segment - T_{10}
3. Lower segment - T_{12}

Reflex arc :

Upper abdominal : Afferent / Efferent } T_8 T_9

Umbilicus:

Lower abdominal : Afferent / Efferent } T_{11} T_{12}

The reflex arc is more elaborate with many interconnecting neurones. The impulses pass up to the motor cortex and then run down the pyramidal tract after local synapses. These connections and their interruption is the reason why the abdominal reflexes are absent in pyramidal damage; they return to normal later, even if the pyramidal lesion persists.

In LMN lesion as the main reflex arc is involved, abdominal reflexes are diminished or absent. They do not return to normal.

Interpretation of the result: A. Absent reflexes due to:

a. Local lesions of the reflex arc (LMN)

b. Pyramidal lesions above the level of the segmental innervation. Commonly occur due to spinal cord lesions or cerebral lesions. In multiple sclerosis the reflexes are lost early.

c. If the abdominal reflexes in a young person get easily fatigued, it. may be a sign of early pyramidal disease.

B. **Exaggerated or absent abdominal reflexes:** In absence of neurological lesions abdominal reflexes may be exaggerated in nervous patients.

The reflexes may not be elicited in patients with a very fat (obese) abdomen after multiple pregnancies, after repeated or major abdominal surgery, or in very tense patients who cannot relax their abdominal muscles.

6. **The Cremasteric reflex:** Stimulation of the inner surface of the thigh results in contraction of the cremasteric muscle leading to upward movement of the testicle and the scrotum.

The upper part of the thigh should be stroked downwards and inwards by an object when the patient is lying down.

Reflex arc: Afferent } L_1
Efferent

The cremasteric reflex is absent physiologically in old people and in patients with previous surgery on the scrotum.

It is lost pathologically in lesions of L_1 reflex arc and in pyramidal lesions.

7. **The Anal reflex:** The external sphincter of the anus contracts when the skin around it is stimulated by pin head.

Reflex arc: Afferent } $S_{4,5}$
Efferent

8. **The Plantar reflex:** (Fig. 15.20) (Pl. 15.17b)

Method of elicitation: When the patient is lying down, the lower limbs are slightly flexed at the knee, The thigh is externally rotated. The patient is told what is to be done, otherwise quite often if not explained there may be a violent jerking of the foot.

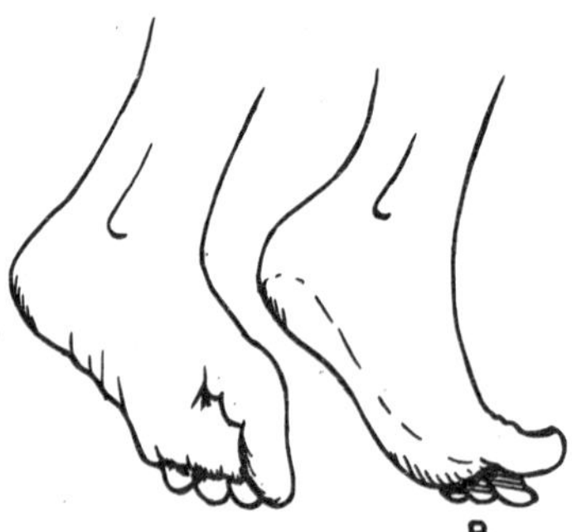

Fig. 15.20
Plantar Reflex
A = Normal flexor response
B = Extensor or Babinski response

The outer aspect of the sole is stroked by a blunt object (key-head is one of the best tools) and after reaching balls of the foot, i.e., heads of metatarsals, it is turned inwards to the medial side of the sole. (PL 15.17 b)

If there is no response due to a blunt object (as often happens in patients who have toughened skin because they work barefoot) a nail file or a sharp object may be required to elicit the response.

The normal plantar response is the flexor response in which the great toe is flexed at the metatarso-phalangeal joint. The other toes are flexed and bunched up or curled together.

The true flexor response is obtained not at the immediate start of the stimulus but after it is drawn up to 1/3rd of the distance, through which is has to travel.

Reflex arc : L_5 S_1 S_2

Interpretation: A normal response confirms the integrity of the local reflex arc of the pyramidal system.

A negative response may be present in patient with very tough skin (common in farmers and due to loss of local reflex arc either on the sensory or the motor side).

The extensor plantar response or the Babinski response:

This consists of extension of the great toe at the metatarso-phalangeal joint and the interphalangeal joint and a fanwise spreading of the other toes with slight dorsiflexion.

This must not be confused with 'the withdrawal reflex'. In sensitive patients any stimulus even with a blunt object results in withdrawal of the foot which includes dorsiflexion of the toes along with dorsiflexion at the ankle. The other toes do not fan out as in the true response and may show even plantar flexion. The withdrawal reflex can be easily recognised after practice. The real clinical difficulty arises in those reflexes which may in the end have to be labelled as equivocal response. The equivocal response consists of only dorsiflexion of the great toe without any change in the dorsi or plantar flexion of the toes. Sometimes the great toe may not contract but there may only be fanning of the toes. The patient with these signs will have to be followed up, to determine its true interpretation.

The extensor plantar response means a pyramidal lesion, It may not be due to structural damage and hence patient in coma or deep sleep may show extensor plantar response.

All the following clinical conditions can give rise to extensor plantar response.

a. Physiologically in infants.

b. In deep sleep.

c. In intoxications (either external: as alcohol poisoning, internal: metabolic comas).

d. After an epileptic convulsion.

e. In apneic conditions.

The dorsiflexion of the great toe which is the cardinal sign in the extensor plantar reflex can also be elicited in many other ways.

If the plantar surface cannot be stimulated for reasons like infection, injury, etc., the following signs can be tried. When they are positive, it means plantar response is extensor.

a. By applying downward pressure along the anterior surface of the tibia : Oppenheim's reflex.

b. By pressing one of the toes down and releasing it suddenly : Gonda's reflex.

c. By pressing the tendo-achillis : Schaefer's reflex.

d. By pressing the calf muslces : Gordon's reflex.

e. By striking around the lateral malleolus : Chaddock's reflex.

In complete transaction of the spinal cord with flexor paraplegia any stimuli anywhere below the level of the lesion results in a flexor response (i.e., bilateral extensor plantars, dorsiflexion of the ankles, flexion of the knees and hips). (Details given under paraplegia.)

2. **Deep reflexes:**

All the deep reflexes are tendon reflexes. They are elicited by a brisk tap on a tendon near a bony point after causing a stretch of muscle. The effect of this is a single short contraction of the appropriate muscles. The first stimulus, i.e., the tap by the percussion hammer stimulates the stretch receptors (sensory end organs) thereby starting the reflex process.

Basic principles involved in eliciting a proper tendon reflex are as follows :

a. The patient must relax his limbs and should not contract his muscles. He should be told 'to do nothing' and lie down passively. Any con- traction of the muscles (which are being tested) either voluntary or due to disease will modify the reflex.

b. The muscle group to be examined should be under a slight stretch but should not be pulled tight. (This tendency on the part of a beginner is most commonly seen when eliciting the ankle reflex.)

c. A good percussion hammer is used. A firm but quick stroke with the hammer will cause the appropriate stretch reflex.

i. **The jaw reflex:** The patient is told to open his jaw slightly (he should be told to allow it to sag rather than open it vigorously). The left forefinger of the examiner is kept below the lower lip and it is tapped with a hammer.

There is a slight upward jerk after the percussion stroke is over. There may be no response in many normal persons.

Jaw reflex is brisk in upper motor lesions above the pons seen in pseudo-bulbar palsy, motor neuron disease and multiple sclerosis.

ii. **The supinator reflex:** The hammer is struck at the lower end of the radius about 4-5 cms above the wrist. The result is a contraction of the brachioradialis and flexion of elbow. There may be a slight flexion of the fingers and contraction of the biceps. The position to elicit the reflex should be as shown in the photograph. Both the hands should be slightly flexed at the elbow, and they should rest lightly over the abdomen. The fingers should be slightly separated from each other. (Pl 15.18 a,b,c,d,e)

Root value : C_{5-6}

iii. **The biceps reflex:** The position to be used is the same as described for the supinator reflex. Also the patient's forearm can rest across the examiner's hand by putting it in a semi-flexed semi-prone position.

The examiner's finger is kept on the biceps tendon and the usual sharp tap is given. The result is contraction of the biceps muscle causing flexion of the elbow.

Root value: $C_{5,6}$

iv. **The triceps reflex:** The patient's arm is drawn across his body by the examiner. The arm should rest lightly across the trunk and then the tap is given on the triceps tendon. This results in contraction of the triceps with extension of the elbow.

Root value: C_{6-7}

v. **The pectoral reflex:** The arm is slightly adducted. The tip of the index finger of the examiner is kept on the tendon of the pectoral muscle near the insertion. The finger is tapped by the hammer to know the response of contraction of the muscle.

Root value: $C_{5,6,7,8}$ and T_1

vi. **The finger flexion reflex:** The patient's hand should rest with the palm upwards and the examiner's fingers should interlock with the fingers of the patient. The fingers of the examiner are tapped with the hammer causing a flexion of the pafient's fingers.

Root value: $C_{6,7}T_1$

vii. **The knee reflex:** The patient who is lying in bed is examined as follows. Both the knees are flexed by putting the examiner's hand below the knee joints and lifting the legs off the bed. The patient is told to relax his legs. The patellar tendon is then tapped with the hammer resulting in a contraction of the quadriceps causing extension of the knee.

The same reflexes can also be elicited easily in a sitting position. The legs are allowed to dangle freely over the edge of the bed. The procedure of tapping the patellar tendon is obviously the same. This may be a better position to elicit pendular knee reflex (in cerebellar ataxia).

Root value. $L_{2,3,4}$

viii. **The ankle reflex:** The leg of the patient should be flexed slightly at the knee and externally rotated. The foot is then dorsi-flexed gently and not vigorously which will cause severe stretching of the tendon.

The tendo-achillis is then tapped with the hammer. The consequent contraction of the gastrocnemius results in plantar flexion of the foot.

Root value: L_5 S_1

Reinforcement:

Absent reflexes are of pathological significance. However, many times there is no contrae tion of the muscles during reflex testing in abnormal person. The 'reinforcement' is used and reflexes can be elicited properly.

Usual cause of such physiological absence is a subconscious tensing of the muscles of the patient or it can even happen in a very well-built muscular individual. If other muscles are put under active strain then the muscles which are being examined relax. This is the basis of the 'reinforcement'.

When the upper limb reflexes are tested the patient should be asked to clench the teeth tightly. If the lower limb reflexes are being tested he should be asked to interlock the fingers and pull them against one another.

Interpretation of deep reflexes:

In general, it can be stated that the reflexes above the level of the lesion are normal, those at the level of the lesion are modified, e.g. (inversion of the supinator) and those below the level are exaggerated. There may be appearance of abnormal reflexes which are not present in a normal person.

Reflexes: are diminished in lesions of

Sensory nerve - Neuropathy

Sensory root - Tabes dorsalis

Spinal cord - Transverse lesion (viral, compression, etc).

Anterior horn cells - Poliomyelitis, motor neuron disease

Anterior root - Compression of the cord, cervical spondylitis

Peripheral motor nerve - Trauma, neuritis

Myoneural junction - Myasthenia gravis

Muscle - Myopathies -muscular dystrophies.

Or absent in :

a. Normal individuals (appear after reinforcement)

b. Lesions in the reflex arc

c. After neural shock : Immediately after a sudden catastrophe of the nervous system, either traumatic or vascular, all reflex activity is suspended for some time (sometimes for weeks).

d. With rigidity (pathological) : In very severe or advanced extra-pyramidal disease, the reflexes are diminished because the patient cannot relax the muscles.

e. In local deformities or contractures : These may follow trauma or disease. Even in advanced spastic paraplegia, this difficulty is encountered. Where the reflexes should be brisk they cannot be elicited due to contractures.

Modification of the reflexes :

a. **Inversion of the supinator reflex :** In C_5 lesions the normal supinator reflex is absent. There is no contraction of the brachio-radialis. However, there is a flexion of the fingers, espe-cially the index and middle fingers. The biceps reflex is absent while the triceps reflex is exag-gerated. As opposed to this, a brisk supinator reflex, flexion of the fingers is exaggerated but the brachio-radialis contraction is also very brisk and hence this should not be mistaken for inversion.

b. **Delayed relaxation in myxoedema:** In myxoedema the relaxation of the contracted muscles is slow and is observed easily in calf muscles.

Exaggeration of deep reflexes:

a. Bilateral symmetrical brisk reflexes with flexor plantar: In nervous individuals. In anxiety states. May be in thyrotoxicosis.

b. Brisk reflexes: (pathological) Due to pyramidal (U.M.N.) lesions.

c. Prolonged reflex: Pendular reflex in cerebellar disease and in chorea : Hung up reflex in chorea and myxoedema. (The involuntary movement is superimposed on the contracting muscles when the reflex is elicited.)

d. Clonus may be present due to marked exaggeration. The muscle which is stretched goes into clonic contractions.

i. Ankle clonus : The leg is flexed at the knee and it is supported by the examiner's hand. The foot is then dorsi-flexed by the other hand sharply and abruptly and a firm (but not too hard) pressure is put on the foot.

A clonic repetitive jerky rhythmic contraction of the calf muscles is seen. In some normal individuals a false clonus is seen by obtaining a few clonic jerks which are not well sustained.

ii. Patellar clonus : The leg is kept extended. The patella is then pushed sharply downwards by the thumb and the fore-finger. The pressure is maintained resulting in rhythmic clonic contraction of the quadriceps muscle.

Other uncommon reflexes:

a. **The Hoffman reflex:** The patient's hand is held with the fingers slightly flexed. The middle finger is then held between the examiner's fingers and a short downward flick is given. When the reflexes (deep) are brisk, the thumb will flex and adduct. This is a helpful diagnostic sign in .unilateral U.M.N. disease.

b. **Wartenberg's sign:** The patient's hand is held by the examiner in a supinated position and the fingers of the patient and the examiner are interlocked. Both then should try to flex the fingers against each other's resistance. Normally, the thumb and the terminal phalanges may bend slightly.

In pyramidal lesions, the thumb adducts and flexes strongly.

c. **Rossolimo's reflex:** The patient lies with the leg extended — the foot is slightly dorsiflexed and the ball of the foot is then tapped with the hammer.

In spastic state, there is a brisk contraction of the toes.

16. Central Nervous System — Common Disorders Encountered

HEMIPLEGIA

Definition: Weakness on one side of the body. Usually lower part of the face, hand and leg affected.

Causes of hemiplegia:

Trauma: Direct - immediately after trauma
Delayed - subdural haematoma
Infection: Encephalitis, meningitis (tuberculous and non-tuberculous); syphilitic basal meningitis, cerebral abscess.
Vascular : Haemorrhage, thrombosis, embolism, hypertensive, encephalopathy.
Tumour : Benign
Malignant : Primary secondary
Degenerative: multiple sclerosis, diffuse sclerosis.
Hysterical.

A proper line of inquiry will enable the examiner to assess the nature and the site of the lesion.

The method of questioning should be adopted as follows (after ascertaining age, sex, occupation).

(A) Motor weakness:

1. When did the weakness start?

2. Whether the weakness has affected all the three components or is the hemiplegia partial? because

a. A dense hemiplegia affecting all the three components will usually mean an internal capsule lesion,

b. Two of the components affected severely and the third only partially will be due to lesion in subcortical area (corona radiata).

c. One component more affected than the other two (monoplegia) or the adjoining component very minimally affected will be due to cortical damage.

The explanation of the above statements can be readily understood if one recalls the anatomy of the pyramidal tracts.

As their origin is in the motor cortex, the areas which govern the face, the arm and the leg are widely separated from each other. Hence, a single lesion produces a pure motor monoplegia.

In the corona-radiata or the subcortical region, the fibres governing these areas come nearer each other but still are widely separated. Hence, a lesion here affects more than one component. These components will always be adjoining, i.e., face and arm or arm and leg and not face and leg because of the relations of the fibres to each other.

As the fibres are densely packed together in the internal capsule, a lesion here produces a dense hemiplegia.

As the immediate relations of these pyramidal tracts are ascending sensory radiation and optic radiation fibres, lesions in internal capsular area may give rise to complaints of cortical type of sensory loss or homonymous hemianopia.

3. Onset: How was the onset of weakness?

a. Instantaneous: The cause will be probably embolism.

b. Very acute: In a few minutes to half an hour. This is likely to be due to cerebral haemorrhage.

c. Gradual : Over a period of hours or one or two days. This is probably possible due to cerebral thrombosis. Rarely, the weakness progresses in a staccato fashion. This is primarily due to both weakness and involvement of the components and is partial. Then it progresses in a stepwise fashion.

This is caused by internal carotid artery thrombosis.

d. Very gradual over a period of days proceeding from one component to the other, due to space occupying lesions.

4. Has the weakness spread from the originally affected parts? Usually seen in space-occupying lesions affecting the cerebral cortex where one component, say the leg, is affected at first and then the arm and later on the face will be affected. This will point towards the way the lesion has progressed.

5. Is the weakness stable from the time of onset? Has the power improved since the onset? If so, in which muscles is it steadily improving worsening?

(a) If the patient suffering from vascular lesion comes to the examiner after a few days, it is quite possible that his weakness has improved. This is either due to relief of the initial cerebral edema or due to improvement in collateral blood vessels supplying the affected part. The muscles governing the movements of fingers and hand improve last, if at all. The prehensile movements of thumb, i.e., movements like picking objects and counting fingers improve last.

In general, the movements of flexion in the upper limbs and extension in the lower limbs tend to recover faster.

(b) The weakness may remain stable without any improvement in a severe vascular lesion or following trauma to the central nervous system.

(c) A spacc-occupying lesion will cause a steadily deteriorating paralysis.

B. H/o. other components of the motor system:

1. Is there any wasting of muscles in affected parts? An upper motor neuron lesion which is the usual cause of hemiplegia does not cause any wasting. However, a disuse atrophy of the affected muscles may be seen in long-standing cases of hemiplegia.

2. Does he complain of severe stiffness of the affected muscles? The patient may answer in the affirmative to this question only after a few days or weeks. In the initial stages, the muscle tone may decrease due to the neural shock or the affected parts may completely paralyse.

3. Usually, tremors or other involuntary movements are not seen in hemiplegia.

C. Sensory system complaints:

1. Is there any tingling or numbness of the affected parts or are there any other parasthesia? Usually, the patient complaints of cramps or stiffness of the extremities due to the accompanying hypertonia of the muscles.

2. Is there any loss of sensations? The loss of sensation in a hemiplegic patient means the lesion is of the cortical origin, i.e., the patient loses the appreciation of passive movements and posture, and sensation of light touch, especially its localisation along with the power of stereognosis. The pain and temperature sensations are usually unaffected.

However, it is very common for patients to complain of diminished sensations on the affected side of the body which should suggest an involvement of ascending sensory radiation fibres.

D. Complaints due to sphincter involvement:

Were there any disturbances of sphincter control, especially at the onset? Was the patient catheterised initially?

The patient may complain of retention of urine in the acute stage for which he had to be catheterised. Usually, recovery occurs within 2-3 days.

H/o. such a complaint will point towards a fairly massive or sudden lesion in acute stage.

E. H/o. Cranial nerve involvement:

Supranuclear facial palsy involving the lower half of the face is almost always present in hemiplegia and H/o. its involvement should always be asked for as mentioned above.

Similarly, hypoglossal nerve involvement causing a supranuclear type of weakness of the tongue on the side of paralysis is also sometimes a feature of hemiplegia.

In addition to this, an inquiry regarding certain specific cranial nerve affection on the opposite side of the paralysis should be conducted carefully.

Any positive history will immediately point towards the site of the lesion. So also a negative history must be mentioned as then the lesion has to be higher in the pyramidal system than the brainstem. (Details given under examination.)

F. H/o. Convulsions:

1. H/o. Jacksonian or focal convulsions: If the history of focal convulsion is present the lesion has to be in cerebral motor cortex. The place where the focal fit starts should be noted as it will indicate whether the cortical lesion is in the area of face, arm or leg. A negative history does not rule out a cortical lesion.

2. H/o. generalised convulsions : These are usually present at the onset and indicate that the nature of lesion is massive or that it is sudden in onset.

G. H/o. coma:

Any cerebral lesion can cause a loss of consciousness at the onset of hemiplegia; but if the patient does not become conscious or if the unconsciousness gradually worsens, it is usually due to either cerebral haemorrhage or space occupying lesion.

H. History which may indicate the cause of the lesion:

1. **H/o. trauma:** This may cause hemiplegia either due to pressure by a depressed skull fracture or by haemorrhage or laceration of the cerebral tissue. Subdural haematoma is not an uncommon cause of hemiparesis and H/o. trauma a few months ago has to be elicited by careful inquiry. This may not be forthcoming if the trauma was relatively minor or if the patient was in an alcoholic stupor.

2. **H/o. infections:** Tuberculous meningitis, and encephalitis are the two common infective disease processes causing hemiplegia. The patient will complain of high fever, headache and vomiting due to these diseases.

3. **H/o. vascular affection:** H/o. hypertension, diabetes mellitus, syphilis and tobacco consumption has to be asked as these will more commonly cause a vascular type of hemiplegia.

H/o. rheumatic heart disease, if present, may point towards an embolus as the cause of hemiplegia.

4. H/o. headache, vomiting, and blurring of vision without fever may reveal space-occupying lesion as the cause. Of course the same symptoms along with fever will point towards either meningitis or encephalitis or cerebral malaria.

Clinical signs in hemiplegia:

These can be divided into the so-called negative and positive signs. Negative signs are those which are due to loss of nervous function, while positive signs are due to overaction of the other centres. This overaction modifies and adds to the abnormality, i.e., paralysis. Hence, they are known as positive signs.

Negative signs:

1. Ocular movements: Conjugate deviation of the eyes away from the side of paralysis. Though the eye movements are governed by bilateral cerebral innervation, there is *temporary* weakness on the affected side. Hence, overaction of the muscles on the normal side pulls the eyeballs away from the side of paralysis.

2. Position of the head: Head is also turned in the same direction as the eyes for the same reasons as given above. In a patient with acute hemiplegia the eyes and the head point towards the side of the lesion, away from the side of the paralysis.

3. Cranial nerves: Weakness of IIIrd, VIth, VIIth, XIIth cranial nerves should be looked for. This is important for localisation of the lesion.

4. Facial movements: Supranuclear VIIth nerve weakness on the side of paralysis.

5. Movements of lower jaw, tongue and soft palate: Affected temporarily on the side of paralysis. Supranuclear XIIth nerve paralysis may persist.

6. Respiratory movementsts: Amplitude of respiratory movement on the paralysed side is

diminished.

7. Movements of limbs : Affected on the paralysed side.

8. Gait: Hemiplegic gait.

Positive signs:

1. Hypertonia : Clasp knife type spasticity due to overaction of extra-pyramidal system (especially of the central reticular formation).

2. Posture: Result of overaction of the more powerful (more spastic) group of muscles.

3. Reflexes: Deep reflexes exaggerated, abdominal reflexes absent on affected side, extensor plantar response.

Localisation of lesion: (Fig. 16.1 a,b,c & d)

Pyramidal tracts can be affected at the following sites :

1. **Cortex:**

(a) Monoplegia,

(b) Monoplegia with slight affection of parts controlled by adjoining cortical area,

(c) Jacksonian convulsions.

(d) No sensory loss — depending on area.

2. **Subcortex:**

(a) Weakness predominant in one of the three members (lower half of the face, arm or leg) but the, adjoining member partly affected,

(b) Cortical type of sensory loss,

(c) Crossed homonymous hemianopia on the opposite side.

3. **Internal capsule:**

(a) Dense hemiplegia (all three members affected),

(b) Cortical type of sensory loss may be present.

4. **Mid-brain:**

(a) Crossed hemiplegia, IIIrd nerve paralysis on the opposite side of hemiplegia condition is called Weber's syndrome.

(b) Supranuclear VIIth nerve palsy on the side of paralysis present.

5. **Pons:**

(a) Crossed hemiplegia.

i. Millard/Gubbler syndrome, VIIth nerve lower motor neuron paralysis on the opposite side of hemiplegia,

ii. Foville's syndrome, VIth and VIIth nerve: lower motor neuron type of paralysis on the opposite side of hemiplegia.

(b) Horner's syndrome on the same side.

(c) No supranuclear VIIth nerve weakness on the side of paralysis.

6. **Medulla:**

(a) Crossed hemiplegia : Jackson's syndrome, L.M.N. type of XIIth nerve and tongue weak-ness on the opposite side of paralysis.

(b) Lesion below the medulla but above the Vth cervical segment.

(c) No facial nerve involvement (UMN or LMN).

7. **Spinal cord:** Spinal hemiplegia due to high cervical lesions:

Hemiplegia will always be dense when the lesion is either in the brainstem or cervical spinal cord as the pyramidal fibres are closely packed together.

Spinal hemiplegia can hardly ever be confused with hemiplegia due to sub-cortical lesion where the involvement of the two components will not be complete or at least one component will be partially affected. In spinal hemiplegia cranial nerves are spared except for cranial accessory.

Importance of involvement of facial nerve in lesions at different levels is as follows.

(a) There will be a supranuclear facial palsy on the opposite side of the lesion (same side as the arm or leg weakness) in mid-brain lesions as supranuclear pyramidal fibres governing the opposite facial nerve nucleus cross at the lower level of mid-brain.

(b) In paralysis caused by pontine lesions or lesions below the pons, there will not be any affection of the face on the side of paralysis as the fibres governing the facial nucleus on the opposite side have already crossed.

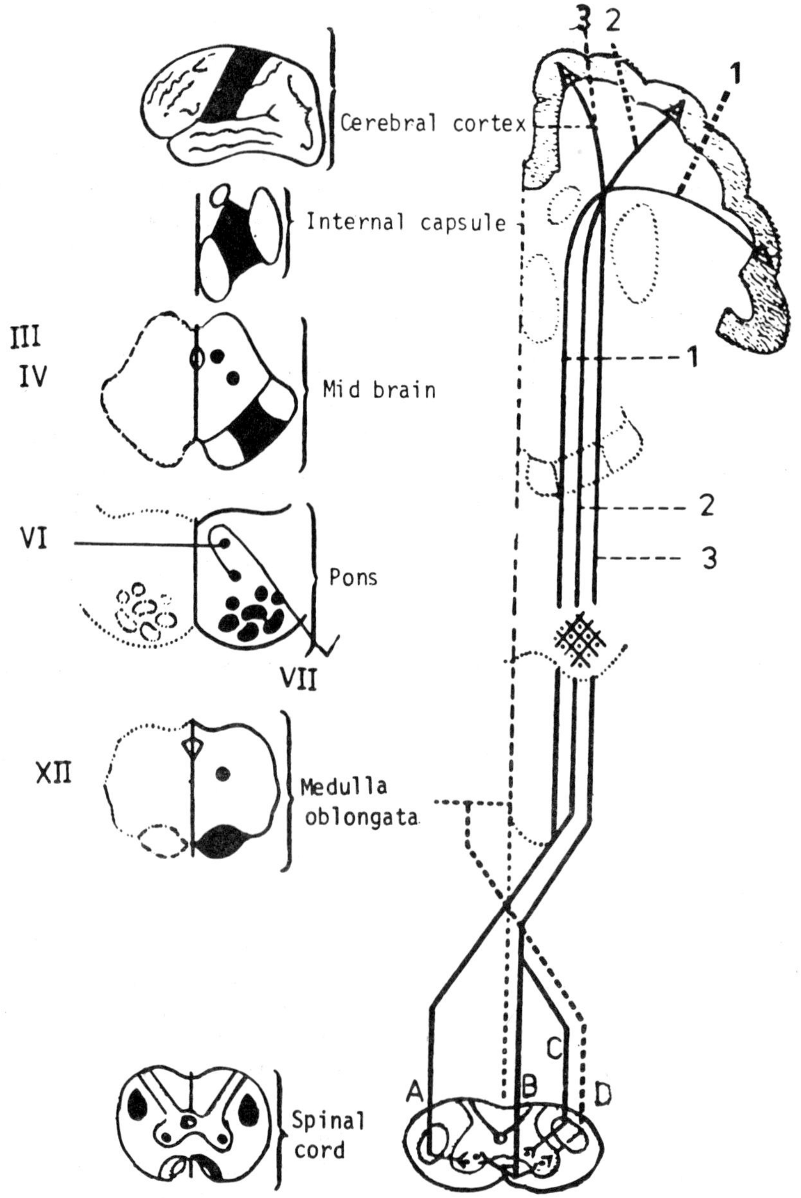

Fig. 16.1 (a)
Cortico Spinal tracts - their origin and course.

1. Fibres for head; 2. Fibres for trunk; 3. Fibres for leg.

A. Crossed fibres - forming lateral cortico spinal tract.

B. Uncrossed fibres - forming anterior cortico spinal tract but ultimately fibres cross to opposite side.

C. Uncrossed fibres - forming lateral cortico spinal tract.

D. Crossed fibres - from opposite side forming lateral spinal tract.

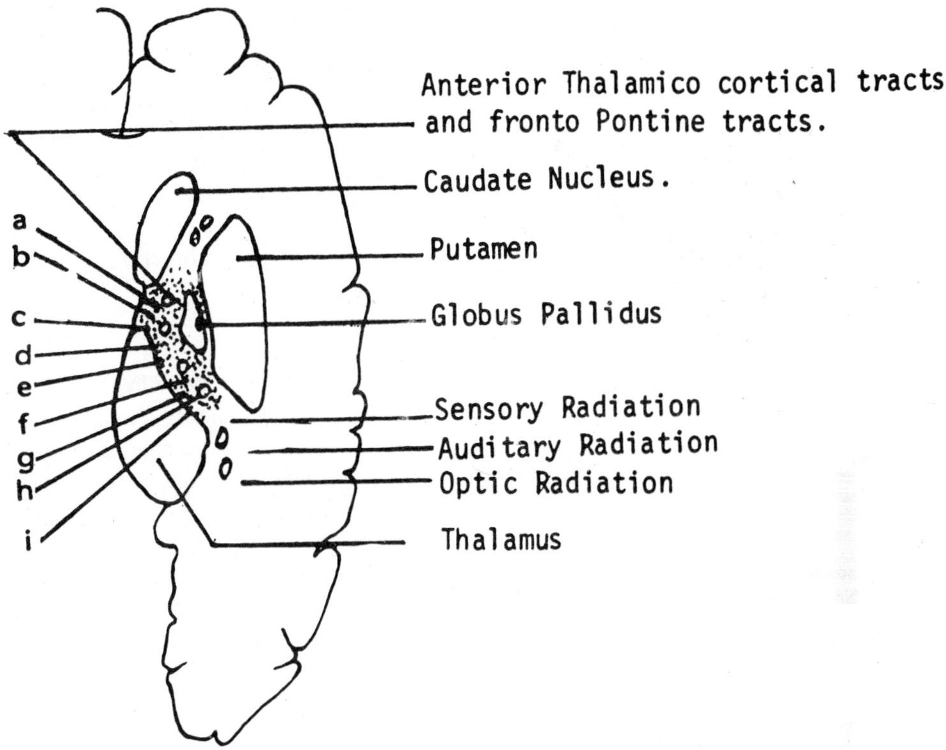

Fig. 16.1 (b)

Horizontal section through right cerebral hemisphere to show interrelationship of basal ganglia, thalamus and internal capsule. Localisation of fibres in the internal capsule is shown.

a- i. Fibres of cortico spinal tracts for different parts of the body.

a. eyes, b. head, c. shoulder, d. arm, e. fingers, f. trunk, g. hip, h. knees, i. toes.

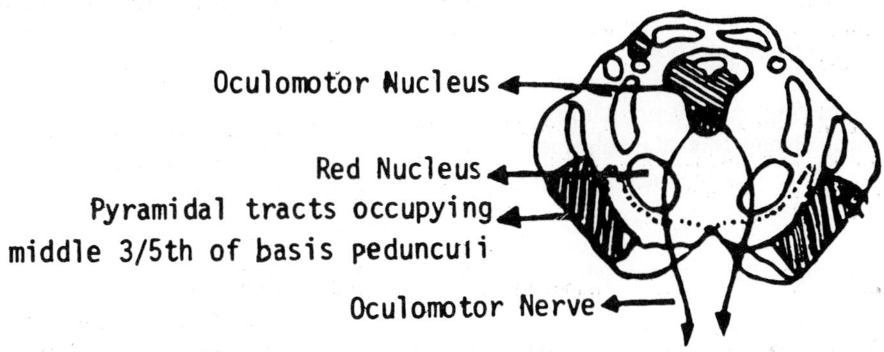

Fig. 16.1 (c)

Cross section of mid-brain at level of superior colliculus to show the close proximity of pyramidal tracts and oculomotor nerves when they emerge anteriorly.

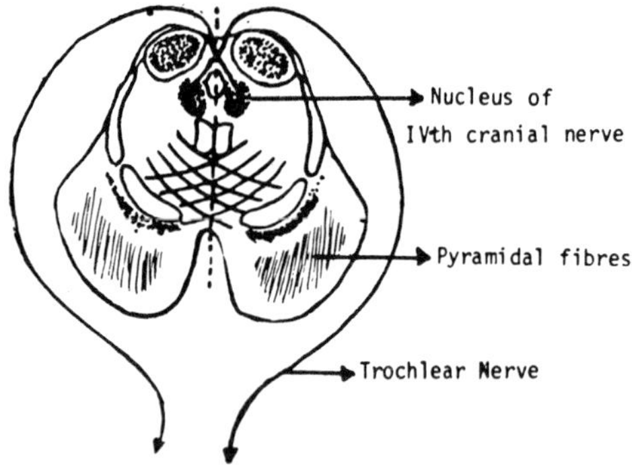

Fig. 16.1 (d)

Cross section of mid-brain at the level of inferior colliculus. Note that the trochlear nerve emerges at the posterior end, goes around the mid-brain to come anteriorly so escapes the injury when pyramidal tracts are involved.

Another important point to be remembered is that only trigeminal nerve motor nucleus (occasionally), facial nerve motor nucleus for lower half of face, and hypoglossal nerve receive unilateral supranuclear fibres from opposite side.

Investigations:

1. **Blood count :** Polymorphonuclear leucocytosis acute cerebral infections.

2. **Urine: Sugar:** may point toward diabetes mellitus. Albumin : Renal involvement in hypertension. Trace of albumin may be present as a result of cerebral irritation.

3. **Blood sugar:** To check for diabetes mellitus.

4. **Blood urea:** As a guide to renal function. Raised in uraemia.

5. **V.D.R.L.:** To check for syphilis.

6. **Fundus examination:** Papilloedema in increased intracranial tension. Diabetic retinopathy; hypertensive retinopathy.

7. **X-ray skull:**

i. Abnormal calcification may be seen in tuberculoma, subdural hematoma of long-standing meningioma, angioma, glioma, etc.

ii. Shift of the calcified pineal body.

iii. Signs of increased intracranial tension. (Erosion of posterior clinoids, silver beaten appearance).

8. **X-ray chest:**

i. Pulmonary tuberculosis. May be present along with tuberculous meningitis.

ii. Presence of secondaries in the lungs may point towards cerebral metastasis.

iii. Cardiac shadow — Valvular disease of the heart may be the source of embolism. Enlarged heart shadow in hypertension. Same may be seen after myocardial infarction. Lesion may be due to embolus from mural endocardium.

9. **C.S.F. :** Will show typical changes in meningitis. Cerebral haemorrhage and cerebral abscess. C.S.F.-V.D.R.L. will be positive in neuro-syphilis.

10. **Serum electrolytes:** Important for management.

11. **Angiography and ventriculography:** For investigation of vascular and space-occupying infarct.

12. **Brain scan:** For localising of space-occupying lesion or cerebral infarct or cerebral haemorrhage and to visualise state of ventricular system.

Management:

General: Maintain nutrition. Care of skin by changing position. Care of bladder.

Specific: Treat the cause, as in meningitis or encephalitis.

Non-specific: Cerebral vasodilators whenever

necessary. Drugs to relieve cerebral edema in acute cases. Treat the cause and symptomatic line of treatment.

After the stage of recovery, occupational therapy, physiotherapy to rehabilitate the patient.

PARAPLEGIA

Definition: Paraplegia means paralysis of both lower limbs.

Causes: Can be classified depending on site or mode of onsot.

Site:

A. **Cerebral causes:** (rare)

1. Meningioma of the falx cerebri.
2. Thrombosis of the superior sagittal sinus.
3. Little's disease (congenital cerebral diplegia).
4. Thrombosis of an unpaired anterior cerebral artery.

B. **Spinal causes:** (common)

1. **Trauma:**

Direct or indirect.

a. Transmitted shock due to fall on buttocks may damage the cervical spine.

b. Fracture, dislocation of vertebrae due to direct trauma.

Lifting of heavy weight can cause acute prolapse of an intervertebral disc.

2. **Infection:**

Acute transverse myelitis.

a. Viral, b.Syphilitic.

3. **Vascular:**

a. Hematomyelia.
b. Haemorrhage in the substance of spinal cord.
c. Multiple sclerosis.
d. Syringomyelia.

4. **Degenerative:**

a. Subacute combined degeneration.
b. Motor neuron disease.
c. Multiple sclerosis.
d. Syringomyelia,
e. Freidreich's ataxia.

5. Compression of the spinal cord.
6. Toxic: Lathyrism, TOCP poisoning.
7. Hysterical.

Paraplegia can also be classified according to the mode of onset. This can be of sudden or of gradual onset.

Causes of paraplegia of sudden onset:

1. Sudden compression from fracture, dislocation of the vertebrae due to trauma.
2. Tuberculosis of the spine due to vascular involvement or due to sudden collapse of the vertebrae.
3. Acute transverse myelitis-viral or syphi-litic.
4. Hematomyelia.
5. Caisson's disease.
6. Hysterical.

Causes of paraplegia of gradual onset:

1. Spinal cord compression — details are given below.
2. Motor neuron disease } Also called non-compressive myclopathies.
3. Syphilitic amyotrophy }
4. Spinal syphilis }
5. Syringomyelia }
6. Subacute combined degeneration }
7. Multiple sclerosis
8. Toxic — Lathyrism, TOCP poisoning

Spinal cord compression:

1. **Vertebral:**

a. Osteomyelitis : tuberculous, pyogenic.

b. Tumours: benign - i. Sarcoma ii. Secondary deposits.

c. Cervical spondylosis.

d. Erosion by aortic aneurysm in thorax or abdomen.

2. **In Vertebral canal:**

a. Extradural metastasis

b. Dural or intradural but extramedullary

i. Meningeal causes, syphilitic pachymeningitis, tuberculous arachnoiditis, infiltration in reticulosis, leukaemic deposits, meningitis circumscripta, meningiomas.

ii. Neurofibromas.

c. Intra-medullary : Glioma, angioma, syphilitic gumma, syringomyelia.

Compression of the spinal cord damages the nervous tissue as follows :

1. Due to direct pressure : Interferes with conduction in the spinal roots and in the cord.

2. Pressure on the ascending longitudinal veins. Causes oedema of the spinal cord below the level of compression.

3. Compression of the spinal arteries leads to ischaemia of the segments which they supply. As terminal branches of these vessels supply the pyramidal tracts, they are the first to be affected.

All the above causes produce spastic paraplegia. Quite often, one encounters cases of paraplegia, slowly progressive and clinically pointing towards diagnosis of spinal cord compression but on myelography or CT scan no compression is detected and CSF also may show no abnormality. These cases are labelled as "Non compressive myelopathies". However paraplegia can also be due to lower motor neuron damage. Causes are as follows :

i. Poliomyelitis.

ii. Acute infective polyneuritis, peripheral neuropathy.

iii. Rarely myopathy — muscular dystrophy.

Paraplegia : History-taking:

The method of inquiry in such a patient should be as follows :

Motor weakness:

1. When did the weakness start?

2. How was the onset?

i. Was it very sudden? This can happen due to fracture dislocation of the spine, haematomyelia, thrombosis of the anterior spinal artery (when it is involved due to disease process of the vertebra) and in hysterical conditions.

ii. Was it subacute i.e. over a period of hours or one or two days? — viral myelitis, ascending paralysis like Guillain Barre syndrome or pressure due to extra-dural abscess may cause a fairly rapid onset of paraplegia.

iii. Was it very gradual? Both compressive and degenerative lesions of the spinal cord usually present with an insidious onset.

3. How did the weakness progress? In this line of questioning both the time factor of the progress of paralysis as well as its mode of spread must be evaluated.

(A) Progress of paralysis (time factor):

i. Was the paralysis total and complete at the onset?

This would indicate paraplegia due to fracture dislocation of the spine which has caused complete destruction of the spinal cord at a particular level.

ii. Did the power in the limbs worsen over a period of hours?

This would indicate an infective lesion like viral myelitis or vascular thrombosis.

iii. Or did it take days or weeks or even months to produce a noticeable weakness? Compressive lesions of the spinal cord usually progress faster than degenerative lesions. So also compression due to malignant deposits in the vertebral column or an extra-dural abscess due to tuberculosis of the spine will result in a more rapid progress than a benign tumour of the spinal cord.

B. How did the weakness progress anatomically?

i. Were both the legs affected simultaneously?

ii. Or was one leg affected before the other? If so, what was the time interval between them? Compressive lesions can produce weakness of one leg before the other and the side where the compression started will be indicated from the history. Infective and degenerative lesions are usually bilaterally symmetrical.

iii. Can the patient make out whether the weakness is more prominent in the distal or proximal muscles? It is difficult to get a voluntary statement on this point from most of the patients. However, a few simple questions are usually enough to evaluate as to which muscles are involved.

a. Is there H/o. stumbling while walking? When the weakness is predominantly in the muscles of foot or around ankles, the patient will complain of stumbling while walking and inability to climb stairs properly due to foot drop.

b. Is there difficulty in getting up from sitting or lying position? When the weakness is more in the muscles around the hip (proximal) joints, the patient will complain of inability to get up from squatting position or from lying down position.

c. Is there any weakness of the upper extremities? Though paraplegia means weakness of the lower limbs, the cause of the weakness is very often due to affection of the cervical cord. Hence following questions must be asked to determine the level of the lesion.

1. Does the patient complain of any weakness of the upper extremities? (If the answer is in the negative the lesion causing the paraplegia will be in the thoracic region or below.)

2. If so, is it of the small muscles of the hand? This manifests as inability to do the finer movements such as buttoning the shirt or writing properly.

3. Is it of the whole arm as such? This will manifest usually as an inability to lift the arm above the head in the early stages.

4. Is the weakness in both the arms or is only one arm affected? This will again point to the side of the lesion in the spinal cord. However, a very patchy and asymmetrical distribution of weakness is positive in both compressive and non-compressive lesions.

5. Has the weakness in the legs improved since the onset? This is possible only in infective viral lesions and in vascular lesions. Otherwise most of the other causes of paraplegia result in a steadily progressive or stable weakness.

6. Does the patient complain of any flexor spasms? Flexor spasms can be described as sudden involuntary flexion of one or both lower extremities with dorsiflexion at ankle, flexion at knee and hip joints. This would indicate that paraplegia in extension is progressing to paraplegia in flexion, i.e., incomplete damage to the spinal cord is progressing to complete damage.

7. Has the patient noticed any wasting or thinness of the involved extremities? If so, what is its distribution? In cauda equina lesions, patient will have bilateral asymmetrical wasting of lower limbs.

8. Inquiry about the sensory system.

i. Are there any root pains? If so, what is the exact distribution of the root pains? This will not only indicate the site of the lesion but also could point to the nature of the causative lesion. Root pains are common in extra-dural lesions, inflammatory lesions such as those due to syphilitic-hypertrophic pachymeningitis. They are usually absent in intra-medullary lesions, viral or vascular lesions of spinal cord.

ii. Does the patient complain of inability to appreciate any sensation in inferior extremities? and/or trunk? Up to what level on the trunk does it extend? The loss of sensations is due to compression of ascending sensory tracts and depending on the degree of compression, there will be partial or total loss of sensations. The loss of sensations can also be due to transection of spinal cord.

Even though the patient is able to point to the exact upper level of sensory loss, it must be remembered that this level does not correspond to the anatomical level of lesion.

iii. Does he complain of any 'band of hyperaesthesia' at any particular anatomical site? This corresponds to the level of the particular spinal segment resulting in a narrow zone where all the sensations are felt more intensely.

iv. Does he complain of paraesthesiac, i.e., subjective sensory disturbances? Does he complain of tight bandage like pain in calf muscles? Does he complain of unpleasant pain especially in distal parts of lower limbs, as may occur in compression of spinothalamic tracts. Paraesthesiae may occur due to compression of spinothalamic tracts. Compression of posterior columns often give rise to sensations like tight bandage or string around limbs.

v. Is there severe continuous local pain over any vertebra? Usually because of tuberculosis of vertebra or malignant secondary deposits.

vi. Are there any sphincter disturbances? Is the patient aware of fullness of bladder? Is there hesitancy or precipitancy or any H/o. retention of urine? Is the passage of urine intermittent and dribbling in nature? Does the patient soil his clothes with urine and stool without any control?

H/o. Causative lesion

I. **Trauma:**

Is there any history of direct injury to the spine associated with either sudden flexion or extension? Direct injury to the spine except a bullet or a knife wound causes either fracture or dislocation or both when associated with sudden flexion or extension of the spine. One such injury in the urban areas is 'whiplash' injury to the cervical spine due to car accident which combines injury with sudden extension of the cervical spine.

Usually a spinal cord injury is caused by transmitted trauma, that is either by a weight falling on the head or by a fall on the buttocks which results in injury to the cervical or lumbo-sacral spine due to transmitted force.

Does the patient give a history of lifting a heavy weight or doing some unaccustomed work following which his complaints started. This can be described as indirect trauma to the spinal cord. A prolapse of intervertebral disc will compress the cord following one of the physical activities described above.

II. **Infections:**

1. Did the patient have high fever with backache and headache at the time of onset of weakness suggestive of viral transverse myelitis?

2. Does he have H/o low grade fever usually associated with upper respiratory tract infection 10-14 days before the onset of weakness?

Conditions like Guillain Barre syndrome or glandular tuberculosis.

Tuberculosis of spine can give rise to paraplegia most commonly by

a. Thrombosis of anterior spinal artery.

b. Arteritis and phlebitis because of tuberculous process.

c. Presence of cold abscess.

d. Prolapse of the vertebrae destroyed by tuberculous infection causing pressure over the cord.

e. Rarely by tubercular arachnoiditis or by

f. Forming intra-spinal tuberculosis.

4. Is there any H/o. exposure in the past? Syphilis can affect the spinal cord and lead to paraplegia in various ways.

a. Syphilitic hypertrophic pachymeningitis common in cervical region and is associated with severe root pains and paraplegia.

b. Acute transverse myelitis.

c. Subacute variant due to meningomyelitis.

d. Erb's syphilitic spinal paraplegia is a rare clinical entity which causes slowly progressive paraparesis.

e. Syphilitic gumma is also a rare clinical manifestation causing intramedullary compression.

5. Is there H/o. conjunctivitis — certain cases of myelitis may be preceded by conjunctivitis.

6. H/o. measles or any infectious disease.

III. **Vascular :**

No specific questioning will elicit any particular cause. However, diabetes, hypertension or rheumatic valvular diseases giving rise to embolic phenomena may rarely be etiological agents causing vascular damage to the spinal cord.

IV. **Degenerative and demyelinating:**

Is there any history of receiving any vaccines or sera in the recent past, e.g., acute demyelination of spinal cord may result due to such sera (e.g., antirabic serum).

V. **Space-occupying lesions :**

Is there any history of systemic carcinomatosis? Secondary deposits in vertebral column can cause paraplegia and on direct questioning primary carcinoma may be found out.

VI. **Toxic** — Alcoholism leading to subacute combined degeneration.

Clinical signs:

1. **Motor changes:** L.M.N. (Lower Motor Neurone) lesion at the site of compression manifests as weakness, wasting and sometimes fasciculation of the muscles innervated by the affected segments.

UMN (Upper Motor Neurone) type of paralysis below the level of the lesion manifests as paraplegia in extension followed by paraplegia in flexion (explained later).

II. **Sensory changes:**

a. At the level of the lesion: Hyperaesthesia and hyperalgesia in the corresponding cutaneous segments.

b. Below the level of the lesion : Loss of pain and temperature sensation on the opposite side if compression is limited to one side. In complete lesions it will be on both the sides below the level of lesion. Posterior column involvement manifests as loss of joint and vibration sensations on the same side in partial lesion. Both sides are affected in a complete compression.

III. **Reflexes:**

Deep reflexes: Lost at the level of the lesion and exaggerated below the level of the lesion.

Superficial reflexes: Cremastric and abdominal reflexes are lost if the level of the lesion is above L_1. Extensor plantar reflex present.

IV. **Sphincters:** Involvement occurs when spinal lesion is at T_{10} or below. Initially precipitancy when the lesion is partial. Retention or automatic bladder in a complete lesion. Constipation usually occurs.

V. **Autonomic symptoms:** Excessive sweating may be present below the lesion.

VI. **Spine:** Local tenderness, angular deformity.

Clinical presentation of a paraplegia

Paraplegia can present in two different clinical ways :

1. As paraplegia in extension, or
2. As paraplegia in flexion.

The former is due to incomplete transaction of the cord while the latter is due to complete lesion.

After an incomplete lesion two antagonistic reflex activities come into play.

1. Hypertonia of the extensors.
2. Flexor withdrawal reflex.

Paraplegia in extension and paraplegia in flexion are two stages of the transaction of spinal cord, incomplete one progressing into complete one. Whenever paraplegia of acute onset takes place, spinal shock is the first stage. After the stage of spinal shock, the stage of paraplegia in extension is short-lived and may be imperceptible and stage of paraplegia in flexion supervenes in extreme lesions. In this respect the integrity of reticulo spinal tracts together with pyramidal tracts play an important role in paraplegia in extension and that in flexion.

Reticulo spinal tracts originate at the level of pons and medulla in reticular formation the fibre travel in close proximity with pyramidal tracts anterior and lateral.

Both pyramidal and reticulo spinal tracts have inhibitory influence on alpha and gamma neurone respectively. Whenever partial spinal cord lesion occurs with intact reticulo spinal tracts but with involvement of pyramidal tracts, extensors predominate the picture due to disinhibition of alpha neurone controlling the extensors. A condition equivalent to decerebrate rigidity developes. At later stage when lesion extends and involves reticulo spinal tracts also; alpha and gamma neurons are disinhibited leading to flexor spasms — under control of spinal reflex arc.

When acute transection of spinal cord occurs due to trauma or infection, reticulo spinal tracts are interrupted from beginning so that paraplegia in flexion follows stage of spinal shock; the stage of paraplegia in extension being imperceptible.

Clinical picture of paraplegia in extension:

1. Position of the lower limbs : Extended and adducted at the hips, extended at the knees. Plantar

flexed at the ankles.

2. Tone : Clasp knife type of spasticity.

3. Sensations : Lost below the level of the lesion. As the lesion is incomplete, the level of the sensory loss may be a few segments below the level of the lesion on one side.

4. The deep reflexes : Exaggerated. Ankle and patellar clonus may be present. Knee reflex may cause contraction of the adductors of the other leg.

5. The superficial reflexes : Lost below the level of the lesion. Extensor plantar reflex.

6. The excretory reflexes : Absent.

Cinical picture of paraplegia in flexion:

1. Position of the lower limbs.

In the severe cases : Feet dorsiflexed, knee flexed, hips flexed.

Patient lying with heels touching the gluteal regions (in extreme cases).

2. The flexor withdrawal reflex :

Before the above mentioned fixed position is reached any irritant stimulus below the level of the lesion results in the following :

i. Upward movement of the great toe with fanning of the other toes.

ii. Dorsiflexion at the ankle.

iii. Flexion of the knee and hip.

iv. Flexion of the other leg also, present in some cases. Spinal shock and urinary infection or bed sores depress this reflex.

3. The mass reflex : Any stimulus of the parts below the level of the lesion will in addition to the withdrawal reflex also cause reflex evacuation of the bladder and rectum with sweating.

4. The excretory reflexes : Reflex evacuation of bladder, automatic evacuation after filling up to 200 cc.

5. Sexual reflexes :

The Dartos
The Bulbocavernosus } reflexes are
The Cremasteric } preserved.

Reflex erection and ejaculation is possible accompanied by contraction of adductors of thigh, flexors of leg and abdominal recti.

6. Deep reflexes: May be present. Not exaggerated.

7. Sensations : Complete loss of all forms of sensations immediately below the level of the lesion.

Investigation of a case of paraplegia

1. **Blood count:** High E.S.R. in infection like tuberculous spine, megaloblastic anaemia in subacute combined degeneration.

2. **Urine : Urinary infection:** Common in patients who have been catheterised for the retention of urine.

3. **X-ray of the spine:** 1. For tuberculosis of spine (Pott's spine). 2. metastasis. 3. Fracture dislocation. 4. Intervertebral disc prolapse. 5. Pedicular erosion in spinal cord tumours (especially neurofibroma).

4. **L.P. and C.S.F examination:** 1. Pressure may be low in subarachnoid block and Queckenstadt's test may not show rise of pressure, 2. Froin's syndrome may be seen. 3. Appropriate changes in viral myelitis, syphilitic pachymeningitis, Infective polyneuritis.

5. **Myelography:** for noting the level of lesion.

6. C.T. scan of spinal cord and MRI to locate the lesion.

Management:

General: Maintain nutrition. Care of bladder catheterisation, bladder wash, prevention of infection. Care of skin - changes of position to prevent bed sores, physiotherapy.

Specific: Treatment of the causes - antituberculous line of treatment in Pott's spine, antibiotics appropriate depending on cause, steroids in case of polyneuropathy and viral transverse myelitis.

Surgery: Indicated in cases of spinal cord compression to remove the causative factor.

NEUROLOGICAL CONTROL OF BLADDER

Neural control of bladder is yet imperfectly understood.

The bladder muscle known as detrusor is made

of bundles of muscle interlacing with each other. These continue along urethra and form the internal sphincter.

A. **Nerve supply is:**

1. Efferent = Parasympathetic / Sympathetic

2. Afferent = Sympathetic

B. **Somatic:** Does not supply bladder but supplies external sphincter, urethra and perineal muscles, included in this context because these fibres are involved in act of micturition.

C. **Higher control:** Afferent - sensations are received by post-central gyrus. Efferent, i.e., 2nd frontal gyrus through hypothalamic and pontine facilitatory centre. (Fig. 16.2)

Details as follows: a. **Efferent:** Parasympathetic + sympathetic form efferent. Parasympathetic fibres arising from cells in sacral 2-3 segments, i.e., the pre-ganglionic fibres (pelvic nerve or nervi erigentis) end in hypogastric ganglia and into vesical plexus. The post-ganglionic fibres arise from the hypogastric ganglia and travel alongwith the sympathetic fibres to innervate detrusor.

Sympathetic fibres arise from connector cells in L_1 L_2 of spinal cord. They travel through the lateral sympathetic chain and end in inferior mesenteric ganglia and then unite to form the presacral nerve. This divides to form two hypogastric nerves which end in vesical plexus on either side of the bladder. They supply mainly blood vessels in the bladder wall and muscles around the bladder neck.

b. **Afferent;** Nerve supply. 1. Fibres mainly pass through sympathetic L_1 L_2, segments and carry sensation of distension through stretch receptors. 2. Same fibres which carry sensation of distention and pain pass to sacral segments of cord via pelvic nerves.

Parasympathetic stimulation results in contraction of detrusor and relaxation of sphincter, i.e., leading to emptying of bladder. The old belief that sympathetic nerves relax the detrusor and contract the sphincter is disproved. The main function of sympathetic fibres is to close the bladder neck at the time of ejaculation.

c. **Somatic supply:** Internal pudendal nerves, i.e., S2,3,4 provide afferent and efferent fibres to external sphincter, urethra and perineal muscles.

d. **Higher control:** The cerebral cortex - 2nd frontal gyrus controls the local nerve supply. The pathway of the afferent fibres is not exactly known but they probably travel in dorsal columns to end in sensory cortex, which is situated in post-central gyrus. The corresponding area in parasagittal regions is in the pre-central or motor cortex (2nd frontal gyrus) which exercises control over parasympathetic centres in sacral region. The fibres from 2nd frontal gyrus travel along with pyramidal fibres on lateral side and relay in centres in hypothalamus and pons. These centres are known as hypothalamic and pontine facilitatory centres.

The function of these higher centres, i.e., cortical and subcortical centres is to initiate micturition whenever convenient. It does so by controlling the local parasympathetic impulses from S2-3 segments.

Physiology of voluntary micturition:

A brief description in this context will not be out of place.

With gradual filling of bladder, intra-vesical pressure gradually rises. The pressor-receptors in the muscles wall are stimulated (stretch reflex) and afferent impulses reach the spinal cord through sympathetic, then to sensory cortex of brain which produces desire for micturition.

If the situation or circumstances are inconvenient, the motor cortex sends inhibitory impulses via efferent fibres which travel with pyramidal fibres. These inhibitory impulses act on parasympathetic spinal centres and the act of micturition is delayed.

As the circumstances are convenient for micturition, inhibitory impulses from motor cortex do not exert inhibitory influence so that local spinal centres are released. The local spinal reflex plays the role and the detrusor contracts and internal sphincter relaxes because of parasympathetic activity. The passage of urine in urethra sends afferent impulses through pudendal (somatic) nerves. The efferent impulses travel through

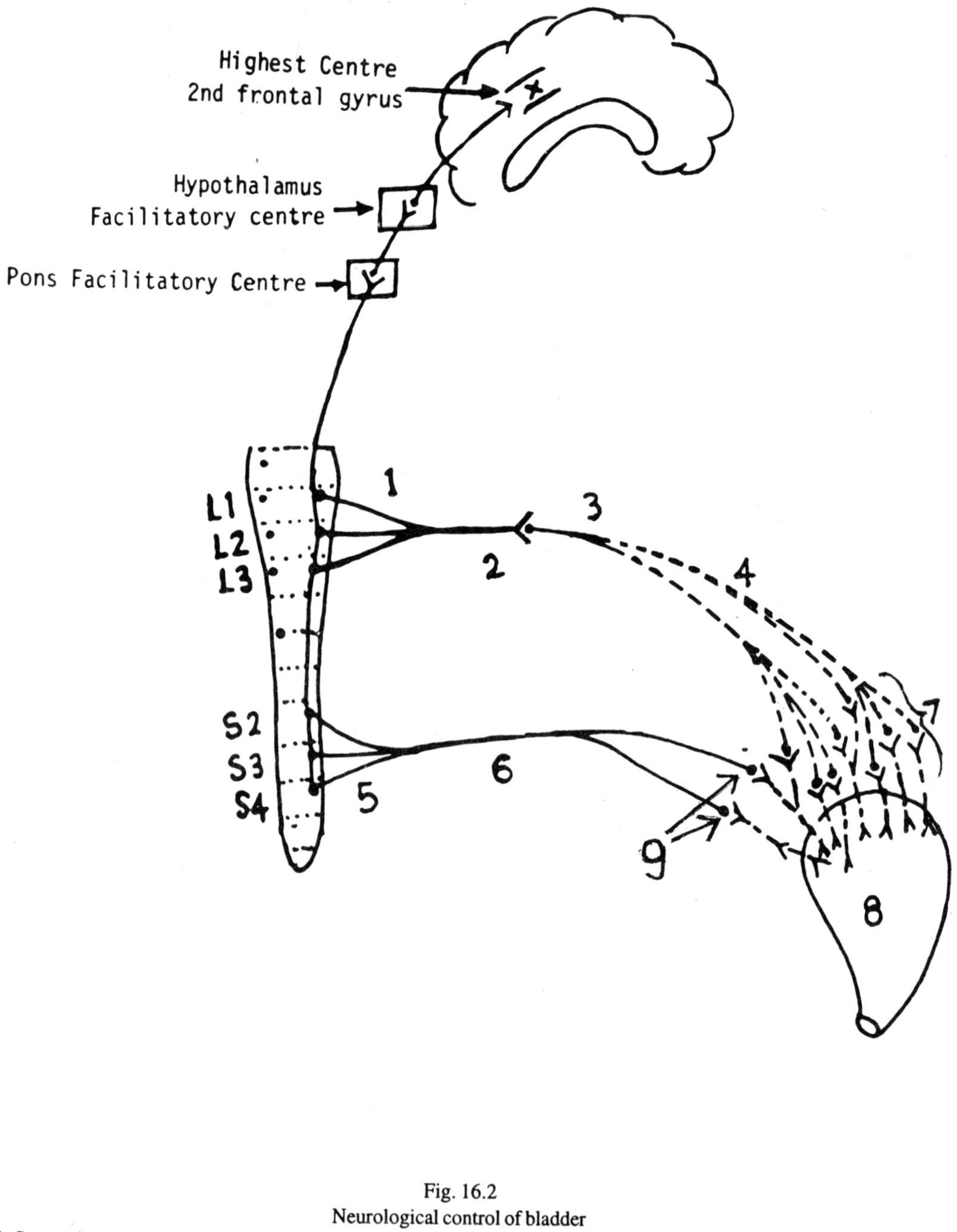

Fig. 16.2
Neurological control of bladder
1. Sympathetic centres 2. Inferior mesenteric ganglion 3. Presacral nerve 4. Hypogastric nerves 5. Parasympathetic centres 6. Pelvic nerves (Nervi erigentis) 7. Vesical plexus 8. Bladder 9. Hypogastric ganglia.

(somatic) nerves and the external sphincter is relaxed (i.e., it is inhibited, reflexly). In addition to the relaxation of sphincter, perineal muscles also contract, diaphragm descends, abdominal muscles contract, i.e., collective effect is, rise in intra-abdominal pressure.

As the intra-vesical pressure starts falling, the local spinal reflex arc does not come into play. The pontine facilitatory centre now plays the role and the act of micturition is continued till the bladder is emptied.

In infants and young children, local spinal reflex arc works and higher centres develop by 2-3 years.

It is obvious from this physiology, that hesitancy, precipitancy, incontinence, inability to stop the act of micturition at will all these symptoms develop whenever the higher centres do not communicate with the lower centres (i.e., when fibres are damaged in between). The other symptoms like associated rectal incontinence, urinary incontinence, impotency, numbness in perineal region occur whenever local spinal arc is disrupted, as in cauda equina syndrome. There can also be various combinations of symptoms depending on lesions.

Neurological disorders of bladder:

1. Uninhibited bladder,
2. Spinal bladder,
3. Automatic bladder,
4. Autonomous bladder,
5. Sensory bladder.

1. **Uninhibited bladder:** The name is self-explanatory. Any lesions involving the cortical centres (i.e., parasagittal meningioma), frontal lobe tumor or dementia can cause this problem. The bladder reverts to infantile variety. The symptoms are urgency at low volumes (in partial lesions) or voiding of urine at any time and anywhere without any control. There is no residual urine in such bladder. (If dementia starts with initial bladder complaints, organic lesions of frontal lobe should be looked for.) The social significance of not voiding urine in public is lost (uninhibited).

2. **Spinal bladder :** Bladder disturbances due to spinal cord lesions. a. Partial lesions: The damage to fibres from motor cortical centre to sacral centres results in hesitancy and precipitancy of micturition. b. Complete lesions : Usually acute in nature.

transverse myelitis — viral / syphilitic

traumatic - transection of cord.

The first reaction of the limbs and bladder is spinal shock. There is retention of urine and when bladder muscle is completely stretched, there is overflow incontinence of urine. When the stage of spinal shock wears off, the local sacral reflex arc takes over the function of bladder control.

3. **Automatic bladder:** This is common sequelae after recovery from spinal shock. If there is no infection in bladder (commonly occurs because of catheterisation during the stage of retention of urine), micturition becomes automatic. The automatic bladder empties suddenly and reflexly as a response to small volumes of urine, (about 250 cc) and the patient is unaware of this act. Usually the bladder contains no residual urine after evacuation. If evacuation is not complete it can be achieved by training. The patient can be trained to evacuate the bladder in such circumstances by massaging the supra-pubic area or stroking inner side of thigh periodically every 2 hours and the bladder will be emptied reflexly.

If infection develops in such circumstance, complete automatic evacuation does not develop and the bladder wall hypertrophies resulting in very markedly reduced capacity and retention persists in such a situation.

4. **The autonomous bladder:** This results as a damage to the motor and sensory components in the cauda equina or pelvic cavity. Usually due to cauda equina lesions, pelvic surgery, pelvic malignancy, spina bifida, lumbar disc lesions.

Due to this, the sensation of bladder distention is lost and the bladder is large with continuous dribbling incontinence. There is associated loss of perineal sensations. Residual urine with high risk infection exists.

If the damage is only to the motor components, the sensations of bladder distention are preserved. But the bladder is large with dribbling incontinence as complete evacuation does not occur at all.

5. **The sensory bladder :** Clinical features are the same as in autonomous bladder but anatomical lesions are different. This occurs as a result of damage to sensory afferent fibres. Though classically it occurs due to diabetic autonomic neuropathy it can also occur due to sub-acute combined degeneration, multiple sclerosis or tabes dorsalis. Striking feature is that the patient is unaware of bladder fullness and the spinal reflex is lost. There is massive retention of urine. This results again in a very large bladder with dribbling incontinence. However, the bladder can be voluntarily evacuated with straining though the evacuation is always incomplete.

Conclusion : Thus whenever spinal cord lesion leads to bladder disturbances the ideal goal is to achieve automatic bladder. It gives maximum benefit to the patient.

DISORDERS RELATED TO THE EXTRA-PYRAMIDAL SYSTEM: (Fig. 16.3)

Anatomical components of the extra-pyramidal system

1. Corpus striatum
   - The caudate nucleus
   - The lentiform nucleus
     - Globus pallidus
     - Putamen
2. The Red nucleus
3. The Substantia nigra
4. The Subthalamic nucleus (body of Luys)
5. The Reticular formation of the brain-stem
6. The Dentate nucleus of the cerebellum
7. Forel's field.

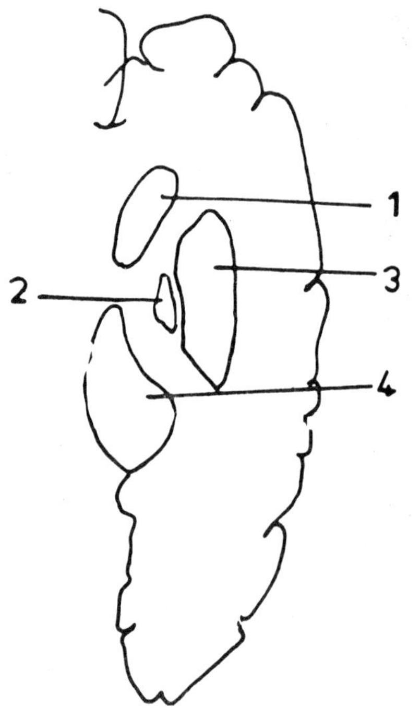

Fig. 16.3
Basal ganglia
1. Caudate Nucleus
2. Globus Pallidus
3. Putamen
4. Thalmus

Parkinsonian syndrome :

Essential features : Disturbance of motor function: 1. Causing slowing and enfeeblement ot emotional and voluntary movements. 2. Muscular rigidity. 3. Tremors.

Causes : 1. Parkinson's disease. 2. Postencephalitic. 3. Atherosclerotic. 4. Symptomatic. (a) Post-traumatic, (b) Carbon monoxide intoxication, (c) Drugs : Reserpine, Phenothiazines, Butyrophenones, (d) Neurosyphilis.

Pathology - failure to sythesize. Dopamine by basalganglia.

Symptoms :

I. **Facies :** Mask like face, wide palpebral fissures, infrequent blinking, immobile facial muscles, staring look.

II. **Attitude :** Moderately fixed attitude of trunk and spine. Limbs flexed and adducted moderately, wrist extended. Fingers flexed at the metacarpophalangeal joints but extended or slightly flexed at the other joints. Thumb usually adducted and extended.

III. **Disorders of movement :** Classically described as akinesia and bradykinesia : Power not impaired : slow movement; Small muscles are affected most (like facial, eye-closure, mastication, deglutition, articulation); Small muscles of the hand most severely affected; Natural swing of arms while walking is lost.

IV. **Lead pipe and cog wheel rigidity :** Increased tone throughout the movement while testing. Cog wheel rigidity is felt when tremors supervene.

V. **Gait :** Shuffling or festinant, propulsion and retropulsion, kinesia paradoxica.

VI. **Tremors :** Usually in the upper limb first. Then in the lower limb on the same side (when unilateral). Classic description pill rolling movements 4-6 tremors per second. Static tremors decrease or disappear during voluntary movement.

VII. **No sensory affection :** Pain due to muscular cramps.

VIII. **Reflexes :** Deep reflexes sluggish due to rigidity.

IX. **Autonomic symptoms :** Flushing of the skin with sensation of heat and unilateral sweating, cold tolerated better than heat.

X. **Mental state :** Normal higher functions. May have mental depression especially because of physical incapacitation.

Treatment:

1. **General :** Maintain physical activity of the patient as long as possible. Any condition like inter current infection due to which the patient has to lie in bed increases the disability of the patient.

2. **Drugs :** Anti-tremors and anti-rigidity drugs.

3. **Stereotaxic surgery :** Usually beneficial in those patients with unilateral disease. Parkinson's disease patients respond the best.

Involuntary movements:

Classification of involuntary movements is given on page 215.

Description of those due to involvement of extra-pyramidal system is given below. Other movements are given in details under involuntary in motor system examination.

1. **Due to involvement of extra-pyramidal system:**

i. Chorea, ii. Athetosis, iii. Choreo athetosis, iv. Dystonia, v. Hemiballismus, vi. Myoclonus, vii. Tremors.

i. **Chorea:**

a. Series of continuous and spontaneous involuntary movements.

b. Mainly involving face, tongue and limbs.

c. Movements are rapid and pseudo-purposive

d. Non-repetitive.

e. Distal joints more affected.

f. Voluntary movements exaggerate the involuntary movements and they are grossly disturbed (e.g., handwriting and buttoning the shirt).

g. Associated movements are grossly exaggerated.

h. Muscular hypotonia.

i. Pendular and 'hang up' tendon reflexes

j. Respiratory muscles also involved in the irregular contraction.

k. Disappear during sleep.

Causes:

i. Sydenham's (rheumatic) chorea.

ii. Huntington's chorea.

iii. Wilson's disease.

iv. Postencephalitic.

v. Phenothiazone toxicity.

vi. Post-kernicterus

vii. Rarely in hyerthyroidism.

ii. **Athetosis:**

a. Means instability of posture.

b. Also known as mobile spasm.

c. Term applied to a disturbance of both the posture and movements.

d. Alteration between postures in the two arms.

e. Occur as spasms, appear on change of posture.

f. Mainly writhing movements.

g. Plantar flexion of the ankle and dorsiflexion of the great toe.

h. Voluntary movement impaired and the movements may increase during voluntary action, or with change of posture.

i. Distal joints more severely affected.

j. Disappear during sleep.

k. Lesion in the putamen.

Causes:

1. Could be congenital or due to post-natal conditions like hypoxia, kernicterus or birth injury.
2. Hepatic coma.

iii. **Choreo athetosis:**

a. Combination of features of both chorea and athetosis.

b. Movements have both slow and rapid elements.

c. May consist of a flick of a single muscle or group of muscles.

d. Movements can be precipitated by a loud noise or on touching the muscle.

iv. **Dystonia:**

a. Related to athetosis.

b. Persistent, maintenance of a posture due to exaggerated muscle tone.

c. Usually either extreme flexion or extension.

d. Lower limbs either flexed or extended.

e. Upper limbs either flexed or extended.

f. May be unilateral or bilateral.

g. Proximal joints affected more severely.

v. **Hemiballismus:**

a. Movements similar to that of chorea.

b. Usually limited to one side of the body.

c. Proximal joints involved to a greater extent than distal joints.

d. Movements mainly at shoulder or hip.

e. Lesion is in Body of Luys.

vi. **Myoclonus:**

a. Involuntary and arrhythmic movements.

b. More rapid than chorea.

c. May involve a single muscle (causing a 'flick') or may involve a group of muscles.

d. Can be precipitated by a flash of light, loud sound or touch.

vii. **Tremors:** Regular oscillation of a part of the body around a fixed point. Rate 3 to 8 movements per second. Usually seen in the distal part of the limbs, the head, the tongue or the jaw, Types: a. Static. b. Action. c. Intention tremor, d. Hysterical tremor.

a. **Static tremor:**

i. Commonly seen in Parkinsonism.

ii. Coarse and rhythmic.

iii. Usually 4-5 C.P.S.

iv. Mostly localised to one or both hands.

v. But may be in the jaw or the tongue.

vi. Willed or voluntary movement temporarily suppresses them.

vii. Gentle and distal tremors in paralysis agitans, wider and proximal in Wilson's disease and post-encephalitis Parkinsonism.

viii. Lesion usually in substantia nigra.

b. **Action tremor:**

i. Tremors are present when the limbs are maintained in a fixed position, i.e., outstretched fingers. Also present throughout voluntary movement.

ii. Increases but does not interfere with fine movement.

iii. Disappears on relaxation.

iv. **Causes:** familial anxiety, delirium tremens, chronic alcoholism and G.P.I. (general paralysis of insane), hyperthyroidism, hepatic coma.

v. Lesion is in red nucleus.

c. **Intention tremor:**

i. Precipitated by voluntary movement.

ii. Absent when the limb is relaxed and during early part of the voluntary movement.

iii. Jerky, rhythmic oscillations with precise movements.

iv. May even persist for a short time after the action is over.

v. Titubation (movement of the head) present occasionally.

vi. Cerebellar disease is usually the underlying cause.

d. **Hysterical tremor:**

i. Bizzare picture.

ii. Does not correspond to any known clinical picture described above.

MOTOR NEURON DISEASE

Syn. - Amyotrophic lateral sclerosis, progressive muscular atrophy.

Definition : A disease characterised clinically by 1. Progressive wasting of muscles, especially those of upper limbs and muscles supplied by lower cranial nerves. 2. Upper motor neuron lesion in lower limbs.

These combinations of UMN and LMN lesion are due to degenerative changes in anterior horn cells, motor nuclei of lower cranial nerves in medulla with degeneration of pyramidal tracts. The pathological changes are most marked in cervical region (Fig. 16.4).

Etiology:

Age : 30 - 60 years

- Familial - dominant and recessive

Sex : Males - Females - 2:1

Trauma and infection have no role in etiology. Degenerative changes occur in inferior cerebellar peduncle, medial longitudinal bundle and reticular formation along with degenerative changes in (a) anterior horn cells of cervical cord and motor nuclei of cranial nerves. (b) pyramidal tracts and (c) motor cortex due to unknown toxin. The degenerative changes in pyramidal tracts are patchy.

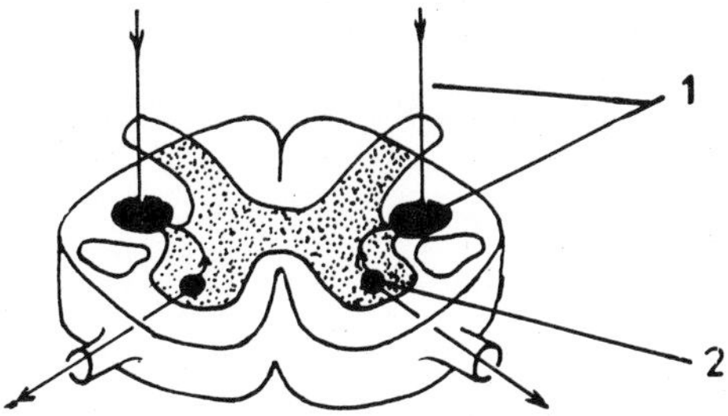

Fig. 16.4
Site of lesion in motor neuron disease
1. Conico spinal tracts
2. Anterior horn cells (Motor neuron)
3. Motor nerve root
Motor neurons are involved at various levels especially cervical cord, lower cranial nerves.

Onset : Subacute to chronic course and insidious onset. Usually starts with wasting and LMN weakness of upper limbs sometimes begins in motor nuclei in medulla manifesting as dysarthria and dysphagia. Rarely it starts with UMN manifestation in lower limbs.

Signs/symptoms: 1. LMN in upper limbs - Weakness, wasting and fasciculation of muscles, clumsiness of movements of hand leading to contractures of hand — clawhand. Flexors suffer before extensors. Weakness gradually spreads forearm, arm and shoulder girdle.

2. Muscles supplied by cranial nerves formerly it was believed that of the motor nuclei of only lower cranial nerves are involved but now it is known that Vth nerve (trigeminal) motor nucleus is involved quite often; then VIIth facial moter nucleus gets involved, though less often. (Surprisingly motor nuclei of IIIrd, IVth, VIth nerves escape). Muscles supplied by lower cranial nerves. IX, XXI, XII are involved simultaneously or shortly after involvement of upper limbs.

IX, X (glossopharyngeal and Vagus): Muscles of pharynx, palate and larynx show weakness manifesting as difficulty in swallowing nasal regurgitation of food, nasal twang in voice and weak voice.

XI : (Spinal accessory) — As it supplies extension of neck, sternomastoids and trapezius, weakness of former leads to head falling forward and that of latter leads to marked head lag and inability to raise shoulders and absence of curve at neck.

XII : (Hypoglossal) — Supplies muscies of tongue therefore weakness manifests as fasciculation, wriggling and shrunken appearence of tongue. Speech is markedly affected leading to dysarthria, words inaudible and slurred.

VII & V : Orbicularis oris and muscles of mastication get weaker — Thus chewing of food is affected, pursing of lips, whistling becomes difficult. Because lips are involved, labial words cannot be pronounced and this adds to dysarthria and misery of the patient's condition as he is couscious of all the changes.

Reflexes:

Gag reflex - poor or absent
Superficial - abdominal reflexes lost
Deep reflexes - jaw reflex}
knee reflex } are exaggerated
ankle reflex}
Plantar - extensor
Sphincters - hesitancy, precipitancy

Investigations: Biochemical change

a. Levels of serum creative kinase (normal 75 IU/L) are raised even up to 400 IU/L - diagnostic.

b. Acetyl cholinestease levels also may rise.

c. VDRL

d. EMG and nerve conduction studies.

Prognosis: poor, patient may survive for 2-5 years after the onset.

Important features: LMN lesion on upper limbs, fasciculation, bulbar muscle involvement, biceps-triceps reflexes may be exaggerated, UMN lesion in lower limbs.

Differential diagnosis: 1. **Infective polyneuritis**, differentiated by absence of fasciculation, sensory changes, diminished or absent reflexes, weakness along distribution of nerve. 2. **Cervical spondylosis** or any tumour in cervical spinal cord-sensory symptoms more predominant, deep reflexes absent or brisk in upper limbs.

Management: Symptomatic - general and physiotherapy.

CEREBELLAR ATAXIA

Ataxia is a symptom and is defined as incoordinated or inaccurate movement which is not due to paresis and characterised by 1. Alteration in tone, 2. Loss of postural sense of involuntary movement. When ataxia is due to cerebellar involvement it is cerebellar ataxia.

Cerebellar ataxias can be classified in two ways : 1. Those occurring in children or hereditary disorders, 2. Those occurring in adulthood or acquired disorders.

Cerebellar ataxias in childhood:

i. Due to congenital malformation

- Arnold Chiari malformation

- associated with meningocele or raised intracranial tension

- ataxia evident when pyramidal fibres get myelinated

- congenital anomalies of brain (congenital stenosis of aqueduct).

ii. Infections

- acute viral cerebellitis,

- complication of exanthem (e.g., post-measles cerebellitis).

iii. Degenerative disorders - usually hereditary ataxia

a. Friedreich's ataxia onset 5-10yrs, degeneration of spino cerebellar tracts, peripheral nerves, pyramidal tracts.

Clinically, signs of
-cerebellar involvement,
-pyramidal lesions,
-peripheral nerve involvement,
-pes cavus,
-scoliosis,
-optic atrophy,

b. Olivo ponto cerebellar atrophy,

c. Ataxia telangiectasia - dysarthria ataxia, spasticity.

iv. Tumours - Medullo-blastoma (posterior fossa tumour).

v. Drugs - anticonvulsants

vi. Metabolic - congenital errors of metabolism.

Cerebellar Ataxias in adulthood:

Hereditary : Friedreich's ataxia, Ramsay Hunt syndrome -

characterised by: insidious onset, 3rd decade, ataxia more marked in upper limbs.

Dejerine - Thomas syndrome - characterised by :

ataxia, dysarthria, sphincter control lost (reason is unknown).

Acquired: toxic - alcoholic (Wernicke's encephalopathy)

- anticonvulsants
- carbon monoxide poisoning

Degenerative - multiple sclerosis

Malignancy -secondary deposits.

Clinical picture:

Symptoms:

a. Ataxia,

b. Dysarthria,

c. Tremors,

d. Those pertaining to the causative factor,

e. Difficulty in performing fine and gross movements due to ataxia, even in absence of muscular weakness,

f. H/o. drugs,

g. H/o. fever (high),

h. H/o. previous infections like measles,

i. H/o. alcoholism,

j. Family history.

Signs:

Hypotonia,

Nystagmus,

Intention tremors and incoordination,

Dysmetria,

Dysdiadochokinesis

Rebound phenomenon,

Gait - wide based and ataxic,

Past pointing - test +ve

Barany's test + ve and Romberg's test -ve.

Reflexes:

Superficial reflexes unaffected,

Deep reflexes pendular

Investigations:

Fundi :

1. Optic atrophy - Friedreich's ataxia,
2. Retrobulbar neuritis - multiple sclerosis,
3. papilloedema - cerebellar tumour.

C.S.F.: May show changes in viral infection and multiple sclerosis.

X-ray skull: Silver beaten appearance in raised intracranial tension (especially, SOL in post-cranial fossa).

C.T. scan brain for posterior fossa tumour.

Treatment: Discontinue drugs in case of drug intoxication-physiotherapy, prevention of respiratory infection.

DIAGNOSIS AND MANAGEMENT OF AN UNCONSCIOUS PATIENT (COMATOSE PATIENT)

Whenever an unconscious patient (comatose patient) is encountered the aim of the examination should be pointed towards the following :

a. To determine the level of consciousness.

b. To identify or to exclude systemic diseases known to cause disturbances of consciousness without primary disease of the brain.

c. If apparently due to a neurological lesion, to determine its site in the brain or brain-stem.

d. After identifying the cause of unconsciousness, the emergency and permanent measures therapeutically to be followed in such patients.

Various stages of consciousness range from a completely conscious individual to a completely unconscious individual. These stages are conscious stage, dazed stage, drowsy or lethargic stage, stuporose stage, semi-conscious stage and unconscious stage.

Causes of unconsciousness:

I. **Causes in brain :** 1. Cerebrovascular lesions : thrombosis, haemorrhage,embolism. 2. Space-occupying lesions: brain tumors, tuberculoma, etc. 3. Traumatic: head injury. 4. Infections - meningitis, encephalitis. 5. Post-epileptic. 6. Encephalopathy - e.g., toxic, hypertensive. 7. Eclampsia.

II. **Metabolic causes:** Uraemia, hypoglycemia, diabetic ketosis, hepatic coma (cholemia), heat stroke, anoxia.

III. **Endocrine causes:** Adrenal crisis, hypopituitarism, myxoedema.

IV. **Intoxications:** Barbiturates, organophosphorous (bug poison), alcohol, opiates, carbon-monoxide, tranquillisers.

To determine what is the cause of coma, a detailed examination is necessary and the points which should be noted will be described below.

Examination of the comatose patient (unconscious patient):

In view of above-mentioned causes, coma is not an independant disease-entity but is always a symptomatic expression of disease. Occasionally the cause is obvious as in a case of head injury. But more often than not, no information about the patient is immediately available when the patient is first seen.

The points of particular interest are:

1. **The mode of onset:** Was it abrupt as in cerebrovascular catastrophes or epileptic states or was it rapid over a period of a few hours as in some cases of intra-cranial haemorrhage or was it gradual over days as in space occupying lesions of the brain.

2. **Premonitory symptoms:** Complete absence of these suggests a primary intra-cranial vascular accident or an attack of epilepsy. Previous similar episodes suggest either epilepsy or the recurrent administration of drugs. Headaches with vomiting, mental changes and increasing weakness or unsteadiness of limbs would suggest a space occupying lesion. Any active infection in the ears, chest or sinuses may suggest intra-cranial infection. H/o. psychological disturbance and availability of drugs may suggest the possibility of drug intoxication. H/o. of any mental set-back as a failure in the examination or any set-back in the young person's life may suggest organophosphorus or any other easily available household poisoning.

Examination of the patient:

The first step is the assessment of the degree of altered consciousness.

General examination of the patient:

After the degree of unconsciousness is assessed it should be immediately followed by the general examination.

Temperature: Elevation of temperature (fever) suggests a severe infection, either systemic like pneumonia, typhoid or bacterial meningitis. An excessively high temperature (40-41^0 C) may arouse the suspicion of heat stroke or cerebral malaria. It can also be seen in pontine haemorrhage. A low temperature reading is frequently observed in alcoholic or barbiturate intoxication, shock or in myxoedema.

Respiratory rate: Very slow breathing rate (4-5/min) is observed in morphine or opium poisoning. It is also seen in barbiturates poisoning or hypothyroidism.

As opposed to this deep rapid breathing suggests diabetic or uraemic acidosis. Diseases that cause severe damage to the brain cause slow, irregular or periodic (Cheyne Stokes) breathing.

Pulse rate: This is less helpful in diagnosis but a slow pulse rate or bradycardia may mean an increased intra-cranial pressure, also hypertensive encephalopathy.

Blood pressure: Severe hypertension is usually present in patients with cerebral haemorrhage and is always a feature of hypertensive encephalopathy.

Hypotension or low B.P. is usual in diabetic coma, alcohol or barbiturate poisoning and also in any coma associated with severe bleeding.

Inspection of the skin: Pallor and sweating

occurs in syncope, blood loss and hypoglycemia. Suffusion (congestion) of the face is seen in hypertension, alcoholism and sometimes in cerebral haemorrhage. Cyanosis means inadequate oxygenation and occurs in peripheral circulatory failure and collapse due to involvement of respiratory or cardio-vascular system, e.g., cor pulmonale or myocardial infarction. Jaundice as seen from the yellowness of the sclera may be the only positive feature pointing towards hepatic coma. A cherry red colour is seen in carbon monoxide poisoning. Bleeding from an ear or nose may suggest the posibility of trauma.

Dry skin may suggest diabetic coma or uraemia. Corrosion of the mouth and lips may suggest corrosive poisoning.

Odour of the breath: Odour of alcohol is easily recognistd. This may occasionally mislead as barbiturates are quite often ingested along with alcohol.

The odour of organophosphorus compounds and allied bug killers can also be recognised easily.

The spoilt fruit odour of diabetic coma, the uriniferous odour of uraemia and the musty odour (compared to the smell emitted by a dead mouse) of hepatic coma can also be identified by the attending doctor.

Examination of the head: Hidden injuries below the hair should be looked for by palpation of the skull which may reveal a fracture line, a depression or 'soggy' area of severe contusion.

Percussion of the skull in children produces a cracked pot note in hydrocephalus.

Signs of meningeal irritation: Neck rigidity and Kernig's sign indicate usually either meningitis or haemorrhage which is in subarachnoid space. Neck retraction is present in children with severe meningitic infection.

The tongue: As post-epileptic coma is one of the common causes, the tongue should be seen for evidence of injury by biting.

Examination of the nervous system: The first step is the attempt to raise the patient to the conscious level and this is done by usually applying pressure over the supra-orbital areas and other sensitive areas. The level of consciousness is thus assessed.

The cranial nerves : As the ordinary routine is not possible (which requires the cooperation of the patient) a somewhat different approach has to be adopted.

Ocular position and movements : These are very important in determining the site of lesion in the brain. In the common carotid artery involvement damaging one cerebral hemisphere, the eyes and the neck are deviated (or are pointing) towards the side of the lesion away from the side of paralysis.

In mid-brain lesion eye balls are turned upwards. In the basilar artery syndrome in lateral pontine lesions the deviation may be towards the same side as the paralysed extremities.

Pupils : Size of each pupil, their comparative size and their reactions should be noted. Very smali pupils occur in pontine lesions and in morphine poisoning. Organo-phosphorus poisoning is another common cause. Widely dilated pupils occur in brain-stem lesions, either in haemorrhage or encephalitis or due to rapidly expanding tumours or blood clots. Unilateral pupillary dilation is usually seen in space occupying cerebral lesions.

Doll's eye movements: Normally brisk turning of head to one side leads to turning of eyes on the opposite direction. This is called Doll's eye movements. This requires integrity of brain stem, fibres from cervical region, medulla, vestibular region and medial longitudinal bundles.

The face: Study of the lines and contours of the face will give valuable evidence. On the paralysed side, naso-labial furrow will be flattened and the angle of the mouth will be drooping. The paralysed side of the face also will be flapping in and out with respiratory movements. Pressure on the supra-orbital notch may produce a grimace and may make the paralysed side evident.

The motor system: The position of the limbs themselves may give a great deal of information.

Curling of the body away from light is seen in meningitis. (Photophobia)

The patient who lies with the head drooped to

one side, one upper limb pronated and adducted and the lower limb of the same side externally rotated is suffering from dense hemiplegia.

When all limbs are extended, the upper limbs pronated and the feet plantar flexed, this represents the decerebrate attitude occurring in the lesions of the brain-stem.

If however, the upper limbs are flexed at elbows and wrists with supination of forearms and lower limbs extended, it is due to the decorticate position resulting from bilateral damage in hemispheres above the level of mid brain.

While examining the motor system, both arms or legs should be lifted and allowed to fall. If there is a paralysis on one side then the arm or the leg on that side will fall very limply as compared to the other side.

Reflexes: Plantars may be absent or they may be bilateral extensors irrespective of the cause and are of little localising value.

Essential investigations (in brief): 1. Urine: For sugar, albumin, ketone bodies. 2. Blood : For blood sugar, blood urea, blood count, ESR. 3. Serum electrolytes. 4. Cerebro spinal fluid : Lumbar puncture should be done only in the absence of papilloedema. CSF may show the presence of haemorrhage or infection. 5. X-rays of skull; The x-ray skull of an unconscious patient may reveal fracture or evidence of increased intra-cranial tension. 6. C.T scan brain for haemorrhage or infarction or SOL.

General management : These patients should be nursed in the semi-prone position with the head on a thin pillow and turned from side to side every two hours to prevent respiratory infections and bed sores.

The respiratory tract : Mouth should be regularly cleaned and pharyngeal suction may have to be used. Air way may be established by intubation. Antibiotics should be used to prevent infection.

Feeding: The patient obviously should not be given any food or drink orally as he is unable to swallow it and any such attempt will result in choking or aspiration pneumonia. A Ryle's tube should be passed and initially a gastric lavage should be done. This may help in cases of poisoning to remove any residual poison. The smell of this aspirate may also point to the diagnosis. The feeding should be maintained through this tube.

The sphincters: Either retention or incontinence of urine may be present which should be dealt with by the presence of an indwelling catheter.

Specific management: (1) Treatment of cause of unconsciousness, i.e., treat hypertension. (2) Treatment of meningitis, encephalitis. (3) Treatment of epilepsy, etc.

17. Central Nervous System - Common Procedures

LUMBAR PUNCTURE (LP) : Method : Always take the consent of the patient or near-relative before undertaking LP. Explain the procedure in brief and reassure the patient.

Position of the patient : (Fig. 17.1) **Lying down :** Spine should be flexed as much as possible without hurting the patient. Sometimes it is difficult in a patient suffering from meningitis. Thighs should be flexed and the knees drawn towards the abdomen. A pillow should be placed in between the knees to get position as shown in the diagram. The head should be flexed so that the chin approximates to the chest. An assistant should hold the patient in this position at the edge of the cot.

The highest point on the iliac crest should be palpated and the line between these points on either side should be checked and the point at which it crosses the spine should be noted. This is usually the space between the 3rd and the 4th lumbar vertebrae. Either this space or one above it should be chosen for puncture.

Skin should first be cleaned with soap solution and then it should be sterilised with successive applications of spirit, iodine and spirit again. Care should be taken to clean the spine first and then the swab should clean the skin on both lateral aspects.

An anaesthetic should be used for local infiltration in the skin. This should be followed by infiltration of the deeper structures.

A LP. needle is then inserted with the cutting edges of the level pointing upwards as the ligamental fibres are running longitudinally. The needle should be pointing slightly upwards. The average penetration required is about 3 to 5 cms. The penetration in the subarachnoid space is felt as 'give' in the resistance when the tip passes through the ligamentum flavum. The stylet is then withdrawn and the C.S.F. then should come out in a drop by drop fashion.

Manometry : Before the fluid is collected a spinal manometer should be attached to it by a three-way connection.

Normal length of the tube is 30 cms. Normal C.S.F. pressure is about 110 to 120 mm of water.

In the absence of manometry one drop of C.S.F. per sec. is the flow when pressure is normal.

Collections : About 3 to 5 cc of fluid is withdrawn from the needle. It should never be aspirated but should be allowed to run on its own.

Indications for L.P. : 1. **Diagnostic :** a. For biochemical, cytological serological and other investigations. b. To measure the C.S.F pressures and note any abnormalities. 2. **Therapeutic:** a. For relief of increased intra-cranial tension (mainly in inflammatory conditions). b. Rarely introduction of drugs (danger of chemical arachnoiditis). 3. **Anaesthetic.** 4. **Introduction of air :** For pneumoencephalograph. 5. **Introduction of radio-opaque substances** for myelography.

Contraindications for L.P: a. Increased intra-cranial tension (especially if due to posterior fossa tumours). b. Local deformity of spine. c. Local skin injection.

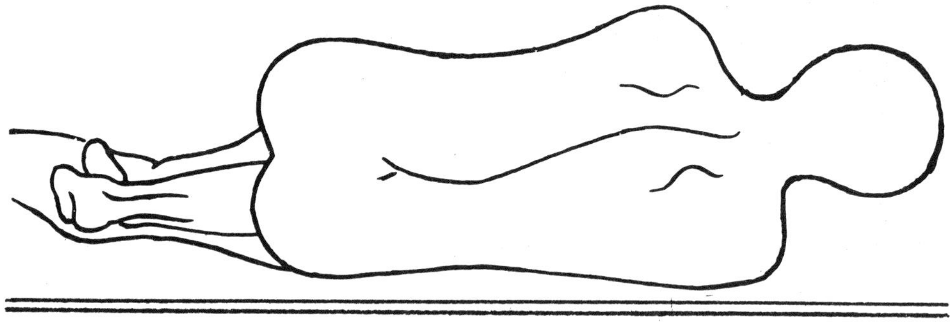

a. Incorrect position of patient - Patient is not at the edge of the cot.

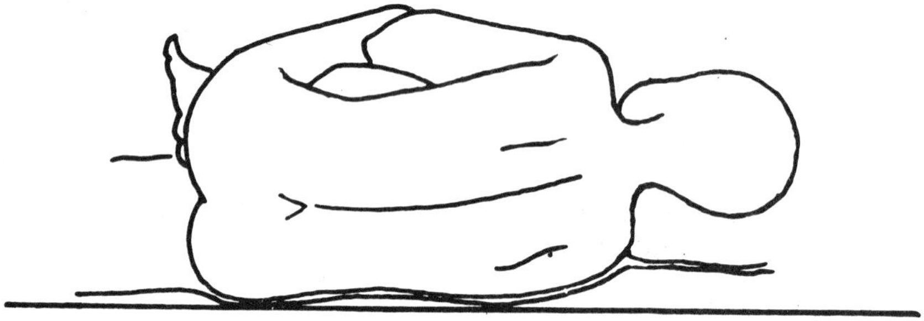

b. Correct position - Patient is at the edge of the cot.

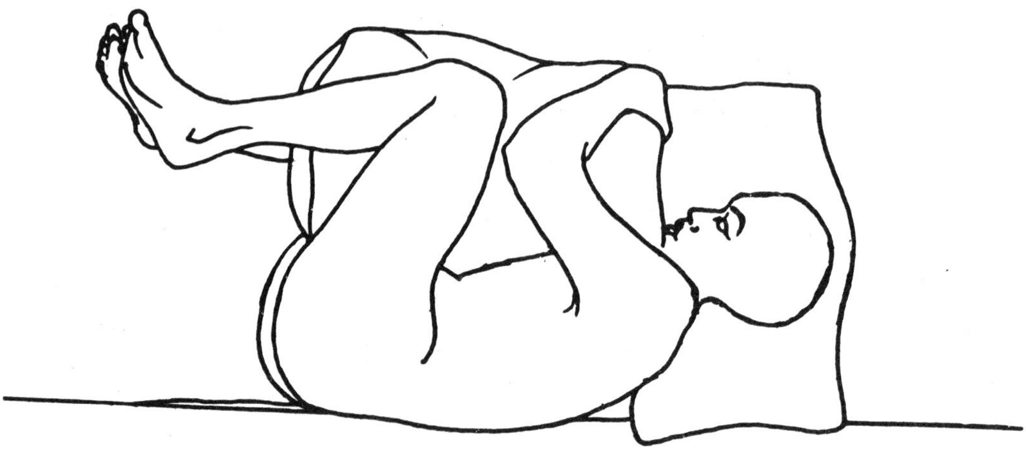

c. Patient in correct position as viewed from above - Note that a pillow is inserted inbetween two knees which are drawn close to abdomen. Head is flexed.

Fig. 17.1 a, b & c

Lumbar puncture

Sequele of L.P : a. Headache. b. Exacerbation of root pains. c. Relapses in demyelinating disorders. d. Meningitis.

Abnormalities detected by L.P :

Abnormalities of pressure: a. Very high pressure in increased intra-cranial tension due to haemorrhage, tumour, hypertensive encephalopathy, hydrocephalus, and meningitis and encephalitis. b. Low pressure following head injury or subarachnoid block in the spinal column.

Queckenstadt's test : If jugular veins are compressed when C.S.F. pressure is being recorded, there is an immediate rise to about 300 mm. This rapidly falls to normal. Variation of C.S.F. pressure during inspiration and expiration are absent. The pressure does not rise whenever there is block in flow of CSF.

Froin's syndrome: In a complete block the C.S.F. picture shows a typical picture : 1. Increase of proteins above normal (up to 1000 mg%). 2. Yellow colouration of the fluid (xanthochromia). 3. Massive coagulation. 4. Cell count normal or slight increase. 5. Queckenstadt's test shows no rise in C.S.F. pressure.

The other points to be noted on C.S.F: examination and the abnormalities are shown in the accompanying table which shows different biochemical and cytological abnormalities in different conditions.

Dry tapping : Failure to obtain fluid.

i. Incorrectly done lumbar tap.

ii. Fluid being too thick does not flow easily through the needle.

iii. Spinal block when C.S.F. below the block is drained.

CSF CHART

	Pressure	Appearance	Proteins and colour	Sugar	Chlorides	Globulin	Pandy's	Cells/c.mm Test	RBC/Organisms
A. Normal	100-120 mms of	Clear Colourless	15-45 mg%	40-65 mg%	720-750 rng%	Not raised	Occasionally weakly +ve if gamma globulins are raised	3-5% lympho-cytes	Nil
1. Pyogenic meningitis	Raised	Hazy	800-2000 mg%	8-10 mg%	650-680 mg%	Increased	+ve	800-2000 cells P-60-80%	Isolated on culture or seen in smear
B. 2. Inadequately treated pyogenic meningitis) 3. Partially treated pyogenic meningitis) 4. Acute fulminating tuberculous meningitis) 5. Miliary tuberculous meningitis)	Raised	Hazy	400-800 mg %	20-30 mg%	650-700 mg %	Increased	+ve	300-500 P-60%	May be isolated in culture
C. Tuberculous meningitis	Raised	Hazy and cobwet present	80-300 mg%	10-40 mg%	610-650 mg%	Increased	+ve	80-200 L-60-80%	AFB may be seen
D. Aseptic meningitis due to any cause	Raised slightly	Clear or hazy	Just increased	Normal	Normal	Normal or slightly raised	+ve	50-80 L. predominant	
E Albumino Cyto dissociation									
1. Froin's syndrome	Normal or raised	Xantho-chromia	1000-2000 mg.%	Normal	Normal	Raised	+vc	10- 15 or normal	
2. Following cerebral haemorrhage	Raised	Xantho-chromia or blood stained	Increased depending on amount of blood	Normal	Normal	Raised	+ve	Increased	
3. Acute viral polyneuritis	Normal or raised	Hazy	600-1000 mg%	Normal	Normal	Raised	+ve may be - ve	Normal or absent	Nil

	Pressure	Appearance and colour	Proteins	Sugar	Chlorides	Globulin	Pandy's Test	Cells/c.mm	RBC/Organisms
F. Cerebral abscess									
1. Rupturing into ventricular svstem			— Picture just like pyogenic meningitis —						
2. Situated near ventricular system	Raised or normal	Normal or hazy	80-100 mg% (i.e. slightly)	Normal	Nornal or increased	Normal or increased	+ve	50-150 P +	
3. Situated away from ventricular system				— Normal CSF —					
G. Encephalitis syndrome (any cause)	Normal or raised	clear or hazy	Normal or raised	Normal or raised	Normal or reduced	increased	+ve	Normal or increased 20-30 cells P +	
H. Lymphocytic choriomeningitis	Increased	Hazy	Raised	Normal	Normal or reduced	Increased	+ve	About 1000 (mono-nuclear majority)	

I. NEUROSYPHILIS

	Pressure	Proteins	Globulin	Cells	Colloidal gold	CSF VDRL	Treponema immoblisa-tion test	Fluorescent treponemal antibody test
Meningo-vascular	Normal	Moderate rise	Increased	Up to 200 Lymphocytes	Meningitis or paretic or leutic	+ve	+ve	+ve
GPI	Increased	Rise 5-100 mg%	Increased	5-50 Lymphocytes	Paretic maximum change in 1st zone	+ve sometimes	+ve occasionally – vc	+ve
Tabes dorsalis	Increased	Slight risc	Slight to moderate rise	Slight rise	Leutic maximum change in mid-zone	+ve occasionally -ve	+ve	+ve

Bibliography

Bannister, Sir Roger (rev. ed.), *Brain and Barrister's Clinical Neurology*, 7th rev. ed., Oxford University Press, London, 1992

Berhrman, Richard E., Robert M. Kliegman, Ann M. Arvin (ed.), *Nelson Textbook of Pediatrics*, 15th ed., W.B. Saunders Co., New York, 1995

Chamberlain, E., and Coln. Ogilvie, *Sign and Symptoms in Clinical Medicine: Introduction to Medical Diagnosis*, John Wright and Sons Ltd., Bristol, 1987

Constant, Jules, *Bedside Cardiology*, 3rd. ed. Little Brown and Co., Boston and Toronto, 1985

Das, Somen, *A Manual on Clinical Surgery*, 4th. ed., S. Das Publications, Calcutta, 1996

Isselbacher et. al. (ed.), *Principles of Internal Medicine*, 13th. ed., McGraw Hill Publications, Singapore, 1994

Patten, John, *Neurological Differential Diagnosis : An Illustrated Approach with 288 Figures*, Harold Starke Ltd., London, 1994

Index